Diagnosis and Risk Management in Primary Care

- words that count, numbers that speak -

WILFRID TREASURE

General Practitioner, Muirhouse Medical Group, Edinburgh

Foreword by

Roger Jones

Emeritus Professor of Primary Care, King's College London
Editor, *British Journal of General Practice*

Radcliffe Publishing
London • New York

Radcliffe Publishing Ltd
33-41 Dallington Street
London
EC1V 0BB
United Kingdom

www.radcliffepublishing.com

Electronic catalogue and worldwide online ordering facility

British Library Cataloguing in Publication Data

A catalogue record for this book is available from the British Library.

ISBN-13: 978 184619 477 1

The paper used for the text pages of this book is FSC®
certified. FSC (The Forest Stewardship Council®)
is an international network to promote responsible
management of the world's forests.

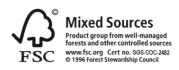

Mixed Sources
Product group from well-managed
forests and other controlled sources
www.fsc.org Cert no. SGS-COC-2482
© 1996 Forest Stewardship Council

Typeset by KnowledgeWorks Global Ltd, Chennai, India
Cover designed by Meaden Creative, Chipping Norton, UK
Printed and bound by TJI Digital, Padstow, Cornwall, UK

Contents

Foreword

It is a great pleasure to write a short introduction to this beautifully written book which I believe will have a major impact on the way that new generations of primary care doctors approach their work. Reading Diagnosis and Risk Management in Primary Care immediately took me back to twenty years ago, and the publication of Clinical Epidemiology: a basic science for clinical medicine written by David Sackett and colleagues – a book which had a profound personal effect on me and massively influenced medical practice in the US, UK and many other western health systems. At the time of publication, diagnosis in primary care was generally based on anecdote and received wisdom, bedside teaching in hospitals often lacked an evidence base and few undergraduate medical curricula included instruction in biostatistics and clinical epidemiology. It was difficult to see the scientia among the caritas.

Now, in the 21st century, medical practice is dominated by the strictures of evidence based medicine, the conclusions of meta-analyses, algorithmic guidelines and checklists. It can be difficult to see the patient amongst the paperwork. What a breath of fresh air, then, to find an author capable of holding these extreme paradigms, along with others, and to put the patient back at the centre of the consultation in which the lessons of clinical epidemiology are synthesised with those of experience, narrative and biography – and who is able to entertain at the same time as he informs and to stimulate critical reflection while, with an enviable lightness of touch, nudging us in the direction of a rigorous approach to diagnosis and the assessment and communication of risk.

It would be a pity if the only readers of this book were family doctors, general practitioners and their teams, because as well as providing learners, teachers and practitioners with a unique source of instruction, many of the pages contain material that needs to be understood by all clinicians. The opening chapter on Diagnosis, for example looks at the multiple processes involved in approaching a diagnosis and the multiple implications of diagnosis-making for the doctor as well as the patient. Residents in the out patient clinic would benefit from having this chapter metaphorically on their shoulder, and it, along with most of the rest of the book, should be required reading for students and trainees. The same goes for statistics – rehabilitating likelihood ratios and odds – *Icebergs, Words that count* – no-one need ever get lost in a consultation again - and the lovely *Pattern design* chapter, which re-opens the diagnostic black box and provides fresh insights into the nuts and bolts of diagnostic decision making.

This isn't an easy read, not because of the writing - which is pretty well faultless – but because it makes demands on the reader. It makes us question our established viewpoints at many levels and opens new avenues of thought which are likely to enhance the consulting and diagnostic skills of the crustiest GP. And it is almost all brand new. Apart from the *Numbers that speak* chapter – a sort of well organised Schott's Miscellany of Medicine, providing facts and figures which constantly surprise, challenge and inform, and which is derived from the literature - the book has been written from the bottom up, drawing its authority from a remarkably wide reading, while reflecting the essence of Wilfrid Treasure's sophisticated and humane stance.

If you need to understand how the health system works, how the NHS runs, what is good and bad about it and where we might be heading in the future, settle down with something warming and simply enjoy chapter 2, on *Healthcare design*. In less pages than are occupied by the executive summary of some Department of Health publications, Treasure tells any willing consumer all they need to know about healthcare – this is the chapter our politicians need to read now and deserves separate publication as a guide for the perplexed on all sides of the political divide.

As resources shrink, lives extend, expectations and costs rise and the information load grows exponentially we need both a scientific and moral compass to negotiate the future of medicine. Medical education, professional training, continuing professional development and policy innovation all have a role to play in securing a future that we can, literally, live with. The wisdom and guidance captured in this book are gold dust which needs to be absorbed and understood by all those involved in shaping medicine in the years ahead.

Roger Jones
Emeritus Professor of Primary Care, King's College London
Editor, *British Journal of General Practice*
London
May 2011

Preface

'It is dangerous to have two cultures that can't or don't communicate. In a time when science is determining much of our destiny, that is, whether we live or die, it is dangerous in the most practical terms.'

Snow CP. *The Two Cultures*. Cambridge: Cambridge University Press; 1959.

'PATIENT: " . . . I'm nearly 45 and I suppose I must be on the change now?"
DOCTOR: "What shall I tell you now?"
PATIENT: (Laughter) "No . . . Women have done it before."
DOCTOR: "Is that what you are telling yourself?"
PATIENT: "That's what I'm presuming . . . I don't know."
DOCTOR: "Mmm, mmm .... " '.

This exchange takes place early in an audiotaped consultation forming part of a seminal mixed methodology observational study conducted by two alumni of the Royal College of General Practitioners and published in 1976.[1] It's moving. The patient seems to be in a fog. She speaks and reaches out for guidance. The doctor says enough to let her know he's heard and he takes her hand but doesn't lead because he doesn't yet know where they're going. Over the next few minutes, the mist clears and they can see their way. Some of the mystery[2] is solved. The consultation might have turned into a discussion about the menopause: instead it becomes an opportunity for the patient to talk about her mother's nervous breakdown. The patient might have gone away pathologised, prescription in hand: instead a woman leaves less worried and more confident—healthier—than before. At the time I read it in 1989, I might have carried from my hospital registrar post into my general practice traineeship the biomechanical model of medicine, and confidently pointed lost patients towards their diseases: instead I was introduced to a gentler touch, a quieter way of observing, more intelligent listening.

Listening intelligently, I realised, didn't mean showing my intelligence. 'What shall I tell you now?' doesn't seem to mean anything. The doctor's speaking to let the patient know he's there.[3] The question hangs in the air between them until an answer begins to emerge. After 20 years of practice—and practising—I understand this a little better.

Consulting requires judicious use of words and numbers. There are other things that matter. But if we can't use words effectively and don't know any figures, we'll flounder. We don't need to be particularly articulate—and certainly not verbose—but we need to be able to hear what the patient is trying to tell us and respond in a way that's comprehensible and comforting. Numbers underlie what we do even though we often don't refer to them directly. In fact, we're necessarily selective in what we articulate—we think more than we say. This book attempts to provide an account of the set of communication skills along with the stock of facts and figures needed to conduct an adequate consultation in general practice.

I think my job as a GP is to give patients the chance to live longer, healthier lives. To do this, I need to combine evidence-based medicine with patient-centred consulting. Is there a tension between being patient-centred and being evidence-based? 'Overall diagnosis', which is one of the aims of patient-centred medicine, includes identifying physical illness using the biomechanical model.[4] And evidence-based medicine uses the individual patient's 'predicaments, rights, and preferences' in decision making.[5] So if there is a tension between the two, it's like the tension in a watch spring that makes the hands turn around.

Cochrane said 'all effective treatment must be free':[6] I would add 'all free treatment must be effective'. To move towards that goal requires the clinician not just to use evidence in the consulting room, but to work with researchers to identify and develop the evidence that's needed.[7] The two cultures considered by CP Snow to have become disconnected were literature and science.[8] The two cultures whose division, I think, jeopardises good healthcare are general practice and medical research.[9]

This book's main title, *Diagnosis and Risk Management*, derives from the first and last chapters. Chapter 1 diagnoses the diagnosis: if we're solving puzzles, we need a rulebook;[10] if we're looking for meaning, we want a phrasebook.[11] The last chapter addresses risk management and argues that practice is safest and the patient most satisfied when we keep our diagnostic minds and our consulting room doors open. Chapter 2 on healthcare design takes the form of a discussion, a device that enables a range of referenced facts and opinions to be presented in a condensed form: it envisages progressive judicious assimilation of technology into traditional holistic general practice. In Chapter 3, it's proposed that statistical stumbling blocks like sensitivity and specificity be replaced with the building blocks of likelihood ratios and odds. Chapter 4 is based on the symptom iceberg[12, 13]—the large volume of distress present in the community of which we see just the tip in our consulting rooms: the examples given are depression, sore throat, and colorectal cancer. Chapters 5 and 6 provide the book's subtitle. Chapter 5 is a repository of numbers that speak: the prevalences of different diseases and the likelihood ratios attached to symptoms, signs, and tests that help us in diagnosis. Chapter 6 is about the words that count: it's a guide to consulting skills, covering a spectrum from the most patient-centred to the most doctor-centred and stressing the importance of reflecting and checking. In Chapter 7, clinical acumen is analysed in an attempt to discover what it's made of and whether it can be learned and taught. Chapter 8 looks at the education of general practitioners from medical school application to retirement: it identifies the objective criteria that have to be met to pass examinations while emphasising the importance of role modelling.

The book is densely evidenced, material from elsewhere sometimes being used unchanged, sometimes developed in different directions from the original. For broad concepts and detailed statistical information, I've tried to track down and refer to the primary source because every iteration—every subsequent commentator's paraphrase—will have changed the meaning. For ideas and statistics that have been usefully summarised, I've referred to the summary rather than to the original. Where technical terms form not a route but a barrier to understanding, I've bypassed them.

The contents of this book are based on what I've learned while consulting, teaching, and working with other members of the team in a large general practice in an area of deprivation in Edinburgh, Scotland. This experience has been supplemented by meetings, discussions, and reading. To avoid a 'pantomime of caution',[14] the provisional and personal nature of the views expressed throughout the book is implied rather than stated explicitly every time. There'll be aspects of general practice—in the UK and certainly beyond—that aren't captured. However, despite differences in health and healthcare around the world, evidence exists for the importance of universal access to sustainable,[15] low-technology management[16] provided in a patient-centred way in primary care.[17] There should, therefore, be material of some use to all primary care doctors anywhere, not least if they're preparing for MRCGP. With that in mind, the RCGP Curriculum,[18] Competence Framework,[19] and General Medical Council appraisal headings[20] are used as the basis for relevant sections of the book and are referenced.

Wilfrid Treasure
May 2011

Some terms used in this book

For readers not familiar with general practice in the UK, a guide to the meanings of various terms might be helpful. A 'general practitioner' is a primary care physician or family doctor; a 'consultant' or 'specialist' is a senior secondary care doctor or internist; a 'specialist trainee' or 'ST' is a junior doctor specialising in general practice through a series of hospital and primary care posts, and working with a dedicated 'trainer' or 'educational supervisor'; a 'foundation year' or 'FY' doctor is a junior in the first year after graduating who spends some time in general practice under a 'supervisor'; a 'medical student' is an undergraduate; 'surgery' refers both to the building in which a general practitioner works and to a consulting session; a 'house call' or 'home visit' is a consultation in a patient's home or institutional residence; a 'follow up' is a repeat consultation serving as a continuation of an initial consultation; 'assessment' is the same as 'evaluation'; a 'district nurse' is a 'community nurse'; and a 'learner' is anyone wishing to improve —I guess that's all of us.

About the author

Wilfrid Treasure graduated from Guy's Hospital Medical School in 1983 and special-ised initially in gastroenterology, becoming a hospital registrar before transferring to general practice. He has worked for 20 years as a full-time general practitioner in Muirhouse Medical Group, a large group practice providing National Health Service care to patients in a part of Edinburgh with a high level of deprivation. He is a trainer and takes part in teaching specialist trainees, foundation-year doctors, and medical students. Before studying medicine he obtained a music degree from Clare College, Cambridge, and continues to play piano in his spare time.

Acknowledgements

I'm grateful to Dr. Susannah McLean; when she was my registrar, I taught her a little about patient-centred consulting and now she's a researcher she's taught me something about evidence-based medicine, helping me to interpret and represent research findings more accurately. That said, any discrepancies between what I've read and what I've written are down to me.

I'll always be indebted to Dr. A. Alan Robertson for what I've gained both professionally and personally from knowing him. I'm glad to have the opportunity to thank Dr. J. Roy Robertson, my other partners, and the staff of Muirhouse Medical Group who've been a support and a pleasure to work with for 20 years. I also owe a lot to junior doctors, medical students, and patients for what they've taught me.

I'm grateful to individuals and organisations in ways too many and varied to detail, including the following: AbeBooks, Alasdair Ball, Andrew Polmear, Anne MacKay of Astley Ainslie Hospital Library, Bill Irish, Center for History and New Media at George Mason University who created the research tool Zotero, Christopher Martyn, the Deprivation Interest Group, Ed Caddick, Google, the Idle Hamsters, ILLiad, Iona Heath, Jenny Reid, John Budd, Jo Wright, Joe Treasure, Kevin Gallagher, Liz Treasure, my Medicine and Literature Group, Michael Blackmore, Nic Robertson, OpenOffice and Oracle, Paul Little, Peter Dorward, Peter Galinsky, Pippa Robertson, RJC Steele, Rob Elton, Tom Schuller, Tom Treasure, my trainers group, the team at the University College London Clinical Operational Research Unit, the staff at the Western General Hospital Library, Wikipedia, Willie Hamilton, and Yassir Hag Musa.

Lastly, I'd like to thank the people at Radcliffe for their help. Jessica Morofke at Radcliffe and Anuradha Mani at Cadmus could not have been more helpful. My editor, Gillian Nineham, has been encouraging throughout; the reader should also be grateful to her for insisting that my photograph should not appear on the cover of this book.

Wilfrid Treasure
June 2011

To Ann, for loving me and criticising my writing.

CHAPTER 1

Diagnosis

'If it is to classify as a puzzle, a problem must be characterized by more than an assured solution. There must also be rules that limit both the nature of acceptable solutions and the steps by which they are to be obtained.'

Kuhn TS. *The Structure of Scientific Revolutions.* 2nd ed.
Chicago: University of Chicago Press; 1970.

'Being ill is not a state, it is a status.'

Kennedy I. *The Unmasking of Medicine: a searching look at healthcare today.*
London: Granada Publishing; 1983.

POWER AND CULTURE

Diagnosis is an exercise of power. Doctors are granted their authority to diagnose, formally by society through its institutions[21] and informally by patients through the consultation.[22] Patients have the freedom to decide what material they bring us and we use our discretion in how we respond. If they assert their own authority by diagnosing themselves, we subject that self-diagnosis to scrutiny and decide whether it's accurate or inaccurate, desirable or undesirable, to be accepted, contested, or rejected.[23]

Use of the term 'wear and tear' by an active old woman who deals with her joint pain by 'just getting on with it'[24] might be regarded as accurate, desirable and acceptable, while an idle young man's conviction that he's unfit for any work because of low back pain[25] might be deemed inaccurate, undesirable, and contestable.

The doctor exerts their authority on the diagnostic process against the background of their own personal and cultural values.[26] The patient comes to the surgery in a state of illness; the doctor may or may not grant the illness the status of a disease.[27, 2] The doctor weighs the patient's knowledge and beliefs against their own knowledge and beliefs and arrives at some sort of synthesis or compromise.[28] One doctor might have the skill and inclination to elicit and explore the patient's perspective,[29] while another may not. The interaction between doctor and patient may be based on paternalism, consumerism, laissez-faire, mutuality, or informed choice.[30] The outcome might be a diagnosis based on the biomechanical or bio-psychosocial models[31, 32] or an account using principles of narrative.[33, 34] The doctor's diagnosis is a proxy for the patient's morbidity: it represents the doctor's attempt to organise unorganised illness.[35] And it's culturally dependent: in primary care around the world, patients' symptoms don't vary by country, but their doctors' diagnoses do.[36]

The diagnostic process is partly governed by external forces.[37] The availability and acceptability of diagnoses—and their evidence-base—are determined by governments, pharmaceutical companies, scientific establishments, and sports bodies. Which areas of medicine become specialties, which diseases are selected for attention, depend on political and economic factors as much as science. Research is sometimes fuelled by fashion[26] and available methodology rather than by clinical need.[37] Microbiology expanded in the nineteenth century to sustain British colonial expansion beyond temperate zones.[38] The emergence of coronary thrombosis in the early part of the twentieth century, although precipitated by the invention of the electrocardiograph, was part of a process by which heart specialists defined their social identity.[39]

The doctor might choose a particular diagnosis for legal or financial reasons rather than medical, and out of concern for people other than the patient being diagnosed. Death certification[40] and notification of infectious disease[41] serve not the individual patient, but society as a whole. A general practitioner will attach more or less importance to a diagnosis according to its effect on their income. And certain diagnoses qualify the patient for particular services, treatments, and financial benefits. In 1972, the United States Congress provided funding for almost all Americans requiring chronic dialysis,[42] and in 2005 the UK government introduced estimated glomerular filtration rate into the Quality and Outcomes Framework.[43] These provisions—which have no equivalents in, say, respiratory or hepatic disease—privilege particular manifestations of renal function and dysfunction. As a result, kidney disease is less worrisome to ill Americans because the state is paying to make them well, and more worrying to well Brits because the state is paying to make them ill.[44]

The exercise of power is evident in the area of mental health.[45] Depression, for instance, is a useful construct for pharmaceutical companies, psychiatrists, health service managers and general practitioners seeking order in chaos, but may not have validity as an entity: it may be more a marker of severity or an epiphenomenon.[46] Some view psychiatry as 'pseudoscience'[47] and regard a disease approach as 'untenable'.[27] In accounts of mental illness,[48, 49] power, autonomy, and helplessness feature prominently. Sufferers might be troubled by irrational fears and inner voices; they also feel victimised, trapped, punished and undermined by a subjective, value-laden diagnostic process.[50]

The principle underlying the *Diagnostic and Statistical Manual of Mental Disorders* is that diagnoses are stable entities. However, symptoms don't always differentiate the normal from abnormal or one disease from another,[51] and psychiatric diagnoses have few pathognomic features.[52] Context is required to distinguish, for instance, sadness from depression.[53] And just as every society is different,[54] so every patient is unique, and a distinction between unusual beliefs and psychosis isn't clear-cut.

Society is powerful, the individual less so. How do individuals exert their influence? They volunteer diagnoses, but they're limited in their choice to those conditions that they've heard about and to those that enjoy official sanction. Publicity can appear to give society's stamp of approval to a disease.[53] Lay awareness of anorexia nervosa, for instance, seems to have made it more prevalent.[55] And twice as many psychiatric outpatients think they have bipolar disorder as meet *Diagnostic and Statistical Manual* criteria.[56]

Power struggles in psychiatry are obvious. They're conducted publicly, everyone has a view, the existential nature of mental illness raises the temperature, and the ambiguity of words such as 'depression', which have different vernacular and medical meanings, generates misunderstanding. Tensions in other branches of medicine are less evident because tests and terminology are sufficiently technical for the public and even many professionals to find themselves quickly out of their depth. The clinical diagnosis of chronic bronchitis has largely given way to a spirometric diagnosis of chronic obstructive pulmonary disease,[57] the diagnostic criteria for diabetes have been changed by international agreement,[58] and research into heart failure has focussed on patients with reduced rather than preserved ejection fraction.[59] These definitions of pathology determine who is and who is not a patient and how much money is spent on them.

When the patient's self-diagnosis doesn't obtain the approval of officialdom, they can't win through strength of force so diplomacy is required: they need to meet the opposition around the negotiating table. The individual seeks societal approbation in the form of medical attention, sickness benefit, or financial compensation. What they can bring to the table are the three elements of physical, mental, and social well-being,[60] surrendering one in order to retain or gain another. Street drug users accept the socially stigmatising diagnosis of dependency—defined as much in social and legal as in medical terms[61]—in order to receive prescriptions. For some disabled people, undergoing a benefits medical examination[62] and meeting the threshold of incapacity under the Personal Capability Assessment[63] represents progress on their path to greater disability. For others, subjecting their bodies and minds to the scrutiny of the International Paralympic Committee[64] and the UK Sports Association for People with Learning Disability[65] is a necessary stage toward achieving their sporting ambitions.

The role of culture is prominent where lifestyle is concerned. Most excess weight in children is gained before five years of age,[66] suggesting that the cause may lie in society rather than in the child. Is the condition due to overeating or lack of exercise or both or neither? Is overeating a type of addiction or just a bad habit, is it compulsive behaviour, or is it merely an enthusiasm for food—a hobby or form of entertainment with risks, just as horse riding or mountain biking have risks?[67] At the other end of the spectrum, variability in the course of the ageing process might be attributed to nutrition or lifestyle (within the patient's control) or to genes, the environment, or chance (outwith their control).[68]

ETHICS

Two millennia ago, Plato contrasted the different approaches doctors took to different classes of patient, criticising the rudeness they showed to slaves and commending the courtesy with which they elicited the views of freemen when taking a history and the use of persuasion when planning treatment.[69] Thus were patient-centred consulting and motivational interviewing born.

Writings attributed to Hippocrates laid down the ethical principles of beneficence and non-maleficence to which autonomy and justice have since been added to form an ethical framework commonly used in medicine.[70, 38] These ethical principles prompt questions that, far from providing a single answer, highlight the complexity of the problem by leading to many mutually incompatible answers. Even the broadest question as to what aspect of health is the proper concern of doctors is an open one.[70]

Medical practice might be informed by other ethical principles, more or less important to different people in different societies: certain actions might be unconditionally prohibited;[71] a person might have an unconditional right not to be harmed; or ethical judgments might be governed by utilitarianism (the greatest good for the greatest number),[72] parsimony,[73] humanism,[74, 75] or religious belief.

The most generic principle of a professional is to subordinate their interests to those of the patient.[70] The neutral stance that this requires can, in certain situations, make doctors—and their patients—uncomfortable.[34] Ethics is clearly relevant to such matters as abortion, euthanasia, torture, ritual genital procedures, and caring for the illegal immigrant or the uninsured. And it has a bearing on whether a revelation about a possible sexual offence should lead to a breach of confidentiality.[76, 77] But ethics also comes into more everyday questions as to whether we regard a sore throat as a self-limiting respiratory tract illness (not needing antibiotics) or a cause of acute nephritis (needing penicillin).

SUMMATIONS OR FORMULATIONS

The diagnosis can take various forms. In the nineteenth century, lesion, cause, and prognosis were considered most important,[38, 51] and this biomedical approach dominated until the 1970s, when the biopsychosocial model was introduced.[31] But practice is variable. The diagnosis might be a paraphrase of the patient's presenting symptoms and this is often what's recorded in the patient's notes by junior hospital doctors.[78] Or it might be a longer formulation of a more descriptive and personal nature.[51]

The acrostics POMR (Problem Orientated Medical Record) and SOAP (Subjective, Objective, Analysis, Plan) signalled attempts in the 1960s to encourage the organisation of records around formal diagnoses.[79] The POMR has since became the main way of structuring the electronic health record.[80] Attempts to standardise verbal communication to maximise patient safety include SBAR (Situation, Background, Assessment, Recommendation).[81] An approach that is useful for quick, safe communication between doctors—and that fosters autonomy in trainees—begins with a commitment to a diagnosis followed by the reasons for doubt and the proposed plan.[82, 83] Recognition of the importance of holistic, multidisciplinary and functional records has led to the use of care plans in residential institutions and patients' own homes: these care plans lead to significant differences in process, but have no effect on outcomes for patients and informal caregivers[84] and their usefulness is unclear.[85] It's possible, however, that they might have a role in routine general practice, especially in the care of patients with complex medical problems.[85]

What we make of a patient, the most important things about them, may be too idiosyncratic to express using a predefined set of parameters. The formulation may not fit the *pro forma*. Once we get to know a patient, we move beyond noting their superficial personality traits, and even beyond understanding their personal values: we get to know them as a person with their own unique story.[86] In my practice, these personal nuggets surface when we allocate house calls over coffee in the morning and the patient's usual doctor tries to tell a deputising colleague about a patient.

METAPHORS

Metaphor—using one thing to represent something else[87]—pervades language, perhaps unavoidably.[88] When we use terms like 'low mood' or 'depression', we're speaking metaphorically as if the mental state has a shape or position. Such metaphor can be helpful or harmful. Talking about illness and recovery like a journey is likely to be therapeutic; pointing out that cancer is like a crab eating away is not. The use of the same word 'depression' to describe both low mood and a state of psychosis is misleading: beyond that word, the two conditions have nothing in common.

Further problems can arise when different people interpret the same metaphor differently—or don't understand it at all. We usually use metaphors unthinkingly, and our often-unconscious choice depends on personal leanings and prevailing culture. The use of metaphor might then suddenly come to notice because of a double entendre causing amusement or embarrassment.

Language influences thought—with the result that thought is narrowly restricted within cultures and widely variable between cultures.[3] When we're trying to convey information about something unfamiliar to our listener, we might find ourselves saying less about what the thing is like and more about what it's not like.[37] The development of concepts is possible only when a language exists to convey those concepts. In science, metaphor fills the gaps in our vocabulary and understanding until our knowledge grows and technical terms emerge to convey concepts more precisely.[88] In a sense, we can't acquire understanding through words but only by experience.[89]

So metaphor has its advantages and disadvantages. In the consulting room, it's easy to find oneself replacing the patient's imperfect metaphor not with scientific fact, but with just another imperfect metaphor. The term 'hypertension' is ambiguous. Some patients think of it as 'hyper-tension', a state of excessive tenseness, physical in nature and part of a vicious circle, being caused by and causing emotional tension. This belief seems to persist comfortably alongside alternative beliefs held by the patient and offered by the doctors. Such lay beliefs may seem questionable— but perhaps no more than beliefs held by professionals.[90] The term 'hypertension' refers to either a disease or a risk factor for disease, with a range of possible manifestations or none, which might be acute or chronic, primary or secondary, resulting from any of several putative mechanisms, none of which are fully understood—and heralding any one of many unpredictable outcomes. We know a lot about hypertension: how much more useful that knowledge is to the patient than the notion of 'hyper-tension' is debatable.

MESSAGES

The diagnosis is a form of communication—it's a message to self or to others. The term 'irritable bowel syndrome' implies a cluster of symptoms without increased mortality, clearly defined pathology, or specific treatment. That much of the message is probably widely understood. In other respects, however, the term is inadequate or misleading.

It tells us little about the individual, and tells the individual little about their condition. Use of the word 'bowel' suggests some affinity with, for example, inflammatory bowel disease, whereas in terms of prognosis, pathology, and treatment, irritable bowel syndrome has more in common with tension headache or precordial catch.[91]

The term 'chronic pain' has come to indicate that the patient doesn't have an identified treatable cause and is on a downward spiral of deconditioning, disability, and depression. The patient is searching for an explanation, comparing themself with others, fearful of not being believed and inclined to withdraw from the world.[25] The treatment and prognosis depend less on site and more on psychosocial factors. There's little evidence that analgesics reduce chronic pain and disability beyond six months,[92] and treating it with painkillers may be worse than useless. Acute pain and chronic pain have the word 'pain' in common—but little else.

Another problem with diagnosis as communication is that different people have different interpretations of the same word. Conversation is a process of developing a common language between two people:[3] the consultation has a similar function. Ideally we find a wording for the diagnosis that's helpful to the patient. The process of looking at the problem from different angles might clarify the diagnosis and help apportion responsibilities between doctor and patient.[93] A shared understanding about the cause of the problem is valuable[94] but not always possible: in that case, agreement about what to do—a sort of muddling through—might be all that can be achieved, and often works well enough.[95]

Diagnosis implies an objectivity that is sometimes lacking. Indeed, in a sense the diagnosis is an attempt to persuade[96]—other professionals, the patient, and ourselves. The diagnosis of 'viral infection' indicates that antibiotics are generally not needed because the cause is supposedly viral, but may be needed if there's secondary bacterial infection—a conveniently mixed message. An alternative such as 'self-limiting respiratory tract illness' argues for no specific aetiology or treatment and more clearly indicates a favourable outcome without treatment. The confused and wandering elderly woman who would not be persuaded by me to go into a psychogeriatric ward accepted my colleague's diagnosis of pneumonia along with admission to the acute medical ward where her husband was already an inpatient.

Sometimes messages are conveyed through media other than words. Symptoms of anxiety give a message to the patient; somatisation is a message from the patient to those around them.[97] The taking of medicine defines the person as a patient;[98] taking an antidepressant defines the patient as a depressive; and taking an antipsychotic defines them as a psychotic. This is backward reasoning but also something more: in psychiatry the diagnosis is sometimes an opinion about which drug-induced state is deemed preferable to the patient's untreated morbid state.[52] The drug history that forms part of the Scottish Emergency Care Summary[99] gives the emergency services diagnostic information not easily acquired directly because of concerns about confidentiality.

Drug reactions constitute an area of confusion. Patients may use the terms 'allergy' and 'side effect' interchangeably,[100] whereas doctors distinguish allergy from dose-related adverse drug reaction,[101] two terms with distinct implications.

Identifying the patient with whom we feel despair, anger, or frustration as 'heart-sink' is a message—from the doctor to themself or to other doctors—about the effect the patient has on them.[102, 103] Interactions between doctor and patient are signalled in other ways. The patient whose notes contain a record of repeat prescriptions without consultations might be diagnosed as 'peaceful repeat prescription'. This represents some form of truce:[104] there's a barrier between patient and doctor preventing true human contact through which the repeat prescription represents communication of a sort.[105]

Conveying a message requires a language or code and a set of patterns or symbols with meanings.[106] For a biomechanical diagnosis, the pattern is often contained by the consultation. A more holistic diagnosis requires us to see the pattern of which the consultation is a part.[107] The fragments that form the pattern might be dispersed in time or through families. In traditional family practice, these fragments would spontaneously coalesce or be brought together in family books.[108, 109] Nowadays, with less continuity of care, the pattern they form can easily escape our notice.[110]

In the electronic health record, messages are conveyed by codes. The doctor selects a word, the software selects a code, and the code determines the message.[111] Depending on the code selected, the message might go to a patient summary, a referral letter, or the out-of-hours service; it might activate an electronic aid or trigger payment.[111] In theory, it should facilitate audit and research, but is often inadequate for these purposes.[112, 113, 114, 115] For instance, NHS24 might provide surveillance of pandemic influenza,[116] but the data are of questionable value,[117] and a separate household survey has been launched to do this monitoring.[118]

So the information communicated by a coded message is limited. Certain information about patients is not codeable, transferable, and enduring, but ephemeral and needing context for it to be meaningful.[119] More worrying is the potential for the coded message to convey, unknown to the clinician, something other than that intended.[111, 120] The American Psychiatric Association decided by a vote in 1973 that homosexuality was not an illness:[121] the NHS continues to give it the Read code 'sexual deviation or disorder'[122]—which is apparent only when the Read code hierarchy is explored.

STORIES

People from many cultures seem to need answers to such questions as: What caused this illness? Why did it begin now? What's happening to me? What will happen? What should be done?[90, 28] The answers are told in stories, stories with plots in which events have causes and consequences.[123] We're not necessarily conscious of this creative process, just as we're not aware of the active mechanism by which we assemble an image when light strikes the retina. And it's not an abstract intellectual exercise but a bodily enactment,[124] representing reality just as a dream does, for as long as it lasts.

Storytelling is not primary concerned with truth or untruth. It's an account of events and it's forever being created and re-created. The patient brings experiences together in their mind to make a storyline, an explanation for what's happened and a speculation about possible consequences.[125] This storytelling isn't a one-off process—nor is it one-way. The doctor helps the patient to produce a story[45] that's helpful to them[45]—a sustaining fiction[126] in which the positive outweighs the negative.[34] Creating this story is a starting point, not a conclusion.[34] The creation is not the doctor's but the patient's—or it's a shared venture. We might raise the possibility of a story more helpful than the patient's own, or a range of such stories, or help the patient to develop the ability to create different stories of their own.[34] Ideally, information we obtain from the medical literature should not be presented as a series of disconnected facts but incorporated into the evolving story.[127]

Patients sometimes talk about getting back to how they were, but how you are is something that needs to be produced, not discovered.[45] And for some people, there may be no previous state of well-being: for them, the term 'recovery' is a misnomer.[128] At a lecture I attended recently, one slide indicated that a sexually abused patient with chronic pelvic pain was referred to a gynaecologist for a 'historectomy'. If only it were that simple.

Narrative is a bridge between lay beliefs about lived illness and the medical case history.[129] The doctor sets the patient's story against other patients' stories and accounts from the scientific literature. Acquiring experience for the doctor is partly a matter of collecting a well-referenced library of short stories,[130] some of which will be patient anecdotes and some medical lore.[33]

MANAGEMENT-NAMING

Diagnosis may be a disease-naming exercise or a management-naming exercise.[131] Disease-naming is the more orthodox and encourages explicit formulation of the problem. In primary care where the prevalence of specific pathology is relatively low, often the important question is not 'What's wrong with the patient?' but 'Do I need to do anything?' Sometimes, deciding what's wrong is difficult and deciding whether anything needs done—and if so what—is easier.[132] In that case, the diagnosis may not be explicitly stated but implicit in the management.[133] Sometimes the diagnosis is arrived at by negotiation,[134] a consensus between patient and doctor about what they're trying to achieve.[28]

In time, the diagnosis might be refined, changed fundamentally, or overshadowed by a new diagnosis, depending on which outcomes we're considering. Pravastatin prevents cardiovascular death in the elderly without affecting overall mortality.[135] We might therefore judge it unsuitable for all elderly patients or suitable only for those in whom vascular risk exceeds risk from other diseases. If the patient develops incurable cancer, the risk of dying from that might overwhelm their risk of a vascular death and prompt us to stop their pravastatin.[136] The diagnosis in this situation, therefore, might be 'not for vascular prevention'.

The diagnosis governing severe acute illness in general practice is often not what the cause is but what the prognosis is and what needs done.[109] We're about to send away a young man with a cough until we auscultate their chest, diagnose pneumonia,[137] and prescribe an antibiotic. We arrive at the house of an elderly woman, find her confused and hypotensive, decide she needs to go to hospital, then listen to her chest and diagnose pneumonia again.[138] The label 'pneumonia' is the same for the two patients, but its implications differ. In the young man, it alters management from doing nothing to treating with an antibiotic. In the old woman, it makes no difference at the primary care stage—the patient needs to go to hospital in any case. When the diagnosis is pneumonia, the pneumonia guideline[139] helps. When the diagnosis is 'needs to go to hospital', it doesn't.

A dilemma often faced by the laboratory services is not 'What's caused this abnormal result?' or even 'What treatment is needed?' but 'How quickly do we need to inform the general practitioner?' This is diagnosis as prognosis over a time scale of hours.[140]

The patient with pneumonia or any other such acute disease is unwell and the right treatment makes them better. Often the treatment itself causes adverse effects that may be the price to pay for recovery. The wrong treatment is a costly mistake, such as rest rather than mobilisation following limb injury.[141] In secondary prevention of chronic disease, the patient might be well and the right treatment makes them ill. Patients having dialysis for end-stage renal failure talk not about the effects of the disease but about the effects of the treatment. Dialysis becomes the sickness.[42]

DEGREE OR KIND

Some phenomena are identified as disease because they differ from normal not in kind but in degree, or because they're associated with an adverse outcome. Since trials were first done and the results analysed statistically in the nineteenth century,[38] many associations between indicators and outcomes have been established. These enable diagnosis of a kind—that one individual is at greater or lesser risk than another. Whether the patient is identified as in a high-risk or low-risk group then depends on how the groups are defined:[142] different scoring systems will allocate any one patient to different risk groups and the patient's estimated risk of an event will change accordingly.

Induction in mathematics leads to great advances in understanding and knowledge.[143] Induction in medicine does the same but often needs to be complemented with hypothetico-deduction and falsification to ensure benefit exceeds harm. Inductive use of antibiotics brought order to the management of war wounds, lobar pneumonia and tuberculosis in the mid-twentieth century;[38] but it brought muddle to the management of self-limiting respiratory tract illness that—using hypothetico-deduction—we're still trying to sort out after 60 years.[144] Mathematics is quantitative, medicine often qualitative. It's difficult or impossible to do a controlled experiment on an individual human being. As a compromise, trials are done on groups of people with categories of disease and clusters of risk factors. Then individual qualitative outcomes (such as a variety of vascular events over a period of time among many patients) are pooled and represented as a quantitative outcome (the number of vascular events). The results of such research are impressive in that they exist at all and helpful—though underused—in determining healthcare policy: but for management of the individual patient, their value is limited by their probabilistic nature.[143] Each of the patients in a group has a different risk from the group as a whole.[145, 146] So, being aware of risks attached to groups may or may not help the individual patient.[147]

In the area of mental health, the psychoanalytical view that dominated Western practice in the first half of the twentieth century was that neurotic tension was present to a greater or lesser degree in everyone and that illness was the manifestation of the individual's failure to adapt. In the 1980s, pressure from government and insurers along with pharmaceutical developments precipitated a shift toward a categorical definition of mental illness: a solution was sought in medical nosology and crystallised initially in DSM-III.[148]

But medical nosology is not as clear-cut as it appears. The categorical nature of medical diagnosis is more apparent than real. Cancer, an exemplar for disease that kills if not treated, actually represents a spectrum of conditions. Prostate cancer has widely variable outcome depending on, among other factors, the Gleason score.[149] Ductal breast cancer, now revealed routinely by mammography, invades in half of cases or less.[150] And other cancers—even those of similar histopathological appearance in a single organ—have variable prognoses.[151]

Personality disorders or psychopathies continue to be regarded as variations or exaggerations of normal personality characteristics distinguished from normal by their maladaptiveness with consequential suffering to the individual or their community.[152]

UNCERTAINTY

If disease is a matter of maladaptiveness or of degree rather than of kind, what's the difference between a disease and a risk factor? It's not always clear. The question is side-stepped by using outcome as a marker: it doesn't matter whether we specify a disease as long as intervention does more good than harm.[6, 153] The diagnosis doesn't have to be right as long as it's better than the alternatives.[73] In any case, it's provisional and will change as the clinical picture develops.[109, 154] Diagnosis is not a single event but a process of reducing uncertainty about the nature of the patient's condition.[155]

The majority of new problems the general practitioner sees are non-specific and must be provisionally diagnosed on clinical grounds. Although, for the purposes of research, medically unexplained physical symptoms require, say, three months duration before diagnosis,[156] in day-to-day work, we diagnose such problems clinically and early. In general practice, we'll often see the patient repeatedly and approach the diagnosis step by step. However, if we eventually arrive at a serious diagnosis, patient and doctor might wonder at which of the previous consultations that diagnosis might reasonably have been made. In hospital practice, a diagnosis is a triumph; in general practice, it can easily appear to represent an earlier failure.[134]

A young woman's anaemia might be attributed to menstruation until other features reveal a diagnosis of colorectal cancer.[157] Where there are multiple agencies involved in healthcare, most of which investigate and treat more actively than general practitioners, diagnosis and recovery can be misattributed to perceived better management rather than to the passage of time. Thus the false impression is systematically created that the model of serial primary care consultations is flawed.

It's suggested that general practitioners ask themselves: 'Would you be surprised if this patient died in the next six to 12 months?'[158] With the exception of advanced dementia—which is accompanied by persistently severe disability—itinerary of demise is independent of cause of death:[159] so it's likely that for many patients, this question will have low predictive value. In future, it's a question that's likely to arise with increasing frequency. Average female life expectancy in Western societies is increasing at 2.3 years per decade. For fit elderly people, acute and preventive care should be just as energetic as for younger people. However, since 1950, the extra years have been not healthy but unhealthy: the period of morbidity between disease onset and death has become not compressed but expanded.[68] So we have increasing numbers of elderly patients with multiple morbidities in whom a decision has to be made about starting, continuing, or stopping preventive interventions. How do we set about making this sort of decision? For some prevention, such as statin treatment, benefit and harm both occur early.[160] For invasive procedures, harm precedes benefit and the delay before benefit exceeds harm can be estimated. For colorectal cancer screening in unhealthy people, mortality from screening drops below mortality from disease at two years in 50-year-old men and at eight months in 60-year-old women, and morbidity from screening drops below morbidity from disease at five years in 50-year-old men and at two years in 60-year-old women.[160] This delay needs to be compared with the patient's life expectancy in order to estimate whether or not screening will improve mortality and morbidity.[161]

In each consultation, we have to consider priorities: presenting problem or continuing problems; short term or long term; process or outcome; comfort or cure; morbidity or mortality. The stages of dying from cancer—denial, anger, bargaining, depression, and acceptance[162]—may have their counterparts in other life-changing but not terminal conditions. When treating a patient with heart failure, we need to judge when to titrate beta-blockade and when to make a transition to palliative care.[158] If we misdiagnose a phase of low mood as a wish to die, we move too soon from active treatment to palliation. If we misinterpret an acceptance of imminent death as a disease called depression,[163] we deny the patient a peaceful decline.

LESION OR DISABILITY

The biomechanical model supposes a chain of linear cause-and-effect relationships. As aetiology becomes better understood, the diagnosis—and therefore the action point for treatment or prevention—moves backwards along the chain.[73] Sometimes the diagnosis is defined in pathological terms, near the beginning of this chain, and sometimes it's defined in terms of clinical features, nearer the end.[97] The scientific basis for this, however, isn't always solid. In the elderly, for instance, higher mental function doesn't correspond in a straightforward way to postmortem findings in the brain. Of elderly people with no cognitive impairment, 38% have features of Alzheimer's disease at necropsy and 23% have brain infarction. Of elderly people with Alzheimer's disease, 88% have it confirmed after death but 40% have—also or instead—brain infarction and 17% Lewy body disease.[164, 165]

The diagnosis of dementia and the further specification of Alzheimer's disease are therefore scientifically dubious. And while naming the disease can be a positive step toward provision of an explanation and access to services, it can have negative consequences, jeopardising autonomy, insurance, and driving licence: in some circumstances, a diagnosis of 'memory problems' may be better.[166] Functional needs can be addressed without a disease having to be named,[167] and in the presence of such pathological imprecision this might be a sensible pragmatic approach.[165] Planning care for the elderly would be easier if we had some idea of the likely timing, cause and course of death.[168] Timing can be estimated approximately,[169] but pathological cause and functional course are largely unrelated to each other and are unpredictable.[159]

In psychiatric conditions, it's not clear that basing the diagnosis not on symptoms but on pathology is valid. Many patients qualify for more than one psychiatric diagnosis,[51] and symptoms such as delusions and hallucinations, rather than putative underlying pathology, may be the correct focus for research and treatment.[170]

Lower urinary tract symptoms also illustrate a dichotomy between lesion and disability. Symptoms and disease (such as prostatic hypertrophy or cancer) are separate entities with only a certain overlap between them. The effects of symptoms on quality of life determine whether we treat. Objective information determines what we treat.[171]

Disease can be defined as a failure of adaptation.[172] If that refers to physiological response to the environment, we've moved our diagnosis a long way to the left. If it refers to the capacity for telling new, more helpful stories, we've moved the diagnosis a long way to the right.

PATHOGENESIS OR SALUTOGENESIS

The choice of diagnosis and the discussion of it with the patient can be pathogenic or salutogenic, harmful or healing.[173] If the problem is thought not to fit the medical model, calling it functional rather than medically unexplained suggests diagnostic success rather than failure, certainty rather than uncertainty, something substantial rather than a vacuum, and it's unlikely to offend patients.[174] Volunteering to a patient that their distressing symptoms are normal—however true and helpful that might be if we're thinking about prevalence in the population—might irritate some patients.[175]

Health is the ability to adapt.[172, 97] This concept is particularly applicable to the elderly.[86] Older people, who feel healthy despite having joint problems, might regard 'wear and tear' as a normal part of ageing that they manage by keeping their joints mobile.[24] Frailty, often a feature of ageing, is distinct from disability, which need not be.[86]

Ageing is accompanied by a decline in specific areas only: in the field of cognition, for instance, working and episodic memory and some aspects of semantic memory deteriorate while other functions are preserved; and emotionally there's a decline in negative affect while positive affect appears to remain fairly constant as long as situations are familiar. Of the big five personality traits, neuroticism, extroversion, and openness to experience decrease (although neuroticism may show some increase in very late life), while agreeableness and conscientiousness increase. There's also an increase in wisdom, which can be thought of as a provisional commitment to one chosen truth system with the awareness that alternative systems exist, along with the balancing of thoughts, desires, and emotions.[86]

It's easy unquestioningly to elide health with happiness and confuse ability to adapt with adoption of amiability. The expectation that people should be happy is cultural, not universal. Being principled, righteous, and moral is not necessarily comfortable or pleasant.[86] There might be purpose and meaning in suffering and the response it elicits from others.[46]

ILLNESS AND DISEASE; FUNCTION AND PATHOLOGY

Patient-centred medicine focuses on the person, and illness-centred medicine on pathology.[4] Personal illness is caused by human situations, and disease illness by organic pathology.[97] Illness is the feeling someone has when they're unwell, disease is dysfunction of an organ,[28] and functional symptoms are bodily dysfunctions unexplained by pathology.[174, 176] Dissimulating disorders include malingering (in which symptoms and signs are simulated in order to achieve a goal), factitious disease (which is really a fiction created in the pursuit of patienthood for its own sake), and hysteria or somatisation (in which distress is involuntarily exhibited in physical form).[177] These definitions in isolation might sound convincing, but strung together they reveal their own and each others' inconsistencies. It's tempting to use a term such as medically unexplained physical symptoms.[178] That seems to define something precise but, apart from being cumbersome and negative, it creates the misleading impression that the symptoms referred to might be explained, if not medically, then in some other way. An alternative term, functional illness, has none of those disadvantages and is more acceptable to patients.[174]

But none of this makes it clear what we're talking about.

Patients can't be divided into those with disease and those with functional illness. Nor can the individual patient be split in two, part diseased, part dysfunctional.

Each patient is a complete human being with their own unique assortment of qualities beyond comprehension. The division between disease and dysfunction is a construct. It exists in the doctor's mind, not in the patient's body.

What we have here, then, is a way of looking at patients, a way of thinking and talking about them. And it's useful. It increases our chances of applying the medical model appropriately. Without such a model, clinical findings make no sense.[10] If the model is confused with reality, patients make no sense.

An unhappy woman with chronic obstructive pulmonary disease has peripheral oedema. The three strands of depression, dyspnoea, and dropsy—with their many causal connections—interweave. Clinical assessment might involve teasing out the warp from the weft, the biomedical from the functional, to get a view of the detail, but the cloth has to remain in one piece and be treated as a whole.

The disease construct is based on the biomedical model, while the functional construct isn't. The disease construct includes defined pathology and an evidence base; the functional construct draws on ideas from the social sciences, the humanities and life experience. Evidence-based medicine helps the doctor manage disease, and patient-centred consulting helps the patient to manage their distress. This approach is a prerequisite for appropriate use of medical technology: that's better for the patient and, being parsimonious, is better for a socialised healthcare system.

Early recognition of the functional aspects to a problem that lie outwith the biomedical model is helpful.[179] It's a positive step that avoids medicalisation.[180] Some problems might be unexplained because of lack of knowledge or expertise,[181] so the diagnosis, like all diagnoses, is provisional. Referral is an option but can raise expectations only to disappoint, waste resources, and risk exposing the patient to potentially dangerous tests and treatments. It can also lead to the 'collusion of anonymity' in which the patient is passed from one specialist to another without anybody taking responsibility for the whole person.[182] Follow-up consultations in primary care can provide a safety net: just as all variables approach the mean over time,[183] functional symptoms tend to improve spontaneously. The use of several consultations might be regarded as inefficient, but it's preferable to the costly and dangerous alternative of inappropriate interventions.

The idea that mind and body are separate is an obstacle to holistic care[175] and is erroneous.[184] Mind and body are one. Physical symptoms are not either in the body or in the mind: they're physical symptoms. Unexplained physical symptoms are not due to psychological problems or stress: they're physical symptoms. The distress caused by functional problems can equal that caused by physical disease,[185] and pain is as bad as it feels.[186]

MAKING A DIAGNOSIS

So there are many aspects of the consultation that can be given the status of diagnosis. Being aware of this doesn't generally give us new tasks that have to be squeezed into or extracted from the 10-minute consultation. Rather, they're ways of thinking about the patient and about the consultation that are useful in answering the questions: 'What matters about all of this? What's the problem here? What's going on?'.[187] For any one consultation, we'll come up with more than one answer.

One new task, however, does emerge, and it's one that I expect will be increasingly required of general practitioners: the new task is an explicit weighing of evidence. This has become more pressing with the increasing availability of investigations and treatment with the power for benefit if used appropriately and the potential for harm if not. We need to decide how to combine biomechanical interventions using technology with a more human response to the patient using ourselves in a relationship with them—the drug called 'doctor'.[182] The frail elderly and people with serious comorbidities impairing longevity or quality of life pose a particular dilemma. Preventive interventions should be initiated or continued only in those for whom benefit is likely to exceed harm. The difficulty of diagnosis must not allow the reach of medical technology to extend, by default, beyond the evidence. And the possibility of making sophisticated diagnoses should not deter us from making a simple one, the right one, one that offers the best outcome for the patient.[154]

EXERCISES

Consider a patient you've just seen while they're fresh in your mind. Write down their diagnoses from a functional perspective and from a medical-model perspective.

Consider an elderly patient that you know and are just about to see. Write down what you know of their functional state and life expectancy and what preventive treatment they're on. Estimate the risks and benefits to them of this preventive treatment.

Consider a surgery you've just done. List the computer codes you used. For each one, identify and find out what purpose it serves.

Consider the patients you saw in one surgery, perhaps a month ago, and study their notes. For each patient, make a judgment as to whether, in retrospect, your medical intervention (referral, investigation, and prescribing) was excessive or insufficient. Ask a colleague to give their view.

CHAPTER 2

Healthcare design

'A competition will immediately begin among them, and the market price will rise more or less above the natural price, according as either the greatness of the deficiency, or the wealth and wanton luxury of the competitors, happen to animate more or less the eagerness of the competition.'

Smith A. *The Wealth of Nations*. London: Penguin Classics; 1999.

'Again, there must be no escape into ideology from thought; all depends on the specific case within the larger context.'

Galbraith JK. *The Good Society: the humane agenda*.
London: Sinclair-Stevenson; 1996.

Imagine one of the following situations: you're a junior doctor applying for a specialist training scheme and taking part in a group discussion exercise as part of the assessment procedure;[188] you're a newly qualified general practitioner applying to join a practice and being interviewed by the partners; you're an experienced general practitioner planning for the future at a partnership meeting; or you're representing general practice in a meeting about healthcare service provision in your area. In any of these situations, you might find yourself involved in a discussion about the organisation of healthcare in general and primary care in particular. A good outcome depends not on your powers of rhetoric but on your ability to think critically[189] and to engage in argument for the sake not of winning but of reaching a valid conclusion.[190]

What follows represents an idealised version of the sort of argument you might have if you're able to access, appraise and present evidence with improbable rapidity. It's presented as the script for a play with a storyline.[191] This device makes it possible for arguments to be stated in the first rather than third person, which makes for brevity, clarity, and conviction; it also means that evidence comes thick and fast. You may wish to join with two colleagues to read a part each and use it as the basis for discussion.

CHOICE

AUDREY: Shall I read out the subject for discussion? 'Securing our health in the future:[192] a roadmap for primary care'.[193]

KEN: First, perhaps we need to get a sense of where we are now and how we got here.[194]

VEE: But I think we ought to focus on patients and patient outcomes: those are the things that really matter.[195]

AUDREY: That sounds like a good idea.

VEE: Take something you see often, like a woman with dysuria.

KEN: And she consults us in general practice ...

AUDREY: Or phones NHS Direct[196] ...

VEE: But she might look up NHS Choices,[197] go to a walk-in centre[198, 199] ...

AUDREY: ... or phone a friend.[12] There are many points of first contact.[198]

KEN: Yes, that's true. And they're largely unnecessary. In general practice, we provide open and unlimited access[200] ...

AUDREY: ... though now only in office hours since we stopped doing out-of-hours care.[201]

VEE: But the availability of other agencies[199] gives more choice, something general practice doesn't see as important.[200, 202]

AUDREY: It depends what sort of choice we're talking about: autonomy of the individual as an ethical principle;[70] the demands of consumer groups;[203, 204] or patient preferences elicited in a good consultation.[205, 206, 207]

VEE: I see freedom as the goal of social progress, and also the means by which we achieve that goal and measure progress toward it. It's inherently good.[208]

KEN: And it puts people under pressure to decide things at every turn—which they don't like. They worry about making the wrong decision and regretting it.[209]

AUDREY: Patients might not want choice so much as personal attention.[210] Perhaps they want to talk through options with their doctor without necessarily having to make the final decision.[211] Rather than choice, they just want good evidence-based, high quality care.[212]

VEE: No, patients want choice, and exercise it when they have it. If they can access secondary care directly rather than by way of the GP gatekeeper[213] they do so.[214] If they're offered the choice of a better hospital than their local one, the majority of patients—in all demographic groups—take it.[215]

AUDREY: The way choice is offered affects which option patients choose.[216] Whether or not patients say they want choice depends on how you ask the question.[217]

VEE: But general practitioners often don't ask the question at all.[215] Patients don't like gatekeeping.[218]

GATEKEEPING

KEN: Well, gatekeeping isn't an essential feature of primary care.[200] In general practice in the UK, we took it on in exchange for preserving our autonomy;[219] it allowed the government to hide rationing behind the doctrine of clinical judgment.[204] We now contain demand in various ways—by directing the patient to a non-statutory agency, undertreating, making a service less accessible, delaying action, or deciding that a condition doesn't come within the remit of healthcare at all.[210] We're probably quite good at it.[220] In most organisations, 20% of the output usually requires 80% of the input,[221] whereas in general practice, the 20% of patients who consult most frequently account for only 55% of the consultations.[222] In England during the years 2005–09 consultant-to-consultant referrals increased by 40% while referrals from primary to secondary care increased by only 20%.[223] We steward public resources, resisting the pressure of consumer demand[210] and balancing the needs of the patient in front of us against needs of other patients.[224, 225, 226, 227] And when necessary, we act as our patients' advocates and find them the service they need.[210] We're good at preventing other services from being overwhelmed.[228, 229, 193, 213]

AUDREY: Being a gatekeeper sounds a bit like being a bouncer—stopping people coming in. Perhaps I'm more like a butler or housekeeper, greeting arrivals.[230]

KEN: Yes, that feels more welcoming. In primary care, we provide universal access, equity, and high quality.[231] We diagnose,[200] coordinate care, and provide continuity[232]—we're a familiar and safe base for patients, a sort of home from home.[233]

VEE: But how do you quantify all of that? What little evidence there is shows that mistakes in diagnosis[157] and referral[234] are made, and care isn't always equitable or of high quality.[235]

AUDREY: Interesting as this discussion is, there is a patient with dysuria waiting for a doctor.

POINT OF FIRST CONTACT

VEE: No, she's waiting to see someone about her dysuria—she doesn't care if it's a doctor or not. It's her lunch break, she doesn't have long, and she wants antibiotics. A nurse in a walk-in centre will do fine:[198] the nurse will look up the electronic health record, use clinical decision support software,[236, 237 238] and prescribe:[221] simple!

KEN: And simplistic. We've several management options for dysuria of comparable average effectiveness—diagnosis by symptoms, urinalysis, or culture, and treatment with immediate or deferred antibiotics. Clinical decision support software improves process but doesn't improve quality or lower costs.[236] Even a condition as apparently straightforward as dysuria requires professional judgment.[239]

VEE: I don't see it that way. This woman's urinary problem is routine and should be fixed by following an evidence-based algorithm.[240] Compared with a doctor, a nurse provides the same or better quality of care at no extra cost.[241] There's no benefit to the patient in being seen by a doctor for minor, self-limiting illnesses.[242] A nurse can deal with the presenting problem and then go on to health promotion.[243]

KEN: The Quality and Outcomes Framework gives us GPs the resources and incentives to do that as well. Equity's been mentioned: in deprived areas, achieving high points under the framework is associated by some measures with improved outcomes, so there's the possibility of reducing health inequalities.[244]

VEE: But I can get full payment under the framework without monitoring all my patients—that's the inverse care law in action.[245] Health inequalities due to deprivation would be reduced if I got full payment only for full coverage.[246] Anyway, a nurse in a multidisciplinary centre can liaise with the other health and social services on site:[247, 198] that's an important way of tackling health inequalities.[246]

AUDREY: Services such as walk-in centres might have a place in conurbations. National government is most influenced by problems in the capital city on its doorstep.[194] Elsewhere in the country, is there a need for such things?

VEE: If people had more of a voice in healthcare delivery, they'd tell us.[248]

KEN: And we're back where we started—offering the patient choice. Healthcare is already stretched three ways by the competing forces of access, quality, and cost containment.[210] Choice adds to the tension. It doesn't necessarily improve efficiency and can either improve or worsen equity and quality.[249] It doesn't fit well with continuity[202, 110] and coordination of care.[200, 110] And it undermines loyalty to a public health service:[209] for instance, if patients can get private healthcare, they'll put less pressure on the public service to improve.[250]

QUALITY

AUDREY: You mentioned quality. How is it defined?

KEN: Quality is a composite measure of safety, effectiveness, and experience for the patient.[251]

VEE: But good quality care is also timely, efficient, and equitable.[252]

AUDREY: Are those measures of quality or of something else? Efficiency, for instance, is a measure of output compared with the maximum feasible output using the same resources.[192]

VEE: Okay, but good quality healthcare requires optimum use of resources.[238] I'd regard a quality improvement as a change that raises quality and lowers costs.[238, 253]

AUDREY: That might be called value improvement.[192]

KEN: Does it matter? As clinicians, our main responsibility is not to manage the service but to provide evidence-based,[204] professional[238] care to patients.

AUDREY: I'm not sure you can separate those things out. If I speak to drug reps, I'm likely to prescribe less well and more expensively than I would otherwise.[254] If I'm typical of healthcare professionals, I'm not good at appraising evidence[255] and I adhere to a median of only 34% of research findings.[256] I'd say that was unprofessional and unethical.[257, 238] If I'm not doing a good job, do you think patients can tell?

VEE: It depends what evidence you look at. Patient satisfaction surveys don't discriminate effectively between individual doctors, but measures of patient experience discriminate between practices.[258] Patients making choices look more to friends and family for information and advice than to official data[215]—which they have difficulty understanding, even if it's well presented.[259]

KEN: Patients generally have difficulty with medical information. They're misled by pharmaceutical companies into believing they have—or are going to get—non-existent conditions.[243] And even well-presented non-promotional literature confuses them. If they're shown written information about effects and side effects of drugs, 20–30% of them choose the wrong drug.[259] And if you give people with low educational attainment a decision aid about bowel cancer screening, only 34% understand well enough to make an informed choice.[77]

VEE: But everyone has problems with statistics—patients,[259] surgeons,[260] physicians,[79] researchers,[80] journalists[261]—even statisticians.[82]

HEALTHCARE FUNDING

KEN: Surely, even if they have difficulty assimilating the information, patients are entitled to the basic human rights of autonomy and self-determination.[208] We already elicit patients' ideas, concerns, and expectations in our consultations.[176] We could do more with patient participant groups. They could be more formal, influential,[262] and involved in improving the service.[263] The Alma-Ata declaration proposed a social, community-orientated, politicised model[264] with total transparency: 'nothing about me without me'.[265]

AUDREY: An alternative would be to give patients a louder voice in a more open healthcare market. The market is efficient at optimising total benefit.[208]

KEN: And effective at maximising inequality.[266, 208] Some healthcare interventions—such as infectious disease control—are better managed collaboratively rather than individually.[208] Longevity is positively related to public expenditure in healthcare,[208] and life expectancy to socioeconomic equality.[267]

AUDREY: That makes it sound as if social provision is equitable, which it is not.[268]

VEE: But a market allows people to seek out services for themselves: that's more equitable.[210] The affluent pay for what they want.[269] That has the additional advantage that people see the money they're paying and insist on good value: that drives up standards.[221]

KEN: And we'd be abandoning the NHS founding principle—healthcare available to everyone according to need, free at the point of use.[38, 251] Anyway, healthcare shouldn't depend on ability to pay: that's unethical.[266]

VEE: But public funding means that the state can justify spying on the consultation:[120] that's equally unethical.[270]

AUDREY: Ethics seems to take second place to ideology: people are committed in the UK to socialised medicine,[262] and in the United States to private medicine.[38] Are there just two options, then: a traditional public service listening to what patients need, or a modern global private business listening to what consumers want?[210]

VEE: No. You see, there are differences between competition, choice, privatisation, and marketisation. Competition can take place in a public service. General practitioners in the UK run private businesses selling their own medical skills but they don't run public limited companies with financial obligations to shareholders. Healthcare is different from most commodities traded in the marketplace.[271] A free market in healthcare would require real competition, informed choice, and no cherry-picking.[210] The free market doesn't work when there's an imbalance of power and the potential for harm to the individual or society.[266] Even if a service is privatised, health isn't like commerce, and contracts are never watertight.[210]

KEN: And in a healthcare market, it's unclear what the commodity is. Is it healthcare? Well, the consultation is a desirable commodity. It's a form of treatment—the process of discussion is therapeutic and beneficial in itself.[34] We might feel it has inherent value. Beyond that type of therapeutic consultation, healthcare is unpleasant and harmful and therefore not worth buying—quite the opposite. It's justified only if we have evidence of subsequent likely benefit, improved health: the patient depends on the doctor to advise about the likelihood of that.[242, 259] So healthcare isn't a commodity in the usual sense. Perhaps, instead, health is the commodity. And what's health? Health is possibly a state of well-being,[60] perhaps the ability to adapt,[172] and maybe a capacity for creating meaningful stories.[34] These are inherent qualities of the individual: they can't be bought and sold. Perhaps the commodity is really the patient's body that's passed around the system for profit.[272]

AUDREY: It sounds as if neither a public nor a private system better enables informed choice. Healthcare could become a combination of a modern responsive public service and a traditional regulated market; and there could be a consultative process for distinguishing between wants and needs, and for determining priorities.[273]

AUDREY: The mix of public and private existed before the NHS was founded in 1948. It did not work then—that is why the NHS was formed—and it is unlikely to work now.[210]

VEE: Mixing public with private provision, and ensuring competition and choice, are all very well, but they won't stop the healthcare service being too complicated, expensive,[221] expansionist, and inefficient.[210] I'd simplify it and make it cheaper. Look at it this way. Healthcare can be split into three groups of activities.[221] One group consists of repetitive tasks that use resources but don't directly benefit the patient.[274] An example would be warfarin monitoring. Ideally, those tasks are done right, first time, every time, for less money and paid for on a capitation basis so there's no incentive to do them unnecessarily.[221] Other tasks are different every time. Suppose our patient with dysuria also has abdominal pain. Diagnosing that has to be done by an expert, perhaps involving specialists. The outcome is unknown, and the payment should be by the hour. Tasks forming the third group are again specialised and skilled but they have predefined outcomes, like injection of a joint. They have to be done often enough by the individual practitioner to ensure expertise is developed and maintained.[274] And payment has to be fee for service.[221]

TRANSFORMING HEALTHCARE

KEN: That seems complicated.[275] In general practice, we deal with tasks from all three of these groups in our surgeries:[200] for instance, managing dysuria, diagnosing abdominal pain, and aspirating a knee. In fact, we might do all three in a single consultation, at a push. These are parts of the whole that is general practice.[26]

AUDREY: I wonder if I can mention our waiting patient, the woman with dysuria. While she is waiting, she might make her voice heard through a patient-participation group or through the market. Once she eventually gets her appointment, she might speak to a nurse, using evidence and algorithm, or to a doctor, using experience and problem-solving skills. Does it matter which?

VEE: No. What matters is that we don't look at the situation in terms of professional allegiances.[276, 210, 277] Most countries' systems of healthcare depend on traditional professional groupings and organisational structures.[194] The sharp division between primary and secondary care in the NHS, for instance, is a legacy of class-based antagonism between general practitioners and hospital consultants in nineteenth-century Britain.[219]

KEN: And that's resulted in small, flexible general practices better able than many healthcare organisations to adapt and innovate.[232]

VEE: But general practice doesn't innovate—it doesn't even keep up. Look at e-mail. Rather than wait to see me, a patient should be able to look up my practice Web site and be prompted to give a structured history that I read and respond to within a specified time period, like 24 hours.[278, 279]

KEN: During which time the patient's condition will be different. And, in the consulting room or on the telephone, we listen for the patient to confirm they've understood. For the proponents of e-mail in healthcare, a 'thank you' is just a nuisance.[278]

VEE: But as a GP I can see what changes are needed and can make them.[221]

KEN: True. And if we don't change, we'll have change imposed from above.[210]

AUDREY: Even change from above is not necessarily decisive. Government policy is often internally inconsistent. It is influenced by competing voices—government departments, local organisations, the professionals, the patients. Reform is slow because all of these voices must be listened to.[280, 262] Successful implementation of health information technology systems, for instance, requires an intuitive system that can be adapted for local use, which is chosen democratically and implemented autocratically.[281] For change, an organisation needs to have the necessary size, knowledge, skills, motivation, leadership, quality control systems, and readiness to take risks; and the change must be well-managed.[276] You have to look at economic, ethical, and professional reasons to change[238] and there's only limited evidence for methods that improve speed and success of change.[238, 282] And all changes have unintended consequences that have to be anticipated and addressed.[208]

VEE: But that looks defeatist. Some poor countries have transformed their healthcare systems and their populations' health.[283]

PRIMARY CARE

KEN: And primary care has been at the centre of these changes.[283]

AUDREY: It does sound as if primary care is cost-effective. Specialists providing evidence-based care of a specific disease manage that specific disease better than generalists but they don't improve the overall health of the population.[257] The large benefit to each of the few people likely to benefit may be outweighed by small harm to each of the many people less likely to benefit.[98] Compared with specialists, generalists improve functional status more—and do it more cost-effectively and equitably for both patients and populations.[257] Population health improvements measured by a variety of criteria are associated with strong primary care systems that provide point of first contact for comprehensive, coordinated, long-term person-centred (rather than disease-centred) care in the setting of family and community.[284, 285] It's likely that healthcare can best be provided predominantly horizontally by general practitioners and public health physicians. For complex diseases, GPs can use a patient-centred approach to prioritise management[286] and to coordinate a more vertical, shared-care approach.[257]

KEN: And that depends on maintaining continuity of care. In the UK, continuity of care by GPs never extended to periods of hospitalisation,[214] and it was further weakened when we abandoned of out-of-hours care.[201] We'll lose it completely if we don't actively preserve it.[110]

VEE: Okay, let's look at that. Hospitals, which were necessary in the nineteenth and twentieth centuries to accommodate the technology required for the growth of scientific medicine,[33] are increasingly unattractive. They're expensive, infected, and outmoded. A nurse can reduce readmission rates for patients with severe heart failure by visiting and monitoring the patients at home. This sort of intervention breaks down the barriers between hospital, GP surgery, and the patient's home and is supported by technological advance. Telemonitoring improves peak flow rate and quality of life in asthmatics,[287] reduces admission in severe asthmatics,[288] improves blood pressure in hypertensives[287] and enables a hospital-at-home service.[289] Information can be sent to hospital specialists to help with management—for instance, of skin lesions.[290] Teleconsulting, near-patient testing, electronic image transfer, interactive computer programmes,[291] and self-care are growth areas.[292] All of these changes require better coordination between primary and secondary care, and that interaction itself improves patient outcomes.[293] Sharing clinical expertise improves patient satisfaction, patient retention, clinician behaviour, and use of resources.[294]

KEN: Yes, and we could allow all of these innovations to disrupt continuity of care or we could hold the centre and incorporate these changes under the umbrella of primary care. Throughout medicine, there's a tendency to do too much because we like to feel we're doing something rather than nothing[295] and because we tend to think that more is better.[296] We pile another investigation onto the previous one just to play safe, and the result is the medical equivalent of a top-heavy ship.[297] For instance, we need to get a handle on unexplained variation in referral practice[223] and incorporate evidence-based referral criteria, peer review, audit, and consultant feedback.[223]

AUDREY: A possible 30% of healthcare in the United States might be unnecessary, producing no demonstrable benefit to the patient.[298] Technological advances in medicine improve management for a small number of conditions and patients. They contribute little to the care of the majority of people or conditions and overall these advances have not been paralleled by improvements in diagnosis or outcome. Autopsies from 1959 to 1989 showed that an increase in scanning from 0% to 77% of patients studied did not improve the accuracy of diagnosis during life.[299] In the Netherlands, expenditure on diagnostic tests is growing at the rate of 7% a year without corresponding improvement in health status.[300] If they are doing these tests to please patients, they are failing there as well. For patients with unexplained symptoms, satisfaction and anxiety are not affected by whether or not a blood test is done.[301] Doctors sometimes erroneously perceive simple linear cause-and-effect mechanisms and rush to act when being less active would lead to a better outcome. Occasionally, both patient and doctor can confidently agree about what is wrong and what is to be done; more often, either patient or doctor is uncertain or they cannot agree,[302] and the gap is sometimes filled by useless or harmful activity.

MEDICAL TECHNOLOGY

VEE: But look at chronic disease.[200] The Quality and Outcomes Framework in the UK was part of the new contract in 2004 and resourced general practitioners to take on chronic disease management. Following this, clinical data recording has improved,[238] and the UK has been ranked first in an international survey of diabetes care.[303]

AUDREY: One can use process measures like those, or outcomes such as mortality. In England, the contract had the potential in 2004 to save about 56 lives per 100 000 and actually saved only 11 lives per 100 000.[304]

A third measure is cost-effectiveness. Here it is difficult to separate signal from noise: hospital costs have been reduced by a small amount—it is hard to say how much. Whether those savings are offset by hidden costs in the community is uncertain.[262, 305]

VEE: Okay. Those figures don't show the benefits of technology. But look at cancer. From 1950 to 1995, there was an absolute increase in five-year survival for each of 20 malignancies, ranging from 3% for pancreas to 50% for prostate.[306]

AUDREY: Survival tells one story and mortality another: mortality rates dropped for only 12 cancers and rose for eight.[306]

KEN: And changes in five-year survival bear little relationship to changes in mortality. They probably depend more on diagnostic pathway. Screening means earlier diagnosis with little if any change in outcome.[306] The reduction in death from the condition being screened for is small: breast cancer screening in Norway reduces breast cancer deaths by 2.4 per 100 000 person-years;[307] the number needed to sigmoidoscope to prevent one colorectal cancer death in England is 489;[308] and population-based screening has no effect on prostate cancer death rates.[309] For those three cancers, screening doesn't improve all-cause mortality.[310, 311, 309] Part of the problem is that screening detects only a minority of cancers—23% of breast[312] and colorectal,[311] for instance.

VEE: But cancer in the consulting room is often invisible. It's camouflaged by non-specific symptoms that blend into the background.[313]

EARLY DIAGNOSIS

KEN: The symptoms aren't entirely non-specific. There are symptoms and signs predictive for cancer, and the predictive values of some of them increase when we elicit them more than once during the course of serial consultations.[314, 315, 316] We can use the test of time[317] to help with diagnosis[318] and refer when appropriate.[200] And a greater supply of general practitioners is associated with earlier detection of, for instance, colorectal cancer.[285]

VEE: Maybe, but it looks as if gatekeeping is the cause of late diagnosis[213] of cancer and early mortality from it in the UK compared with other European countries.[319, 320]

KEN: Those figures aren't reliable; they're based on differences in data collection rather than in management.[321, 322] And anyway, delay in cancer diagnosis is associated with worse, better, or the same outcome for different cancers and in different studies.[313, 151]

AUDREY: Those findings are based on observational work; they don't prove that
            delay doesn't matter.[151]

KEN: That's true. We just need to be confident that we have evidence for ini-
            tiatives with the potential for harm, such as raising awareness, refer-
            ring, and investigating.[320]

AUDREY: So, cancer diagnosis either by screening or by symptoms and signs
            is difficult. Not much has been said about prevention—of cancer or
            of any of the big killers. Primary prevention is one of the roles of
            primary care.[200]

PREVENTION

VEE: I ought to show individual patients how they should change their
            lifestyle.[323, 324] But whatever individual difference I make, I won't see
            much difference at a population level.[98, 325]

KEN: And there's the risk that people forget to live while they worry about
            the risk of being at risk.[326]

VEE: But you're looking at it negatively. I see preventing illness as preserv-
            ing health.[327]

KEN: Healthcare reformers are over-optimistic about the possibility of
            health gains. We're all on an inevitable descent to illness and death.[328]

VEE: But that's too pessimistic.

KEN: We need to be realistic. In hospital clinics, different juniors spend
            a few minutes with the patient at a series of stopping-off points on
            their itinerary. In primary care, a single doctor accompanies them for
            long parts of their journey.[329] We need to be wary of allowing health
            promotion[330] and secondary prevention[262] to outweigh other aspects
            of healthcare. There's a misplaced emphasis on targets instead of car-
            ing.[262] Items-of-service payments distort priorities, lead to gaming,
            and increase costs.[208] They might have a place[238] alongside profes-
            sionalism. That means subjugating ourselves to an ethical code and
            then, rather than hiding behind professional bodies and guidelines,
            taking personal responsibility[263] for shouldering some uncertainty
            on behalf of our patients and guiding them through their journey.

VEE: That's paternalistic.[70]

AUDREY: Or paternalistic libertarianism.[216]

KEN: 'Pastoral' perhaps.[331] In general practice, we're using our relationship
            with the patient[264, 332, 333] to modify expectations, to influence behav-
            iour,[334, 335] to witness, to hold, to help patients cope,[172] and to give
            them the opportunity to create different stories for themselves.[34] The
            mystery of general practice[2] isn't understood by hospital specialists,[336]
            managers, and politicians[125]—they're too much in the grip of the new

medical-industrial complex.[271] The totality of individual specialist recommendations exceeds available resources,[337] and what can't be measured is squeezed out.[338]

VEE: But medicine is a science.

KEN: And general practice is the application of science.[339, 25, 172] The science we're trying to apply is flawed, but even where it's robust, it covers only a part of what we do in general practice.[340] Consulting involves a series of judgments[25] using knowledge, skill, and experience in a context of uncertainty, often requiring compromise and half measure.[203] General practice has a high complexity density per hour.[341] A risk factor is like being offside in football: it only matters if it affects outcome.[342] That's a matter of judgment for the referee in one case and the physician in the other. Medical science is reaching a dead end. Advances in medicine have depended on testing theory against practice. Modern risk-based statistical preventive healthcare can't be tested in the same way.[343] Once a form of prevention has become widespread, it becomes impossible to research its effectiveness. We mustn't medicalise everyday life and turn science into dogma or superstition.[213]

THE FUTURE

AUDREY: Meanwhile, our patient with dysuria is still waiting. Should she make an appointment for the nurse, the doctor, the pharmacist?

KEN: She could make an appointment for the future.

AUDREY: That rings a bell: the future is the subject of this discussion.

VEE: But we haven't discussed it.

AUDREY: Or maybe we have. Let's see whether we've got answers to the following questions: Might provision be publicly or privately funded? How many points of first contact might there be? How might primary and secondary care relate? What will happen to general practitioners' gatekeeping role? What will be the role of technological innovation? Might nurses substitute for doctors? How will information be managed? What form will clinical governance take? and How will we educate the next generation of doctors?

KEN: A publicly funded service will give us the most secure future. It enables systemic rather than piecemeal development paid for on a capitation basis.[221] And it's likely to be the cheapest way of providing high quality, equitable, universal coverage.[208] A single point of first contact would preserve the traditional role of GP as gatekeeper, but that's unlikely to sit comfortably with societal changes. A shared electronic patient record will enable agencies to provide coordinated care—and that coordination should be done by the GP.[110]

VEE: I see a place for more rapid transfer of patients from primary to secondary care and back again in person, as now, but also virtually.[274, 290] Again, information technology will allow everyone involved to see what's happening to the patient. But technological innovation will also be evident in other areas, especially diagnostics.[221] You'll see fewer patients in hospital and more at home being monitored and possibly treated using telemetry.[287, 289]

KEN: The most important attribute we generalists have is the ability to wear two hats, the holistic hat and the medical-model hat and the robustness to distinguish between self-limiting conditions and potentially dangerous ones. To help with this, we need better information about the predictive value of increasingly sophisticated diagnostic tests. Nurses as a profession don't have these skills or knowledge and can supplement, but not substitute for, general practitioners.

VEE: I envisage clearer recommendations about management to appear on the GP's computer. Initially this'll be generic information as now, but presented in a format more applicable to the clinical setting.[344] Later it'll use information from the electronic health record to provide patient-specific advice which will be visible to both doctor and patient. As a GP, I'll no longer have to look up and assess research data. Instead I'll be provided with results in a form that I can apply in practice. My job will then be to mediate between that information and the patient's needs and preferences. Dichotomous disease labels will be replaced by assessments of risks and benefits. Treatment will be directed at risk factors to improve mortality and morbidity, and at symptoms to improve morbidity and quality of life.[165]

AUDREY: Vociferous patients will call for the best care medicine can provide. In turn, doctors—and politicians—might tell them more about the harm that medicine can do. There will be more discussion about balancing of risks against benefits of tests and treatments.[298] Publicly available audit data will improve performance a little by guiding patient choice and a lot by hurting professional pride.[215] How about education of future doctors? Increasingly good understanding of risk will pervade medical education along with patient-centred care, teamwork, and continual improvement.[345] Skills will be learnt in simulated environments probably with interactive computer programmes for learning clinical skills. General practitioners will teach junior doctors how to apply these skills in practice.

KEN: And whatever changes in technology and service delivery take place, the ill will continue coming to see their family doctors, speaking to them, and being heard, touched, and treated—as patients and as people.

EXERCISE

Take a bundle of letters and results from agencies outside your practice and think about how many of them would reach the patient's usual doctor. For a patient with many such documents, is there room for making their management more coordinated?

CHAPTER 3

Statistical building blocks

'... without theory practical medicine is blind, and theory of medicine without practical medicine is lame.'

Adler RH. Engel's biopsychosocial model is still relevant today.
Journal of Psychosomatic Research. 2009; 67(6): 607–11.

'For we shall find that since the time of Hume, the fashionable scientific philosophy has been such as to deny the rationality of science ... But scientific faith has risen to the occasion, and tacitly removed the philosophic mountain.'

Whitehead AN. *Science and the Modern World.*
Cambridge University Press; 1946.

INTRODUCTION

In a tutorial, my trainee and I discuss the part of the curriculum of the Royal College of General Practitioners recommending health promotion and disease prevention.[18] We then surf the Internet and discover risk factors ranked according to the contribution they make to mortality worldwide: high blood pressure, smoking, high cholesterol, childhood underweight, unsafe sex, low fruit and vegetable intake, adult overweight, physical inactivity, alcohol use, and indoor smoke from solid fuels.[346] And we come across an article saying that if we manage to prevent all cardiovascular disease, our 50-year-old patients will have their life expectancy increased by 13 years.[347]

We agree to audit a surgery each, concentrating not on patients' presenting problems, but rather on our opportunistic health promotion.

My first patient, Abe, is a 50-year-old office worker whom I encourage to exercise. Next is Bea, a generally healthy and fit 40-year-old nurse worried about her high cholesterol: I give her a low-fat diet leaflet. The third consultation is for a married couple, the Cedars—both 47-year-old unemployed overweight smokers on benefits. I tell them that their lifestyle puts them at high risk of cancer and vascular disease and that they should attend our health promotion clinic. The next patient, Dean, says he's started dieting to lose weight and wonders if exercise would help—I say 'yes'. After him, there's a woman called Eve planning to stop smoking and I recommend she attend our smoking cessation clinic and get nicotine replacement therapy. The last patient, Fergus, is a diabetic business executive whom I encourage to increase his self-monitoring.

Pleased with how much I've fitted into my consultations,[338] I choose audit as my core category for appraisal and present the results to my appraiser.[348] She says that I haven't referred to any criteria by which to judge quality and that I should look up evidence for what I've done in the literature—which I do.

Among 50-year-old men like Abe, life expectancy is about 30 years and starting exercise increases it by 2½ years, from, say 80 to 82½ years of age.[349] Dietary change has no demonstrable effect on mortality or cardiovascular events in people at low risk such as Bea.[350] Mortality rises with body mass index above 25[351] and with smoking,[352, 349] but multiple risk-factor interventions such as health promotion clinics don't reduce all-cause or cardiovascular mortality for people like the Cedars.[353] Shared decision aids,[354, 355] while possibly improving the process of care by prompting and facilitating discussion, don't improve outcome.[356] Using fear to prompt lifestyle change is ethically questionable.[357] Attempting risk-factor reduction in socioeconomically deprived individuals doesn't necessarily work; structural change such as prohibiting smoking in public places is more likely to be effective.[358] Compared with diet alone, intense exercise by someone like Dean is associated with additional weight loss—but only of 1.5 kg.[359] Fewer than one in five smokers such as Eve attempting to stop smoking use nicotine replacement;[360] 80 to 90% of smokers trying to give up don't get professional help; most of those who quit on their own used a 'cold turkey' approach; and 48% of those who try to stop unaided are successful, compared with 24% using cessation programmes.[361]

If I adhered to U.S. Preventive Services Task Force recommendations, primary prevention for patients like my first five patients would lengthen my working day by at least two hours.[19] If my last patient, Fergus, were to follow guidelines on diabetic self-care, it would take him two hours a day for the rest of his life.[362, 98] Patients don't always comply with medical advice;[357] they need reminders, leaflets, follow-up appointments at times convenient to them, and encouragement to do their own monitoring[363]—and even all of that doesn't work very well.[364]

So preventive activities require considerable resources and have variable benefit. How do we clinicians appraise the evidence on which we base this part of our work?

ANSWERING CLINICAL QUESTIONS

The Royal College of General Practitioners requires general practitioners to be able to identify the questions arising from a consultation, then to find and appraise the relevant scientific literature.[18] Appraising research on the basis of publications[365, 366, 344, 9, 367, 261, 260, 368, 369, 370, 371] is difficult: general practitioners aren't good at finding evidence-based answers to questions—they end up with the wrong answer half the time.[255] Judging whether publications accurately represent the results of research by studying protocols and re-analysing patient-level data[372] is beyond the resources of most clinicians. So general practitioners need to rely on reviews and guidelines.[344, 373, 374] This is reflected in the policy adopted recently by the *British Journal of General Practice* and the *British Medical Journal* of publishing full research papers on the Web while, in print, having abridged reports accompanied and followed by commentary and debate.[375]

It's important to keep this in perspective. There are divisions of labour throughout medicine: just as, traditionally, we've had physicians, surgeons, and general practitioners, we now also have statisticians, qualitative researchers, and systematic reviewers. What's needed is communication between specialties, and there are two ways in which general practitioners contribute to this dialogue.

Firstly, we continue to study original research papers. This isn't primarily in order to keep up-to-date or to find out the right thing to do: in fact, we might easily waste our time and harm our patients by following researchers along promising avenues that turn out to be blind alleys.[367] By reading and commenting on original papers, we're reminded of—and remind researchers and editors of—the strengths and limitations of medical science: we help them identify questions that matter to patients [9] and work with them to supply the answers.

Secondly, we question orthodoxy. The research establishment uses large resources, high levels of skill, and narrowly defined methodologies in a strictly governed ethical framework[376] to pursue narrow questions with results that, for the general practitioner, are essential in some areas and useless in many others. What medical research achieves is necessary for clinical practice but not sufficient. With it behind us, we're a science-based profession; without it, we're quacks. There are other complementary areas of enquiry. Conventionally, research is discovering the right thing to do and audit discovering if we're doing the right thing,[377] but the distinction between the two isn't as clear-cut as it might appear. On a small scale, prescribing is an experiment by the doctor, and taking medicine an experiment by the patient:[378] these n-of one trials are being conducted many times a day.[379] The results are systematically biased. Patients who are satisfied and get better consult us again with their next illness, those who are dissatisfied or don't get better consult someone else, and those who are disgusted or dead leave our practice list. Such bias can be removed by comprehensive data collection and follow-up. On the other hand, large-scale data collection fails to capture the individual tailored good that's done in the one-to-one encounter. Perhaps the enthusiastic talk about lifestyle change coming through my consulting room wall from the health promotion clinic next door tells me something positive that the negative research results miss.[353]

So what's called research is only part of the process by which we learn about general practice. The way even that fraction is conducted and reported is imperfect.

Published scientific literature is an unreliable guide to the truth.[380, 381, 382, 383] Some research isn't published because its conclusions are commercially embarrassing for pharmaceutical companies or uninteresting to researchers and publishers, so what is published is not representative of the whole. Authors are required to disclose competing interests only of a financial kind: disclosure of other kinds of competing interest is discretionary.[384]

Much research isn't relevant to clinical practice,[385] and many relevant research results aren't translated into practice.[386, 385] A lot of publicly funded and professionally motivated research is published for profit and sold back to publicly funded libraries and professionally motivated researchers; only a portion is freely available online.[387] And there's disagreement about how to interpret evidence, even in relation to major national programmes such as breast screening.[388]

Despite guidelines for authors,[389, 390, 391, 392, 393, 368, 391] scientific papers don't always tell us what we need to know in order to be able to put research findings into practice. Non-drug interventions might not be described in sufficient detail for the practitioner to reproduce them.[394] Rating scales may be under copyright.[395] Benefits might seem large because they're given in relative terms and harms small because they're given in absolute terms.[260, 261] Surrogate markers (such as HbA1c) that aren't necessarily related to patient-orientated outcomes (such as macro-vascular events in diabetics) are used because evidence can be accumulated relatively easily.[396] Even if the research results are valid, well presented, and applicable to my group of patients, they might not apply to the patient in front of me.[145] A middle-class vicar in a working-class area has different risks from the parishioners. And reproducibility of clinical findings is poor: clinicians often don't agree as to whether a sign is present or absent.[397]

STATISTICAL STUMBLING BLOCKS

Statistics are an obstacle for all groups involved in healthcare—patients,[259] surgeons,[260] physicians,[398] researchers,[399] journalists[261]—and even statisticians.[400] Sensitivity and specificity are the most prominent stumbling blocks: the sensitivity of a test is the proportion of patients with a particular condition having a positive test result; the specificity is the proportion of patients without the condition having a negative test result.[401] They tell us the likely result of the test once we know whether or not the patient has the disease.[367] It's hard to imagine why a clinician should want to know that. It's like asking how to walk from A to B and getting directions for driving from B to A. We want to know whether we should do the test and whether the patient has the disease once we know the result.[366] Predictive values are sometimes given. The positive predictive value of a test is the prevalence of the disease in patients who test positive. The negative predictive value is the prevalence in those who test negative.[366] These are useful, but only if the disease prevalence given in the paper[261, 260] is the same as in our own practices:[153] we often don't know if this is the case.

STATISTICAL BUILDING BLOCKS

I suggest replacing these stumbling blocks with two building blocks: odds and likelihood ratios. These are no harder or easier to grasp than sensitivity and specificity—the difference is that they're helpful to clinicians. Odds and likelihood ratios do three things: first, they give us an idea how useful or useless a test is; second, they help us make a diagnosis; and third, they indicate how certain or uncertain our diagnosis is. The next two paragraphs are probably best read through fairly quickly, then reread more slowly. They show how the building blocks of odds and likelihood ratios fit together, so it's important to get an idea not just of the parts, but also of the whole.

Odds are ratios of events to non-events.[69] If we take 100 people with headache, 11 will have migraine and 89 won't.[402] That corresponds to odds of 11:89, which is about 1:8. (1:8 is said as 'one to eight', not 'one in eight').

The likelihood ratio[403, 366] is a number attached to a test indicating how much the test result changes the probability of disease being present. We clinicians need know nothing about where this ratio comes from: we just need to know how to use it. And we use a likelihood ratio as follows. If we consider our patient with headache, we've seen that their odds of having migraine are 1:8.[402] Suppose they meet all the criteria in a migraine clinical decision aid that has attached to it a likelihood ratio for definite migraine of 6.[402] We multiply 1:8 by 6 to get 6:8. So, using the two building blocks of odds and likelihood ratios, we find that the odds of definite migraine have increased from 1:8 to 6:8, close to even.

Once you're sure about these two building blocks, odds and likelihood ratios, and how they fit together, you'll have a firm foundation on which to build. Let's look next at the strengths and weaknesses of odds and likelihood ratios.

The information conveyed by odds is usually stated in terms of probabilities.[404, 405] If we take headache as an example again, we can represent the differential diagnosis as a pie chart. There's a migraine slice representing 11% of the pie and a tension headache slice representing 40%.[402] But this pie is a fudge. Firstly, we only make the pie complete by including a slice labelled 'other', containing not only rare diagnoses, but also anything we haven't thought of. Secondly, we've taken no account of the 5% of people with both tension headache and migraine.[402] Odds, like clinical practice, represent different diagnoses as separate entities and there's no assumption we've exhausted all diagnostic possibilities or that patients can't have two diagnoses. That better represents the messiness of clinical practice. Odds also make us aware not only of those with disease who benefit from investigations, but also of those without disease who are harmed by investigations. After using our clinical decision aid and finding the odds of migraine are 6:8, for every 6 patients we subject to the benefits and harms of an anti-migraine drug, we subject 8 to the harms without the possibility of benefit. The only danger with odds is that we might start discussing them with patients and convey the opposite of what we intend. A doctor says the odds of someone with headache having migraine are '6 to 8'. The punter, expressing the same odds, would say '8 to 6'.[406]

We've seen how we can multiply the initial odds of migraine (1:8) by the likelihood ratio attached to a migraine questionnaire (6) and obtain new odds (6:8). If we discover that attacks are precipitated by physical activity, a feature with a likelihood ratio of 4,[407] we can multiply 6:8 by 4 and get new odds of 24:8, which equates to odds of 3:1: for every 3 patients in whom we correctly diagnose migraine, we diagnose it incorrectly in 1 patient. So we can build up the evidence for the diagnosis layer by layer. We can also use what's called the negative likelihood ratio, the number attached to a negative result, to build up evidence against the diagnosis.

So far we've considered tests with only two results, positive or negative. Many tests, however, have a numerical result. In that case, we can have a range of likelihood ratios corresponding to the range of possible numerical results. The more the result deviates from normal, the greater the likelihood ratio. For example, if we use prostate specific antigen in the diagnosis of prostate cancer, the higher the antigen level, the higher the positive likelihood ratio, and the greater the probability of prostate cancer. These figures are not—in my experience—provided by laboratories, but they're available in research literature and quoted with other such data in Chapter 5.[408]

Likelihood ratio is a number attached to a test but is influenced by other factors. Firstly, we need to be sure that the test is the same whatever the context. Mammography has various positive likelihood ratios for breast cancer: 3 in women with bloody or watery discharge or with a lump; 13 in women with other breast symptoms; and 15 in women with no symptoms.[409] This might be explained by different physiological and physical properties of the breast. So mammography is not a single reproducible test. Imaging of a breast in one physiological state is not the same test as imaging of a breast in a different physiological state. The second factor affecting a test's likelihood ratio is the prevalence of the condition in question. This is a matter not of biology but of arithmetic. As the prevalence changes, the positive likelihood ratio will change most when specificity is high, and negative likelihood ratio most when sensitivity is high. So we must be cautious in transferring likelihood ratios from, say, secondary to primary care: the most accurate likelihood ratio is one derived from research in a setting similar to the one in which we're practising.

Another problem with likelihood ratios is that the results of different tests are not necessarily independent of each other, which means we can't use their likelihood ratios serially to approach a diagnosis. Consider our patient with odds of migraine of 3:1 based on a migraine decision aid plus exercise-sensitivity. Nausea has a positive likelihood ratio for migraine of 19 but it isn't valid to multiply 3:1 by 19 to arrive at revised odds because nausea is a component of the decision aid.[410] In practice, you would have worked through the decision aid, would realise that nausea had already been taken into account, and would not use that information twice. On the other hand, further research might reveal that patients with high decision aid scores are all exercise-sensitive: that would invalidate our serial use of the decision aid and exercise-sensitivity. Lack of independence of symptoms in this way can only be discovered empirically.

Sensitivity and specificity are building blocks for pathologists and form a foundation for scientific research. If the sensitivity is near 100%, we have a SnNOut: a Sensitive test with a Negative result rules the diagnosis Out. If the specificity is near 100%, we have a SpPIn: a Specific test with a Positive result rules the diagnosis In.[411] If neither is near 100% and their sum is near to 100%, the test is useless. If their sum is near 200%, the test is likely to be helpful. If their sum is near 0—an unusual situation—again the test is likely to be helpful but indicating the opposite of what was expected, a negative result suggesting no disease rather than a positive result implying disease.[412]

Sensitivity and specificity, therefore, are building blocks for the infrastructure of medical science—but they're stumbling blocks for clinicians. The building blocks we need are likelihood ratios. Likelihood ratios have no disadvantages that sensitivity and specificity don't have and they have unique advantages for the clinician. They're often not given in research papers but they can be calculated quickly using mental arithmetic or by scribbling in the margin. We then have numbers that, unlike sensitivity and specificity, tell us whether the test is likely to be useful in clinical practice. The formulae,[401] using sensitivity and specificity expressed as percentages, are given in Figure 3.1.

In the extreme case, likelihood ratios make clear what sensitivity and specificity obscure: for instance, that ischaemic heart disease is less likely when the patient clenches their fist in describing the pain,[413] and that foreign body aspiration in children[414, 415] is less likely[416] when dyspnoea is present.

Perhaps one day Internet-based decision aids might use information imported directly from the patient record to give us a differential diagnosis with odds attached.[410] A necessary condition for these tools to be helpful is involvement of general practitioners in their design. For now, we can use our understanding of odds and likelihood ratios to inspect our medical knowledge infrastructure, use what's robust as foundations for our clinical practice, and identify gaps needing to be filled.

$$positive\ likelihood\ ratio = \frac{sensitivity}{100 - specificity}$$

$$negative\ likelihood\ ratio = \frac{100 - sensitivity}{specificity}$$

FIGURE 3.1 Likelihood ratios

Primary care must remain generalist at heart. Vertically delivered screening or prevention may be valuable for certain conditions. It might be best delivered in primary care. But it doesn't substitute for holistic care. Multiple morbidity means that there's often more than one diagnosis to deal with in each consultation. Multiple morbidity also means that the risks attached to medicalisation multiply. We must keep our holistic hats on while performing these mechanistic, single-issue tasks.

Below are the features of the ideal general practice research paper identifying features that, I think, can be assessed by a general practitioner with no specialist research or statistical knowledge. Ideas are incorporated from the various sources referenced earlier in this chapter.

AUTHOR
- there's no pharmaceutical funding, affiliation to a special interest group, or empire building
- for general practice literature, at least one of the authors is a practising general practitioner

AIM AND METHOD
- the question matches your patient-centred question
- the method addresses the same question
- disease, symptom, sign and test are all clearly defined and relevant to your clinical practice
- there's a single relevant endpoint—death is a good one, unless quality of life is more important

WORDING
- expressions like 'may, 'can', 'up to', 'as much as', or 'as little as' are used to indicate uncertainty rather than to mask ignorance

REFERENCE STANDARD
- this is reliable, appropriate and used for all subjects—if it's not used in patients apparently without disease, we learn nothing about false positives

COMPARATOR
- this is clinically relevant

PATIENTS STUDIED

- these are like your patients
- the method and rate of recruitment indicate inclusiveness rather than selectiveness
- all patients are accounted for

STATISTICS

- categories are not treated as numbers and are not redefined during the study ('very good' doesn't equal 5, 'good' doesn't equal 4, and the two together don't equal 4.5)
- the same denominator or natural numbers are used throughout
- graphs include 0 on both axes
- framing is both positive and negative (e.g. both survival and death)
- prevalences and likelihood ratios are quoted or calculable

RESULT

- the paper answers the original question
- subgroup analysis gives not answers but further questions
- significance of results is clinical (not just statistical)
- association is not taken to mean causality
- causality prompts not clinical implementation but a trial

REFERENCES

- statistics cited are from primary research papers or systematic reviews, not commentaries.

EXERCISES

Take a paper that might be relevant to your practice and use the checklist above to assess it.

Take any sensitivity and specificity and calculate positive and negative likelihood ratios.

CHAPTER 4

Icebergs

'Patients get hip fractures because they fall.'

Welch HG, Schwartz LM, Woloshin S. *Overdiagnosed: making people sick in
the pursuit of health.* Boston, Massachesetts: Beacon Press; 2011.

*'Men can be provincial in time, as well as in place. We may ask ourselves whether the
scientific mentality of the modern world in the immediate past is not a successful example
of such provincial limitation.'*

Whitehead AN. *Science and the Modern World.*
Cambridge: Cambridge University Press; 1946.

In Chapter 3, I began with prevention of disease and ended with a set of tools for
the clinician to use when appraising the literature. This chapter concerns treatment
of disease and draws particularly on one of these tools: using natural numbers or
keeping the denominator constant. That means that comparisons are always made
to the whole group of patients rather than to successively smaller subgroups. If
we take any one condition, we find an iceberg, most of which is submerged in the
community and the tip of which is visible in the consulting room.[12] Let's apply this
notion to three conditions—depression, sore throat, and colorectal cancer—and
set what we do in the consulting room against what's happening among our entire
patient population.

DEPRESSION

If I were to ask members of the public closed questions about symptoms, 23% would
report at least one physical, mental or behavioural symptom in the previous two
weeks for which they didn't seek professional advice, even though they considered
the pain extreme, the disability severe, or the symptom serious. These people would
bring 34% of their physical symptoms and 17% of their mental symptoms to the
doctor.[12] So there's an iceberg of symptoms of which the tip is seen in the consulting room. On the other hand, almost 10% of people say that in the last two weeks

they've consulted about a symptom causing no pain, disability, or worry. So I can find myself dealing with what appear superficially to be trivia.[12]

Physical and mental symptoms are therefore common in everyday life and bear a linear relationship neither to consulting patterns nor, possibly, to presence of disease.[52] If we're not aware of this, we might misuse resources, mistreat the well, and, particularly in areas of mental health, maltreat the vulnerable. For the patient surrendering themselves to the care of a specialist, seeing a surgeon and losing their appendix represents an isolated threat to their autonomy, but seeing a psychiatrist and losing their mind has existential ramifications.[33] If I joined 26 other general practitioners to watch a consultation on video and we independently decided on the main mental health problem, we would arrive at eight different diagnoses from the International Classification of Diseases and seven from the International Classification of Health Problems in Primary Care; and our prognoses would vary widely.[417] How do we make these assessments?[418] The Quality and Outcomes Framework prompts us to use two questions to screen for depression.[419] But the evidence[420] is based on an assessment made by psychology graduate students using the National Institute of Mental Health Diagnostic Interview Schedule as a proxy for DSM-III criteria. So, diagnosis of mental illness is an uncertain process.[47]

Suppose I look further into this by taking figures from the literature and converting them to round numbers on the sort of scale I might be dealing with in practice (*see* Figure 4.1). Imagine that I work part-time and that my notional list includes about 500 adults of whom I see about 120 a month and discuss a handful over coffee with my partners. Suppose for the sake of argument that I accept, more or less, that there is such a thing as depression for which antidepressants are useful and that I'm typical of the average general practitioner in the way I diagnose and treat it.

If I were to phone up adults in Scotland, 15% of them would say that they had felt depressed in the last month, and 4% would say they had consulted their doctor about this.[421] So of my 500 adults, 75 have felt depressed in the last month and 20 have consulted about it.

Of patients consulting in general practice, around 10% have depression according to standards such as the *Diagnostic and Statistical Manual*. The diagnosis by general practitioners has a sensitivity of 20–80% and specificity of 60–90%.[422] So of the 120 adults I see in a month, I diagnose depression in 20 of the 108 who don't have depression and in six of the 12 who do. That means I diagnose depression in 26 patients.

When patients are diagnosed in general practice with depression, 30–42% are given antidepressants.[423] So, I'm likely to prescribe antidepressants for 10 of my 26 patients.

Some 28–74% of patients improve on antidepressants compared with 16–35% on placebo;[424] and 27–30% of patients prescribed antidepressants withdraw because of side effects.[425] So, of the 10 patients for whom I prescribe antidepressants, three

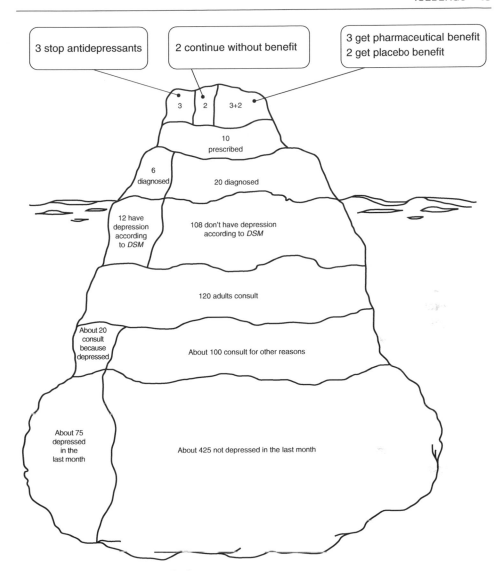

3 stop antidepressants

2 continue without benefit

3 get pharmaceutical benefit
2 get placebo benefit

3 | 2 | 3+2

10
prescribed

6
diagnosed

20 diagnosed

12 have
depression
according
to *DSM*

108 don't have depression
according to *DSM*

120 adults consult

About 20
consult
because
depressed

About 100 consult for other reasons

About 75
depressed
in the
last month

About 425 not depressed in the last month

FIGURE 4.1 The depression iceberg

stop taking them, two continue without benefit, and five continue with benefit, of whom two would have benefited from placebo.

By taking this overview, approximating where necessary and using natural numbers, I get the following picture. I've diagnosed depression correctly in six people, diagnosed it incorrectly in 20, and missed it in six. Antidepressants have produced pharmacological benefit in three people and been unhelpful or harmful in three who stop taking them and two who continue without benefit.

What do we learn? Whether or not antidepressants are beneficial for the individual, the contribution they make to relieving distress on a population level is small. If we want to decide whether or not to use antidepressants, perhaps we should base our decision on the finding that they're more beneficial than placebo only in patients with a Hamilton Rating Scale score ≥25.[426, 427, 428] That replaces the diagnosis of depression with a judgment that a drug-induced state is likely to be preferable to the existing morbid mental state.[52]

It's possible to spend a lot of time in the consultation and in educational sessions considering the advantages and disadvantages of antidepressants. But it's probably more important to make time to find out what differentiates the patient who's consulted from the many in the community with low mood who haven't consulted,[12, 421] and respond holistically. Any symptom, sign or abnormal test result is more likely to improve than to worsen over a short time scale.[183] Our expertise, manner, personality, and relationship with the patient—even after only a few minutes of acquaintance—have been called the drug 'doctor'.[182] This drug, perhaps repeated at a follow-up consultation, might be the main treatment and the one with most benefit.

We can prescribe, or not. Whichever, we should do it efficiently, safely, positively, and engagingly and allow time and energy to concentrate on other important matters.

SORE THROAT AND TONSILLITIS

I've developed an overview of depression in my imagined practice. It's possible to do the same sort of thing with other conditions and other practices. Suppose you have 4000 patients on your practice list and decide to look at your management of sore throat and tonsillitis (*see* Figure 4.2).

Sore throat and tonsillitis are common, and the best management is a matter of debate. Antibiotics are sometimes used in treatment and are the subject of much research. They reduce the risk of suppurative complications (otitis media, sinusitis, and quinsy) and old studies show that they reduced the risk of carditis but no research has demonstrated reduced risk of nephritis.[429] It remains an open question whether you should generally use an antibiotic for treatment of sore throat and tonsillitis. Suppose, for the sake of the exercise, that you're typical of UK general practitioners in your use of antibiotics.

If you ask middle-aged people in Scotland, 9% will tell you they've had a sore throat in the last month and 2% of the total consult a general practitioner for it.[421] So, among your 4000 patients of all ages, something in the region of 200 middle-aged people have a sore throat every month and 40 of them consult.

Sore throat or tonsillitis is diagnosed by UK general practitioners 26 to 39 times a year for every 1000 people in their patient population.[430] So in your practice of 4000 patients, you and your partners will diagnose sore throat or tonsillitis in about 11 patients a month.

In the UK, general practitioners prescribe an antibiotic for 60 to 88% of cases of sore throats and tonsillitis.[430] So of your 11 patients, eight are prescribed an antibiotic and three are not.

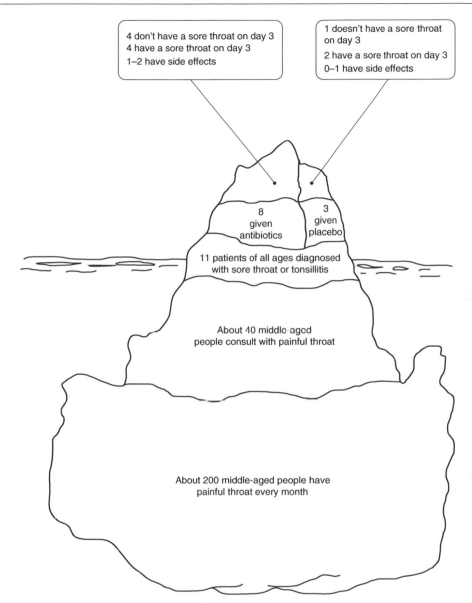

4 don't have a sore throat on day 3
4 have a sore throat on day 3
1–2 have side effects

1 doesn't have a sore throat on day 3
2 have a sore throat on day 3
0–1 have side effects

8 given antibiotics

3 given placebo

11 patients of all ages diagnosed with sore throat or tonsillitis

About 40 middle-aged people consult with painful throat

About 200 middle-aged people have painful throat every month

FIGURE 4.2 The sore throat and tonsillitis iceberg

The percentage of patients getting relief from their painful throat after three days is 51% on antibiotics and 34% on placebo.[431] So out of your eight patients given antibiotics, four have relief after three days; and, of the three not given antibiotics, one has relief at three days.

The rate of side effects is similar with antibiotics (18%) and placebo (15%).[432] So none of your patients is likely to be harmed by the antibiotic but one or two of them feel they get side effects.

Non-steroidal anti-inflammatory drugs reduce pain by 25–93%,[431] and 10–12% of patients have mild side effects.[433] So if 11 patients take them, their pain will be reduced on average by about 50% and one will have mild side effects.

You can see that sore throat is common and only a minority of sufferers consult. Antibiotics play only a small part in relieving the burden of symptoms in the community, make only a small difference to the patients in the consulting room, and, perhaps, confer less benefit than non-steroidal anti-inflammatory drugs. Whether or not you prescribe is probably not a major determinant of outcome. The process of discussing this might be an important part of building your relationship with the patient but, I guess, only if it broadens rather than narrows the discussion. Finding out what has prompted the patient in front of you to consult unlike the others in the community who have not consulted might be as important as anything else.

COLORECTAL CANCER

As a cause of death in high-income countries, colorectal cancer is one of the top 10 diseases and, among malignancies, second only to lung cancer.[434] It's hard to diagnose clinically because the features—including rectal bleeding—are relatively non-specific.[435] I'll illustrate the difficulties of diagnosing it clinically and then discuss the place of screening.

Using approximations: in a population of 6000 adults, there are six people with undiagnosed colorectal cancer;[436] 1000 have rectal bleeding in any one year, 150 for the first time; 50–100 report it to their general practitioner; and a diagnosis of cancer is made in 1–3.[437] The proportion of consulters referred for investigations is unknown, but the prevalence of colorectal cancer among adults referred with rectal bleeding is 5–7%.[436] Cancers not diagnosed by symptoms and elective investigations come to light in other ways—following emergency admission, screening, and so on.

Colorectal cancer is thought to arise in polyps and to have an annual progression rate of 58% from Duke A to B, 66% from B to C, and 86% from C to D.[438] Sixty per cent of colorectal cancers are at or distal to the splenic flexure[314] and a trial of screening flexible sigmoidoscopy in people aged 55–65 years in the UK resulted in a reduced rate of colorectal cancer, although the number needed to sigmoidoscope to prevent one colorectal cancer was 191 and to prevent one colorectal cancer death was 489, with no change in all-cause mortality.[308]

Screening by testing for faecal occult blood and then further investigating those with positive results detects a quarter of cancers.[311] This process becomes cumulatively less selective. After repeated cycles over a number of years, more than half of people screened will have colonoscopy at some point.[439] The Scottish bowel screening programme[440] involves postal invitations every two years to people aged 50–74y to return faecal specimens in the mail. The accompanying literature recommends that if there's frank blood in the stool, a general practitioner should be consulted but does not advise against continuing with screening, so presumably some respondents coincidentally have frank rectal bleeding. Participants whose specimens are positive for occult blood by guaiac-based testing are invited for colonoscopy.[440] The programme began as a pilot in 2000 and was fully operational throughout Scotland in 2007. This means that data are based partly on prevalence (among people who had colorectal neoplasia for some years leading up to their first screen) and partly on incidence (among people developing neoplasias during the two years between screens).[441] The figures relating to prevalence are, however, small compared with those relating to incidence.

Let's apply data from the Scottish programme and other sources to a notional group of 4000 people aged 50–74y on the list of a group practice in Scotland (*see* Figure 4.3).

So far 53% of invitations to colorectal screening have resulted in the return of analysable faecal specimens.[441] So of our 4000 people, 2120 return specimens and 1880 don't.

Of returned specimens, 2.1% test positive for occult blood.[441] So in our group there are 44 people with positive stool specimens.

Of people with positive stool samples, 74% accept and undergo colonoscopy.[441] That's 33 of our group.

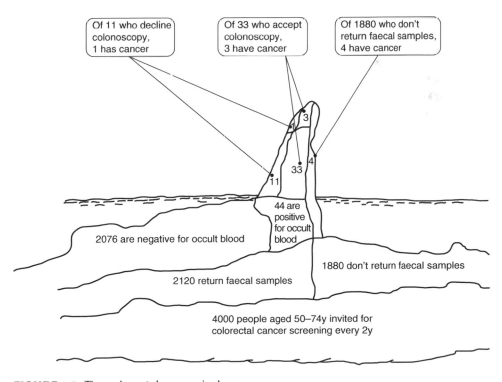

FIGURE 4.3 The colorectal cancer iceberg

Among people with positive stool samples, the rate of detection of cancer is 8.6%.[441] That means, for our group, screening detects cancer in three. (Small adenomata aren't detected by faecal occult blood testing[439] and are detected coincidentally in 0.5% of people returning stool specimens.[441] That means, in our group, nobody has adenomata detected).

The colonoscopy complication rate—requiring admission after the procedure—is 1.1%,[441] and the colonoscopy death rate is 0.025%.[442] Death and complications will therefore affect 0.4 people from our cohort. Colonoscopy misses 4–5% of cancers.[443] It also misses small, flat, or serrated adenomata.[439] In our cohort, therefore, another 0.1 people will have cancer undetected at colonoscopy.

Unrehydrated guaiac-based faecal occult blood testing as used in the Scottish programme[444] has a sensitivity for colorectal cancer of 56%.[445] And non-compliance with screening is highest among men with high deprivation scores who have the highest risk of colorectal cancer.[441] So for every four cancers in those who returned stool specimens, we can expect four cancers in those not returning specimens. In sum, we find that of eight colorectal cancers, three will be detected by the Scottish Bowel Screening Programme and five will present clinically.

Detecting these cancers offers the chance of cure. However, the necessary investigations and treatment have associated risks—possible complications of colonoscopy and then minor hazards from other investigations plus the dangers of surgery. These risks must be less than the corresponding risks from undiagnosed cancer if screening is to prove worthwhile. In weighing one set of risks against the other, we must consider not only their size and nature, but also their timing. The risks of investigating and treating cancer are immediate but, because of the natural history of the disease, the benefits are delayed. The time period before benefits outweigh risks is least in a healthy 80-year-old man for whom it is five years; the time period increases to 10 years and beyond in people with lower risk of colorectal cancer (such as younger women) or higher risk of complications of investigations and treatment (such as those with severe systemic disease).[442]

What can we learn? Whether or not screening is useful depends on healthcare systems, economics, societal and personal values, and the estimated delay in the individual before benefit exceeds harm. General practitioners might be able to spare patients with short life expectancy investigations for which estimated risks outweigh likely benefits. For reducing specifically colorectal cancer mortality, it's cost-effective in developed countries to expand screening and in developing countries to expand treatment.[446] But screening hasn't been shown to reduce all-cause mortality: in fact, that would be hard to demonstrate since elimination of all malignancies in any bodily site would increase life expectancy at birth by only 2½ years.[347] Clinical diagnosis on the one hand and detection by screening on the other are not mutually exclusive but complementary. There continues to be a place for diagnosis based on symptoms and signs not only among those unscreened, but

also because of false negatives among those screened. But clinical diagnosis is difficult. Symptoms and signs are relatively non-discriminating.

Rectal bleeding is a puzzle. When occult, and detected by faecal testing in the
population, its positive predictive value is 6.5% in primary incidence screening and
11% in prevalence screening.[447] When frank, its positive predictive value is 0.1% in
the community, 2–3% once presented to primary care, and 5–7% once referred.[436]
Frank bleeding probably has a lower positive predictive value than might be
expected because it often has benign local causes such as piles. I wonder if positive
predictive value is even lower than evidence suggests. In the clinical context where
many symptoms and signs are uncertain, frank rectal bleeding is one of the features
most easily defined as present or absent. Other features along with gut feeling—on
the part of doctor or patient—might play more of a part in diagnosis than we have
yet been able to ascertain.

As with any condition, we can use our understanding of the natural history
of disease to weigh the probability and consequences of missing or delaying the
diagnosis against the probability and consequences of harming, by irrelevant investigation, someone with a different disease or no disease at all. There's sometimes a
place for using time as a diagnostic tool.[317]

EXERCISES

Take a surgery perhaps a month ago and for each patient with a self limiting
respiratory tract illness (otitis media, laryngitis, pharyngitis, rhinitis, sinusitis, sore
throat, tonsillitis, tracheitis, bronchitis) and note: Did you prescribe an antibiotic?
Did the patient return during the same illness episode?

During your next surgery, make a point of trying to find out what made that
patient consult unlike the other patients with apparently similar symptoms who
did not.

CHAPTER 5

Numbers that speak

'… we academics devote ourselves to research; we write up the results as articles for journals; we referee the articles in the process of peer reviewing; we serve on the editorial boards of the journals; we also serve as editors (all of this unpaid, of course); and then we buy back our own work at ruinous prices …'

Darnton R. The Library: three Jeremiads.
The New York Review of Books. 2010 Nov 23.

'Bet only when the time is right and the conditions are suitable.'

One of Richard Birch's golden rules of betting, quoted in
Quinn J, Cremin J. *The Definitive Guide: A–Z of betting.*
Newbury, Berkshire: Raceform; 2008.

INTRODUCTION

This chapter is a list of recipes. They tell us what dishes can be made from the ingredients that the patient has brought. We weigh each ingredient according to the recipe and do some calculations to get the proportions right. But we don't follow the recipes blindly: we use our judgment. This is cookbook medicine with doctor as chef, checking and making adjustments along the way, and patient as gourmet, prepared to send back to the kitchen what they don't like.

I'll give three examples, below each of which there are references to the literature. Before you start, you'll need to know two definitions.

Firstly, 'the odds[403] of a patient having a disease' is a short way of saying 'the number of patients who have the disease compared with the number who don't'. If one patient has the disease for every three who don't, we write, 'the odds are 1:3' and say 'the odds are 1 to 3' (not '1 in 3').

For instance, a worried man of 60 whose wife has just been diagnosed with bowel cancer consults, asking to be tested for this himself. His age and sex give him initial odds of colorectal cancer of 1:1000.[448] That means one such man will have colorectal cancer for every 1000 that don't.

The second definition you need is for likelihood ratio.[403] Likelihood ratio is a number attached to a symptom, sign or test that tells us whether a particular diagnosis is more or less likely. If you multiply the initial odds by the likelihood ratio, you get the revised odds. The likelihood ratio will be described as positive or negative, depending on whether the symptom, sign, or test is positive or negative.

Think again about our worried 60-year-old man with initial odds of colorectal cancer of 1:1000. He has constipation with no other symptoms or signs. For colorectal cancer, constipation has a likelihood ratio of 2.[449] So, you multiply 1:1000 by 2 and find that his revised odds of having colorectal cancer are approximately 1:500. That means that one such man will have colorectal cancer for every 500 that don't. You might consider this risk low enough to wait for further developments. You choose to find out a little more about his wife's presentation and diagnosis with a view to reassuring him and checking how he and his wife are coping.

Take another example.

A woman of 50, who rarely comes to the doctor, consults you because she's found a lump in her breast. Her initial odds of having breast cancer are 1:24,[450] which is said as '1 to 24'. That means that one such woman will have breast cancer for every 24 who don't. When you examine her, you can't confirm a lump. For breast cancer, clinical breast examination has a negative likelihood ratio of 0.4.[451] When you multiply the initial odds of breast cancer, '1 to 24', by the negative likelihood ratio of 0.4, you get '1 × 0.4 to 24', which is '0.4 to 24', which equals '1 to 60'. So her revised odds of having breast cancer are 1:60. That means one such woman will have breast cancer for every 60 who don't. You might consider odds of 1:60 for breast cancer a high enough risk to warrant a follow-up appointment or a referral.

Notice that when we talk about a negative likelihood ratio, we don't mean that it's a negative number: we just mean that it refers to a negative symptom, sign, or test. We clinicians don't have to understand where these numbers come from: we just have to know our multiplication tables. And likelihood ratios can be multiplied one after another, as in the next example.

A non-pregnant woman of 20 in a stable relationship telephones complaining of a new troublesome painless vaginal discharge. Her initial odds of having bacterial vaginosis are 1:2 and of having thrush are 1:3.[452] That means that one such woman will have bacterial vaginosis for every two who don't and one will have thrush for every three who don't. You ask whether the discharge smells—which it doesn't—and whether it itches—which it does. For bacterial vaginosis, smell has a negative likelihood ratio of 0.1 and itch a positive likelihood ratio of 0.7.[453] So, you multiply 1:2 by 0.1 and then by 0.7 and find that her revised odds of having bacterial vaginosis are 0.07:2, which is about 1:30. That means one such woman will have bacterial vaginosis for every 30 who don't. For thrush, smell has a negative likelihood ratio of 2 and itch has a positive likelihood ratio of 1.5.[453] So you multiply 1:3 by 2 and then by 1.5 and find the revised odds of thrush are 3:3, which is 1:1. That means one such woman will have thrush for every one that doesn't. You consider that thrush is the likeliest identifiable cause for her discharge and that, from the medical point

of view, consequences of a wrong or delayed diagnosis are acceptable. You offer her imi-
dazole pessaries and—if the discharge doesn't resolve—a face-to-face consultation (with
possible vaginal examination),[454] *and check what she thinks about that plan.*

EXPLANATORY NOTES

I suggest you read this section only briefly, making sure you don't get bogged down in technicalities, then return to it after you've browsed through some of the statistics in the rest of the chapter.

There's no satisfactory way of classifying medical information for clinical use. The statistics below are organised by Royal College of General Practitioners curriculum heading,[18] which applicants for MRCGP might find helpful, but I think the index at the end of the book will prove the best way of finding the information needed for clinical practice.

The statistics are incomplete: for many conditions, the necessary research hasn't been done or has eluded me; and for other conditions, there's so much information relating to so many different contexts that I've limited what I've presented. I've included any evidence relating to diagnosis in its narrowest orthodox sense of pathology or lesion that I think is likely to be helpful in the general practice consultation. I've sometimes also included evidence relating to diagnosis in its other senses such as management-naming but generally stopped short of results of trials. As more research is done and more results are presented in a suitable format, databases such as this can be extended.

The term 'initial odds' corresponds to the more formal terms, 'prior odds' or 'anterior odds', and the term 'revised odds' corresponds to 'posterior odds'. (Odds ratios, often mentioned in research papers, are something different and not relevant to this book). These initial odds refer to the eventual diagnosis. The odds are then revised serially as we go through the stages of history, examination, investigation, and follow-up. The initial odds in this chapter represent a good starting point for a doctor new to general practice. However, within seconds of assessing a patient—and then over years of acquiring knowledge and experience—the general practitioner's own initial odds for a particular patient might rightly differ from those cited.

Likelihood ratios vary between patient groups,[409] between the general population and primary care consulters, and between primary care attenders and hospital clinic patients.[153] How much they vary isn't known. Where possible in this chapter, the source of data is specified.

To change the odds of a diagnosis from 1:10 to 10:1, the positive likelihood ratio needs to be 100. For a test to be useful for rare conditions in general practice, its positive likelihood ratio needs to be over 5 (preferably over 10). To change the odds of a diagnosis from 10:1 to 1:10, the negative likelihood ratio needs to be 0.01. For a test to be useful for rare conditions in general practice, its negative likelihood ratio needs to be under 0.2 (preferably under 0.1). These figures are rare: tests are often less helpful than we think and less helpful than the literature seems to suggest. However, for common conditions, symptoms and signs with more modest likelihood ratios can be helpful.

I've rounded numbers to the nearest number compatible with mental arithmetic and omitted confidence intervals so that we're not overwhelmed by numbers that we won't use in practice. Odds are followed by prevalence in brackets expressed as a percentage. For a given parameter, the odds and prevalence might appear not to tally exactly. This is because I've taken a number from the original source to derive odds and probability individually, and then made an approximation to each. For instance, an original probability of 6.4% might be approximated to 1:15 (6%) and an original probability of 5.6% might be approximated to 1:17 (6%). Where odds are quoted followed by a qualifier, the range of odds is spread around the odds quoted: for instance, 'the odds were 1:2, increasing with age' means odds were less than 1:2 in younger patients and greater than 1:2 in older patients.

Gold standards (such as histopathology) are rare, so reference standards (such as expert assessment) are often used as a proxy.[455] I've used past tense when citing results of individual studies and present tense for reviews. Decision aids are sometimes summarised in the text. Those that the doctor might want to copy are provided where possible at www.darmipc.net.[428] Where there is copyright protection, other relevant sources are indicated. Databases complementing this chapter are found in print[171, 456] and on the Internet.[457, 458]

LR+ stands for positive likelihood ratio and LR− for negative likelihood ratio. PPV stands for positive predictive value and NPV for negative predictive value. The section numbers correspond to the RCGP curriculum.[18]

EXERCISES

Before an investigation, referral, or prescription, consider the initial odds, likelihood ratios, and revised odds of the various possible diagnoses.

Pair up with a colleague and quiz each other on the content of this chapter. Make sure you write down your answer before the true answer is revealed.

Find in the medical literature a statistic not provided in this chapter that's relevant to your practice.

THE NUMBERS
The Consultation (RCGP curriculum 2)

Among patients consulting in English general practice, the odds of their being in the top 20% and 50% of attenders were, respectively, 1:1 (55%) and 6:1 (86%).[220]

Among first attenders at a Swiss hospital consulting with doctors trained for one hour in active listening, the odds of the patient's initial spontaneous talking time exceeding two minutes were 1:4 (22%).[459]

Among patients with a new problem consulting a general practitioner known to them in Slovenia and Croatia, the average time taken by the patient to reply to the doctor's question translated as "What can I do for you today?" was 29 seconds.[460]

Among patients presenting with perceived illness (rather than for service delivery) in UK general practice in 1974, the odds of their being undiagnosed at the first consultation were 2:3 (43%); of those undiagnosed at the first consultation, the odds of not re-attending for the same complaint were 3:1 (72%).[461]

Among patients with no definite diagnosis in UK general practice, the odds of not returning within a month were 72% (3:1); the odds of getting better were 1:1 (58%).[295]

Among U.S. angiography patients asked electively about hypothetical vignettes, the odds of different role preferences were: for problem solving (diagnosis, options, determining risk and benefit, probability), handover to the doctor 3:1 (78%), share 1:4 (20%), retain 1:50 (2%); for decision making (weighing risk and benefit, what to do), handover to the doctor 1:3 (22%), share 1:1 (48%), retain 1:2 (30%).[462]

Among 'sicker adults' (people who had recently been hospitalized, had surgery, or reported health problems) in the UK, Australia, Canada, Germany, New Zealand, and the United States, the odds of self-reports were as follows: having received advice on diet and exercise from any health professional in the past year 1:1 to 2:1 (45–65%); doctor having explained medication side effects 1:1 to 2:1 (49–65%); doctor having reviewed and discussed medication 1:1 (50–59%); regular doctor involving them in treatment choices 1:1 (43–59%); and regular doctor giving them clear instructions such as symptoms to watch out for 3:1 (68–82%).[463]

Among doctors in a range of settings in the United States, odds of probing for contextual problems (inability to pay for prescriptions, responsibilities as carer, incapacity to self dose, inadequate access to food) were 1:1 (51%). Odds of appropriate treatment plan were 1:3 (26%) when problems elicited and 1:20 (5%) when problems not elicited.[464]

In Japan, South Africa, the UK, Germany, Canada, and the United States, the public's view on who should be mainly responsible for risk-related health decisions were: doctor gives options and lets patient decide 2:1 (51–69%), doctor gives options and their opinion 1:2 (26–38%), doctor makes decision 1:13 (3–10%), not sure 1:100 (0–2%).[465]

Among general practitioner consultations, the odds of patient not mentioning something relevant even though the patient thought the doctor did not know were 2:1 (61–69%).[100]

Among consultations in England, the odds of a patient being able to remember the key points correctly in the three areas of diagnostic-significance, treatment-action, and preventive-action were 13:1 (90–95%).[100]

Among U.S. public given information about a drug in a table quantifying outcomes with and without the drug, the odds of understanding effectiveness were

2:1 (70%); the odds of understanding side effects were 4:1 (80%); the odds of choosing the correct drug were 2:1 (68%).[259]

Among patients on anti-epileptics, the odds of omitting at least one dose on any one day (assessed by microprocessors in pill container caps to record each opening) were 1:3 (24%) overall, 1:7 (13%) on once daily regime, 1:4 (19%) on twice daily, 1:3 (23%) on thrice daily, 3:2 (61%) on four times daily; neither pill counts nor drug levels were predictive.[466]

Patient safety (RCGP curriculum 3.2)

Among patients in Netherlands primary care, the annualised odds of error with actual or potential harm were 1:5 (when assessed by random patient record check) and 2:1 (when wrong appointments and lack of respect were reported in patient questionnaires).[467]

Among New Zealand primary care doctors in 2001, the odds of ever having received a complaint were 1:1 (46%), increasing with male sex, higher degree, and number of years since graduation.[31]

Among general practitioners in England in 2002–07, the annual odds of poor performance requiring remediation or reporting to professional body were 1:25 (4%).[468]

Among general practice and NHS24 patient contacts, the odds of a complaint reaching the Scottish Health Services Ombudsman in 2007–08 were 1:3 000.[33]

Among UK general practitioners, the odds of being suspended in 2009–10 were 1:500 (0.2%).[469]

Odds of incorrect coding of smoking status in the primary care electronic patient record are 1:6 (14%) for those coded as having smoked ever, 1:3 (30%) for those coded as being current smokers, and 2:3 (40%) for those coded as being former smokers.[470]

Odds in 2010 of adults not filling prescriptions or of skipping doses in the previous year because of cost were: 1:7 (12%) in Australia; 1:9 (10%) in Canada; 1:13 (7%) in New Zealand; 1:50 (2%) in the UK; 1:20 (3–7%) in some other European countries; and 1:4 (21%) in the United States.[471]

Evidence-based practice (RCGP curriculum 3.5)

Among quantitative therapy trials, the odds of being out-of-date were: 1:13 (7%) at time of publication; 1:6 (15%) after 1y; and 1:3 (23%) after 2y.[472]

Among primary care patients in England, the odds of their death having being prevented by UK primary care pay-for-performance programme (Quality and Outcomes Framework) adherence were as follows: in 2004, with actual adherence, 1:10 000 (0.007–0.016%); if adherence had been total, 1:2000 (0.029–0.081%); in 2006, with actual adherence, zero; if adherence had been total, 1:3000 (0.03%).[304]

Among U.S. schoolchildren, odds of red-green colour-vision defects were 1:16 (6%) in boys and 1:180 (0.6%) in girls.[473]

Among photographs viewed by U.S. volunteer healthcare workers or healthcare students in their thirties with red-green colour blindness, the odds of recognition of blood in stool were 2:1 (70%), blood in urine were 9:1 (90%), and blood in sputum were 4:1 (78%).[474]

Teaching, mentoring, and clinical supervision (RCGP curriculum 3.7)

In the AKT for MRCGP in 2009, the pass rate was 87% at the first attempt, falling to 56% at the fourth (the maximum allowed[475]); it ranged from 92% for female UK graduates to 55% for male European Economic Area graduates, from 95% for white UK graduates to 42% for black European Economic Area graduates, and from 97% for East Scotland to 69% for Oxford.

In the CSA in 2009, the pass rate was 84% at the first attempt, falling to 61% at the fourth (the maximum allowed[475]); it ranged from 97% for female UK graduates to 55% for male international medical graduates, from 97% for white UK graduates to 35% for black European Economic Area graduates, and from 97% for Northern Ireland to 73% for Northern England. (Some subgroups are small and differences not necessarily statistically significant).[476]

Management in Primary Care (RCGP curriculum 4.1)

In Netherlands primary care, among patients having blood tests, the odds of abnormal result were 2:1 (64%) overall and 2:1 (69%) when done to reassure patient; among blood tests, odds of abnormal result were 1:4 (21%) overall and 1:7 (13%) when done to reassure patient.[477]

Among patients presenting for first time with fatigue in primary care in the Netherlands, the odds of limited range of blood tests giving true positive were 1:16 (6%) and giving false positive were 1:3 (22%); the odds of extensive range of blood tests giving true positive were 1:12 (8%) and giving false positive were 1:1 (56%).[478]

Among people aged 18–60y in the UK, in the previous 2w, the odds of feeling tired/run down were 2:3 (41%).[479]

Among U.S. primary care patients who had been assessed acutely for fatigue, the odds of investigation leading to diagnosis not revealed by history and examination were 1:10 (9%); the odds of identifying physical cause were 1:7 (13%); odds of improvement were 1:1 (47%).[480]

Among patients presenting with general weakness or tiredness in Dutch primary care, the odds were: general weakness or tiredness 2:3 (38%), self-limiting respiratory tract illness/viral 1:4 (20%), psychosocial 1:10 (9%), and iron deficiency anaemia 1:28 (4%).[137]

In family practice in the United States, in 249 patients with average age 26y and isolated lymphadenopathy, no patient initially followed by observation later developed serious illness, and serious or treatable causes were always suspected at first encounter; odds of firm diagnosis were 1:2 (36%); odds of biopsy were 1:30

(3%); odds of serious disease (depending on definition) were 1:24 (3–5%); and odds of malignancy were 1:120 (0.8%).[495]

Healthy people: promoting health and preventing disease (RCGP curriculum 5)

U.S. Preventive Services Task Force recommendations concerning primary prevention are graded A, B, and C according to the level of evidence. Providing or overseeing A and B, which are recommended as part of the periodic health examination of the symptomatic individual, requires 7h/d of physician time; providing or overseeing A alone requires 2h/d.[337]

Among people in England and Wales in 2005, the odds of death within the next year were 1:100 (1%). Among deaths in England and Wales in 2005, causes with odds were: cardiovascular disease 1:2 (34%); malignancy 1:3 (26%); injury and poisoning 1:30 (3%); infectious and parasitic diseases 1:100 (1%); and diabetes 1:100 (1%).[481]

Among people in low- and middle-income countries in 2001, the odds of death within the next year were 1:100 (0.9%); causes with odds were: cardiovascular disease 1:3 (26%); infectious and parasitic diseases 1:4 (21%); malignancy 1:10 (9%); injury and poisoning 1:10 (9%); and diabetes 1:70 (1.5%).[482]

Among Scottish people >35y in 1995–2003, the odds of tooth-brushing less than once daily were 1:20 (5%), the higher odds being among older, lower socio-economic group men.[483]

In worldwide population of non-smokers in 2004, the odds of exposure to secondhand smoke (at home or at work) were 2:3 (40%) in children, 1:2 (men 33%, women 35%) in adults. Among worldwide deaths, the odds of death being attributable to secondhand smoking were 1:100.[484]

In the population, the odds of being a smoker are: Europe 1:2 (33%); UK affluent 1:6 (14%); UK deprived 1:2 (34%); and the United States 1:4 (21%).[485]

In newly recruited asymptomatic middle-aged smokers given smoking cessation intervention, the odds for quitting at two years were 1:4 (17%); for quitting, pharmacological therapy (nicotine replacement or bupropion) had LR+ 50, LR− 0.4, and positive attitude to cessation intervention had LR+ 1.5, LR− 0.1.[486]

Nicotine replacement therapy is associated with a relative increase of smoking cessation as follows: any route 60%; gum 40%; patch 70%; inhaler 90%; oral 100%; and nasal spray 100%.[487]

Among UK male doctors, stopping smoking was associated with the following life-years gained: 10y after stopping at 30y; 9y after stopping at 40y; 6y after stopping at 50y; and 3y after stopping at 60y.[488]

The delay before colorectal cancer screening benefit exceeds harm is ≥10y in a woman aged 40y, falling to 5y in a man aged 80y. The delay is greater in people for whom colonoscopy is riskier (with severe systemic disease or warfarinised), greater in people with lower risk of colorectal cancer (on aspirin, NSAIDs, or HRT), less in healthier people, and less in people with greater risk of colorectal cancer (inflammatory bowel disease, smoking, obesity, heavy alcohol, diabetes, positive family history).[442]

In the 27 member states of the European Union, life expectancy was 75y (range 65–78y) in men and 81y (range 74–84y) in women.[489]

Among (mainly white European) middle-aged women with a mean age of 56y followed for 10–12y, the odds of death were: overall 1:10 (9%); alcohol >14 IU/w 1:9 (10%), 7–14 IU/w 1:12 (8%), 1–6 IU/w 1:13 (7%), teetotal 1:6 (14%); physical activity ≥15 h/w 1:13 (7%), <15 h/w 1:7 (12%); BMI <18.5 kg/m² 1:4 (20%), 18.5–25 kg/m² 1:11 (8%), 25–30 kg/m² 1:10 (9%), ≥30 kg/m² 1:9 (10%); non-smoking 1:16 (6%); and smoking 1:8 (12%).[352]

Among people in England and Wales aged 16–59y in 2009–10, the odds of illicit drug use were 1:2 (36%) ever, 1:10 (9%) in the last year, and 1:20 (5%) in the last month; the odds of Class A drug use were 1:6 (15%) ever, 1:30 (3%) in the last year, and 1:70 (1.4%) in the last month.[490]

Among men aged 50y in Sweden, the odds of death after 35y of follow-up were 3:2 (62%) in the highly active and 4:1 (81%) in the inactive; life expectancy was 2.3y greater in the highly active compared with the inactive. Among men aged 50y in Sweden, mortality after 10y of follow-up was 50% less if activity increased from inactive to highly active; 40% less if smoking ceased. Being highly active was self-assessed by positive answer to either: 'Do you engage in any active recreational sports or heavy gardening at least three hours every week?' or 'Do you regularly engage in hard physical training or competitive sport?'[349]

Among residents of an urban slum in Brazil, the odds of head lice adults or nymphs found by professional wet-combing were 1:1 (44%): self-diagnosis had LR+ 10, LR– 0.2; professional visual inspection had LR+ infinity, LR– 0.7.[491]

Among white non-smokers, annual deaths per thousand people according to BMI in kg/m² are as in Table 5.1.[351]

TABLE 5.1 Annual deaths per thousand white non-smokers

BMI (kg/m²)	15–18.4	18.5–29.9	30–39	40–49
50–59y	5	4–5	6–8	11
60–69y	12	8–9	11–15	19
70–84y	27	16–22	20–26	31

Among healthy U.S. non-smokers aged 30–74y, relative risk of death increased by no more than twofold from BMI 19 to BMI 30, with maximum relative risk in 30y old women; at >75y, relative mortality was constant for BMI 19–30.[492]

Care of acutely ill people (RCGP curriculum 7)

Among adults having out-of-hospital cardiac arrest in the United States, the odds of hospital discharge with good or moderately impaired cerebral function

(Cerebral Performance Category 1 or 2) were 1:23 (4%) overall; 1:30 (3%) if given no cardiopulmonary resuscitation; 1:20 (5%) if given lay bystander conventional cardiopulmonary resuscitation; and 1:12 (7.5%) if given lay bystander compression-only cardiopulmonary resuscitation.[493]

In UK intensive care units, the odds of refusal by relatives for organ donation were 1:2 (35%) when deceased white and 2:1 (70%) when deceased non-white.[494]

Care of children and young people (RCGP curriculum 8)

Among live births, the odds of dying in infancy are 1:12 (8%) in India, 1:9 (10%) in sub-Saharan Africa. Among children, the odds of undernourishment are 1:1 (40–60%) in India, 1:2 (20–40%) in Africa.[208]

Adults attending a Californian primary care clinic in 1995–97 were surveyed about childhood physical abuse and asked: 'Sometimes parents or other adults hurt children. How often did a parent, stepparent, or adult living in your home (1) push, grab, slap, or throw something at you or (2) hit you so hard that you had marks or were injured'? A respondent was defined as being physically abused if the response was 'often' or 'very often' to the first part or 'sometimes', 'often', or 'very often' to the second part). Odd of physical abuse were 1:2 (30%) for males and 1:3 (27%) for females.[496]

Adults attending a Californian primary care clinic in 1995–97 were surveyed about sexual abuse during childhood and asked: 'Some people, while they are growing up in their first 18 years of life, had a sexual experience with an adult or someone at least five years older than themselves. These experiences may have involved a relative, family friend, or stranger. During the first 18 years of life, did an adult, relative, family friend, or stranger ever (1) touch or fondle your body in a sexual way, (2) have you touch their body in a sexual way, (3) attempt to have any type of sexual intercourse with you (oral, anal, or vaginal), or (4) actually have any type of sexual intercourse with you (oral, anal, or vaginal)?' A 'yes' response to any of the four questions classified a respondent as having experienced contact sexual abuse during childhood. Odds of sexual abuse were 1:5 (16%) for males and 1:3 (25%) for females.[496]

Among children <17y presenting to GP or A&E in Belgium with acute illness for <5d, odds of serious infection were: 1:130 (0.8%) overall; 1:12 (8%) if parent thought 'illness is different', 1:6 (15%) if doctor thought 'something is wrong', and 1:15 (6%) if dyspnoea/tachypnoea present; ≤1:200 (≤0.5%) in the absence of these features.[497]

Among children <5y with diarrhoea, vomiting, or poor intake presenting as emergency in Pennsylvania: odds of >5% dehydration were 1:2 (34%); score 1 for each of capillary refilling >2s, dry mucous membranes, absent tears, altered general appearance; for dehydration >5%, score ≥2 had LR+ 6, LR– 0.2.[498]

Care of older adults (RCGP curriculum 9)

Among institutionalised people (mainly >65y, some catheterised) in Canada with fever, the reference standard for cause was antibody rise in paired sera. Odds for causes were: unexplained 2:3 (43%); respiratory 2:3 (40%); urinary 1:13 (7%); gastrointestinal 1:16 (6%); and soft tissue 1:30 (3%). Initial odds of bacteriuria were 1:1 (50%) in all residents and 2:3 (40%) in uncatheterised residents. For urinary tract infection, bacteriuria in uncatheterised residents had PPV 11%; clinical diagnosis of urinary tract infection had PPV 43%.[499]

Among U.S. people living in the community (outwith institutions) aged >50y, probability of dying in next 4y[161] and the declining exponential approximation of life expectancy[442] could be estimated using Table 5.2 (which can be downloaded from www.darmipc.net).[428]

TABLE 5.2 U.S. people living in the community (outwith institutions) aged >50y: estimation of probability of dying and life expectancy

Criterion	Potential score
Age:	
60–64 years	1
65–69 years	2
70–74 years	3
75–79 years	4
80–84 years	5
≥85 years	7
Male	2
BMI <25	1
Diabetes	1
Cancer (other than non-melanocytic skin cancer)	2
Chronic lung disease limiting usual activities	2
Heart failure	2
Smoking	2
Difficulty bathing	2
Difficulty with finances	2
Difficulty walking several blocks	2
Difficulty pulling or pushing living room chair	1

Total score	4y odds of death	Life expectancy
≤10	<1:2 (<30%)	≥10 years
11–13	1:1 (44–57%)	4–7 years
≥14	≥2:1 (66%)	<4 years

For English-speaking Americans >70y with average age 84y, initial life expectancy >12m, without needing help from another to complete four activities of daily living (bathing, dressing, rising from sitting, and walking) but skewed toward slow gait and living in the community, the odds of dying within 10y were 1:1 (54%). There were five distinct trajectories in the last year of life (the denominator being the total cohort): persistently severe disability 1:8 (11%), catastrophic disability (from 3m before death) 1:9 (10%), accelerated disability (from 10m before death) 1:10 (9%), no disability 1:10 (9%), and progressive disability 1:12 (7%). Causes of death were frailty 1:6 (14%), organ failure 1:8 (11%), cancer 1:9 (10%,) advanced dementia 1:13 (7%), sudden death 1:70 (1.3%), and other 1:12 (8%). Trajectory was independent of cause of death except that persistently severe disability accompanied advanced dementia, and no disability accompanied sudden death.[159]

Among white rural Swedish women ≥70y, the FRAMO (FRacture And MOrtality) index gave the results shown in Table 5.3. (which can be downloaded from www. darmipc.net).[169, 428]

TABLE 5.3 FRAMO index

Criterion	Standard	Potential score
Age	≥80 y	1
Weight	<60 kg	1
Can you rise five times from a chair without using your arms? (Try if you want.)	No, I must use my arms to rise.	1
Radiologically evident fracture after age of 40y of wrist, arm, hip, or vertebra.	Yes	1
Actual score	2y hip facture risk	2y mortality risk
0–1	1:100 (1%)	1:30 (3%)
2–4	1:20 (5%)	1:3 (24%)

In a year of modest influenza activity and incomplete vaccine match, immunisation of healthcare staff in long-stay settings costs ≤ £274 (€407; $542) per patient life year gained.[500]

Women's health (RCGP curriculum 10.1)

In women ≥20y presenting to primary care with breast lump or mass, odds of breast cancer are ≥1:20 (≥5%).[501]

In Dutch general practice, for a woman presenting with breast symptoms, odds of breast cancer were 1:30 (3%) (increasing with age), comprising odds for the following symptoms: breast lump 1:12 (8%); nipple complaint 1:50 (2%); fear of breast cancer 1:70 (1.4%); pain 1:100 (1%); and other 1:60 (1.7%).[502]

For a woman aged 40–70y with breast symptoms consulting a U.S. primary care physician, odds of breast cancer were 1:22 (4.5%) (independent of age).[450]

For breast cancer, clinical breast examination has LR+ 9 and LR− 0.4.[451]

The number needed to invite for screening mammography to prevent one death from breast cancer is 1900 at 39–49y, 1300 at 50–59y, and 380 at 60–69y.[150]

For breast cancer, mammography in Australia had the LRs shown in Table 5.4.[409]

TABLE 5.4 LRs for mammography in diagnosis of breast cancer

	LR+	LR–
Women with lump or with watery or bloody discharge	3	0.3
Women with other breast symptoms	13	0.4
Women with no symptoms	15	0.3

Among women of reproductive age in Scandinavian primary care with vaginal discharge or offensive odour, initial odds were: bacterial vaginosis 1:2 (34%); no specific pathogen 1:3 (25%); thrush 1:3 (23%); Chlamydia 1:6 (15%); Trichomonas 1:10 (9%), genital herpes virus 1:13 (7%), *Neisseria gonorrhoeae* 1:100 (1%).[452]

Among premenopausal women in primary care with vaginal symptoms, LRs are shown in Table 5.5.[453]

TABLE 5.5 LRs for premenopausal vaginal symptoms

Symptom	LR+ for bacterial vaginosis	LR– for bacterial vaginosis	LR+ for thrush	LR– for thrush
Smell	1.6	0.1	0.5	2
Itch	0.7	1.6	1.5	0.5
Increased discharge	2	0.6		
Cheesy			2	0.5
Watery			0.1	1.5
'Another yeast infection'			3	0.7

Among women aged 17–65y seen by general practitioners or gynaecologists in Germany with 'relapsing' vaginitis (defined as seeking further medical help for identical symptoms), none of itching, burning, redness, discharge and odour was associated with the microbiological cause; for bacterial vaginosis, clinical diagnosis had LR+ 2, LR– 0.5; for thrush, clinical diagnosis had LR+ 1, LR– 1.[454]

In woman aged 75–84y in primary care with a computer code of postmenopausal bleeding, odds of endometrial cancer are ≥1:20 (≥5%).[501]

Among women referred to a hysteroscopy clinic in Europe with postmenopausal bleeding, odds of endometrial cancer were 1:20 (4%) with subgroups shown in Table 5.6. Ultrasonic endometrial thickness ≥5 mm had LR+ 1.2 and LR– 0.8; positive hysteroscopy had LR+ 14 and LR– 0.3.[503]

TABLE 5.6 Initial odds (probability) of endometrial cancer among women referred with postmenopausal bleeding

	On HRT	*Not on HRT*
<60y	1:500 (0.2%)	1:100 (1%)
≥60y	1:40 (3%)	1:8 (13%)

In U.S. women, mean age of menopause was 48y and duration of menstrual irregularity 4y. After 12 months of amenorrhoea, odds of spontaneous menstruation were 1:50 (2%).[504] Odds of perimenopausal or postmenopausal status were 1:2 (33%) at 40y,[505] 2:3 (40%) at 45y, 3:1 (75%) at 50y, and 50:1 (98%) at 55y.[504] Table 5.7 shows LRs for menopause within next 3y.[504]

TABLE 5.7 LRs for menopause within next 3y

Feature	LR+	LR-
Self-rating	2	0.3
3–11 months of irregular or absent periods at age 45–55y	3	0.4
hot flushes	3	0.7
night sweats	2	0.8
vaginal dryness	3	0.9
FSH ≥24 IU/L	3	0.5

Among women having pregnancy tests done in U.S. emergency departments, the odds of positive results were 1:40 (2%). For positive pregnancy test, 'Do you think you might be pregnant?' had LR+ 11, LR– 0.5; 'Is there any chance you could be pregnant?' had LR+ 3, LR– 0.1; self-reported use of no birth control had LR+ 2, LR– 0.5; last menstrual period 'not normal' had LR+ 2, LR– 0.7; period late had LR+ 2, LR– 0.6; and a history of sexual activity had LR+ 1.4, LR– very low.[506]

After previous birth, risk of adverse perinatal outcome is least when conception is 18–59 months later.[507]

After previous miscarriage, risk of adverse pregnancy outcome in Scotland was least when conception was <6m later.[508]

Among women in Amsterdam presenting to general practitioners with bleeding at <16w of pregnancy, outcomes and odds were as in Table 5.8.[509]

Among women presenting to primary care in England, the odds of having ovarian cancer were: intermittent abdominal bloating presenting once 1:300 (0.3%); presenting twice 1:50 (2%); sustained abdominal distension presenting once 1:40 (2.5%); and presenting twice 1:20 (4%).[316]

TABLE 5.8 Outcomes with odds (probability) after bleeding at <16w of pregnancy

Outcome	Odds (%)
Ultimately viable	1:1 (45%)
Complete miscarriage	1:3 (25%)
Non-viable	1:4 (22%)
Ectopic	1:24 (4%)
Mole	1:100 (1%)

Among couples with sub-fertility, causes are sperm problems 1:2 (30%); anovulation 1:3 (25%); unexplained 1:3 (25%); and tubal infection 1:4 (20%).[510]

Among couples trying to conceive, odds of conceiving naturally were 1:2 (38%) within one cycle; 2:1 (68%) within three cycles; 4:1 (81%) within six cycles; 12:1 (92%) within 12 cycles;[511] 20:1 (95%) within 48m; and very low thereafter.[512]

Among couples with unexplained infertility, the odds of achieving pregnancy are similar with and without treatment.[512]

Among women in Europe using natural methods of family planning, the odds of pregnancy resulting from intercourse during 0–5d before ovulation were ≥1:20 (≥5%) and on other days of the cycle <1:20 (<5%). Odds of pregnancy resulting from intercourse 2d before ovulation (fertility peak) were 1:1 (50%) in women aged 19–26y, falling to 1:3 (30%) in women aged 35–39y [513]

In Canada, among screened women aged 30–69y, the odds of cervical intra-epithelial neoplasia grade ≥2 were 1:250 (0.4%), for which liquid-based Papanicolaou testing had LR+ 18, LR– 0.5 and human papillomavirus testing had LR+ 16, LR– 0.05.[514]

Among women presenting with at least one symptom of urinary tract infection, the odds of proven urinary tract infection are 1:1 (50%);[515] among non-pregnant women aged 18–69y presenting in English primary care with possible urinary tract infection and no alternative likelier diagnosis, the odds of urinary tract infection defined as >1000 cfu/mL were 2:1 (66%) and defined as >100 000 cfu/mL were 1:1 (50%).[516] LRs for symptoms and signs[515] and for dipstick test results are shown in Table 5.9.[516]

In English primary care, women 18–70y with suspected lower urinary tract infection had mean duration of moderately bad or worse symptoms after consultation of 3.5d (with 8% having symptoms for >7d).[517] Whether management involved empirical immediate antibiotics, delayed antibiotics, culture, dipstick, or symptom score, there were no significant differences in mean duration or severity of symptoms. Antibiotics were taken by 97% of women in the immediate group and 77% in the delayed group; the delayed group re-consulted less. Women who actually deferred antibiotic use by 48h had symptoms for a mean of 5d rather than 3.5d and re-consulted less.[518]

TABLE 5.9 LRs for urinary tract infection

Feature	LR+	LR−
Dysuria	1.5	0.5
Frequency	1.8	0.6
Haematuria	2	0.9
Fever	1.6	0.9
Lower abdominal pain	1.1	0.9
Back pain	1.6	0.8
Loin tenderness	1.7	0.9
Vaginal irritation	0.2	
Vaginal discharge symptom	0.3	
Vaginal discharge sign	0.7	1.1
Dipstick		
Blood haemolysed trace or greater	1.7	0.5
Leucocyte esterase + or greater	1.6	0.3
Nitrite positive	5.5	0.7

In urinary tract infection, the odds of resistance to antibiotic are 1:2 (19–40%) in previously untreated patients, 2:1 for 1m after treatment, 1:1 for 6m after treatment, and 2:3 for 12m after treatment.[227]

Among patients whose urine samples were analysed by one laboratory in Ireland in 2004–08: if the initial sample showed *E. coli* infection resistant to nitrofurantoin, the odds of resistance to nitrofurantoin after 2w–3m were 1:4 (20%) and after 9–12m 1:17 (6%); if the initial sample showed *E. coli* infection resistant to ampicillin, co-amoxiclav, ciprofloxacin, or trimethoprim, the odds of resistance to the respective antibiotic at 2w–12m were >2:3 (>43%).[519]

Among the general population, the odds of urinary calculi are probably about 1:40 (2–3%).[520] Among patients admitted to hospital in Finland with acute abdominal pain, for urinary calculi, LRs are as in Table 5.10.[521]

TABLE 5.10 LRs for urinary calculi of various features

Feature	LR+	LR-
Appetite normal	1.8	0.7
Duration of pain ≤12h	2	0.5
Loin tenderness	30	0.8
Haematuria (at least +)	75	0.25

Among non-dialysed or transplanted adults in the community in Canada who had had at least one blood creatinine and one urine dipstick or albumen:creatinine ratio done, annual odds of death were 1:100 (1%); for the same eGFR, mortality with proteinuria ≥2+ was approximately double mortality with no proteinuria, and mortality with albumen:creatinine ratio ≥34mg/mmol was approximately double mortality with ACR <3.4 mg/mmol.[522]

Among dialysis patients in Australia and New Zealand, the odds of death during first 4y of dialysis were 1:2 (37%).[523]

Men's health (RCGP curriculum 10.2)

Among male urology clinic patients in the United States, midstream sampling produced less contamination than initial sampling; in combination, midstream sampling, cleansing, and circumcised state produced less contamination than initial sampling, no cleansing, and uncircumcised state.[524]

Among well men ≥35y and women ≥55y having screening in California in 1980 using Multistix, the odds of microscopic haematuria were 1:20 (4%); for urological cancer, microscopic haematuria had LR+ 1, LR− 1.[525]

Among UK men having routine health checks, the odds of microscopic haematuria detected by Labstick were 1:40 (2.5%). Of 76 subsequently selected by their GP for further investigations, odds were: bladder cancer or dysplasia (1:25) (4%) and benign urological disease 1:4 (18%).[526]

After presentation in primary care in England with macroscopic haematuria, the odds of having no specific diagnosis by 90d were 4:1 (82%) and by 3y were 3:2 (63% in men, 58% in women);[527] the odds of having urinary tract cancer by 3y were 1:12 (7%) for men and 1:28 (3%) for women.[528] Among patients in primary care in Belgium with macroscopic haematuria, the odds of urological cancer were 1:6 (14%) in men and 1:20 (5%) in women, rising with age from zero at <40y to 1:4 (22%) in men ≥60y and 1:11 (8%) in women at ≥60y.[529]

In patients ≥60y presenting to primary care with macroscopic haematuria, the odds of urological cancer are ≥1:20 (≥5%)[501]

In men ≥40y presenting to primary care with malignant prostate on digital rectal examination, the odds of prostate cancer are ≥1:20 (≥5%).[501]

Among healthy American men >55y, for prostate cancer, prostate-specific antigen (ng/mL) at various thresholds had LRs as in Table 5.11.[408]

Among men aged 45–96y being screened for prostate cancer, the odds of prostate cancer are 1:20 (1–7%); digital rectal examination malignant has LR+ 10–20, LR− 0.4.[530]

Among unscreened men aged 55–74y in the United States with clinically local prostate cancer managed with observation or androgen withdrawal, the odds of death were as in Table 5.12.[149]

Among unscreened men >40y seen in general practice in England, the odds of prostate cancer were as follows (the risks for combinations of features should not be

TABLE 5.11 LRs for prostate cancer

Prostate specific antigen threshold (ng/mL)	LR	Any prostate cancer (versus no cancer)	Gleason ≥7 (versus <7 or no cancer)	Gleason ≥8 (versus <8 or no cancer)
>1	LR+	1.4	1.5	1.5
	LR−	0.4	0.2	0.2
>2	LR+	2	2.3	2.5
	LR−	0.6	0.4	0.2
>3	LR+	2.4	3.3	3.6
	LR−	0.8	0.5	0.4
>4	LR+	3.3	4	4.6
	LR−	0.8	0.7	0.6
>6	LR+	3	6	10
	LR−	1	0.9	0.8

TABLE 5.12 Odds of death within 20y among men with localised prostate cancer

Gleason score	Odds of dying from prostate cancer	Odds of dying from other cause	Odds of dying
Overall	1:3 (29%)	2:1 (64%)	13:1 (93%)
2–4	1:13 (7%)	4:1 (81%)	7:1 (88%)
5	1:6 (14%)	3:1 (76%)	9:1 (90%)
6	1:3 (27%)	2:1 (67%)	16:1 (94%)
7	1:1 (45%)	1:1 (53%)	50:1 (98%)
8–10	2:1 (66%)	1:2 (33%)	100:1 (99%)

added): none 1:300 (0.35%); macroscopic haematuria presenting once 1:100 (1%) and presenting twice 1:60 (2%); loss of weight presenting twice 1:50 (2%); any lower urinary tract symptoms such as frequency, urgency, nocturia, and hesitancy 1:30 (2–5%); impotence 1:30 (3%); abnormal digital rectal examination considered benign 1:30 (3%); and digital rectal examination malignant 1:8 (12%).[315]

Among men in the United States, the odds of complete impotence were 1:20 (5%) at 40y and 1:6 (15%) at 70y.[531]

Among U.S. primary care patients who had been assessed acutely for impotence, the odds of investigation leading to diagnosis not revealed by history and examination were 1:6 (15%); the odds of identifying physical cause were 1:4 (21%); and the odds of improvement were 1:1 (56%).[480]

In a meta-analysis of men and women, the odds of sexual dysfunction associated with various drugs were as follows: bupropion, moclobemide, and nefazodone 1:13

(4–10%); placebo 1:6 (14%); fluvoxamine, mirtazapine 1:3 (24–26%); duloxetine, escitalopram, and imipramine 2:3 (37–44%); and citalopram, fluoxetine, paroxetine, sertraline, and venlafaxine 3:1 (70–80%).[532]

Among men with erectile dysfunction, Modified Leiden Impotence Questionnaire[533] and LRs for cause being functional or physical can be downloaded from www.darmipc.net.[428]

Sexual health (RCGP curriculum 11)

For human immunodeficiency virus infection, a rapid HIV test had LR+ 166, LR– 0.004.[534]

Care of people with cancer and palliative care (RCGP curriculum 12)

For patients with metastatic cancer, the odds of surviving 1y and 5y are: breast 1y 1:1 (49%), 5y 1:7 (12%); lung 1y 1:2 (33%), 5y <1:20 (<5%); colorectal 1y 1:1 (49%), 5y 1:30 (3%); and prostate 1y 4:1 (82%) 5y 1:2 (30%).[136]

Among deaths in England, the odds of their occurring in hospital were 1:1 (55%).[535]

Care of people with mental health problems (RCGP curriculum 13)

For bipolar disorder among psychiatric outpatients in the United States, a self-reported history of bipolar disorder had LR+ 5, LR– 0.3.[536]

Among people aged 18–60y in the UK, in the previous 2w odds of feeling nervous/anxious were 1:4 (19%) and of feeling depressed were 1:5 (17%).[479]

Among adults attending primary care at 15 international sites, the odds were: depression 1:8 (12%); depression not recognised by GP 1:17 (6%); anxiety 1:9 (10%); and anxiety not recognised by GP 1:19 (5%).[537]

For (mainly) DSM and ICD anxiety and depression, the Hospital Anxiety and Depression Scale cut-offs for depression of 8 and for anxiety of 8 have approximately LR+ 4, LR– 0.25 (the scale is copyright).[538]

Among patients attending New Zealand general practitioners, the odds of major depression (assessed by lay interviewer using the composite international diagnostic interview that has κ = 0.58–0.97 concordance with ICD-10) were 1:20 (5%). For major depression, a written questionnaire (which can be downloaded from www.darmipc.net[428]) asked 'During the past month have you often been bothered by feeling down, depressed, or hopeless?' ('yes/no'); 'During the past month have you often been bothered by little interest or pleasure in doing things?' ('yes/no'); and 'Is this something with which you would like help?' ('help today, help but not today, no help') and had the following LRs: all 'no' 0.05; at least one 'yes' and 'no help' 4; at least one 'yes' and 'help but not today' 4; at least one 'yes' and 'help today' 18; and GP, having seen completed questionnaire and patient, making diagnosis of depression had LR+ 13, LR– 0.2.[539]

Among cognitively intact patients >65y in nursing home in Italy, the odds of DSM-IV depression were 1:1 (48%) and a five item version of the Geriatric Depression

Scale had LR+ 3, LR– 0.1 (available for download from www.darmipc.net[428]). Questions asked were as follows: (1) Are you basically satisfied with your life? (2) Do you often get bored? (3) Do you often feel hopeless? (4) Do you prefer to stay at home rather than going out a doing new things? (5) Do you feel pretty worthless the way you are now? 'No' in Q1 and 'yes' in Q2–5 score 1 and a total score of 2 was positive. Mean administration time was 1 minute/patient.[540]

Among postnatal women in England in 1999, the odds of finding screening for depression unacceptable were 1:1 (54%).[541]

Among mothers in Wales 6–8w postpartum, the odds of DSM-III major depression were 1:6 (15%); Edinburgh Postnatal Depression Scale ≥13 had LR+ 14, LR– 0.05.[542, 543, 428]

Antidepressants have clinically significant superiority over placebos, according to NICE criteria when Hamilton Depression Rating Scale score ≥25.[426, 427, 428]

In patients with no, or partial, response to an antidepressant, there is no good evidence that either switching to another class or increased dosage (above fluoxetine 20mg, paroxetine 20mg, sertraline 100mg) increases response; there is limited support for augmentation with another antidepressant. Discontinuation of antidepressants shows odds of relapse over 1–3y of 2:3 (41%) on placebo and 1:5 on antidepressant.[544]

Among adults ≥25y in the community in Scotland, the odds of chronic pain (pain or discomfort present either all the time or on and off for three months or longer) were 1:1 (46–54%); annual odds of recovery were 1:20 (5%); among those with chronic pain initially, odds of chronic pain after 4y were 4:1 (79%); among those without chronic pain initially, odds of chronic pain after 4y were 1:2 (33%); among those with chronic pain at both 0y and 4y, odds of same chronic pain grade were 1:1 (50%), of higher grade 1:2 (29%) and of lower grade 1:4 (21%).[545]

The pain relief attributable to opioid or nonsteroidal anti-inflammatory drug administration for up to three months is a maximum of 8–12 out of 100 units and to placebo a mean of 15–18 out of 100 units. Effect is less after 6w and in uncontrolled studies insignificant after 3m. The odds of stopping analgesics because of side effects or lack of effect are 1:2 (33%) for opioids and 1:3 (25%) for non-opioids.[546]

Among UK GP consulters in 1999, odds of DSM-IV/ICD-10 personality disorder were 1:3 (24%).[547]

In primary care consulters, odds of personality disorder are 1:14 (5–8%) as main diagnosis and 1:2 (29–33%) as comorbidity.[152]

Among people aged 18–60y in the UK, in the previous 2w odds of difficulty sleeping were 1:3 (28%).[479]

Among U.S. primary care patients who had been assessed acutely for insomnia, odds of investigation leading to diagnosis not revealed by history and examination were nil (0%); odds of identifying physical cause were 1:30 (3%); and odds of improvement were 1:1 (50%).[480]

Among patients in Hong Kong with a first episode of non-affective psychosis controlled with quetiapine without previous relapse, odds of relapse after 1y were 2:3 (41%) on quetiapine and 4:1 (79%) on placebo.[548]

Among people treated in hospital in Sweden for attempted suicide by the following means, odds of completed suicide by any means within 1y were: poisoning 1:30 (3%); cutting or piercing 1:30 (4%); gassing 1:9 (11%); hanging, strangulation, or suffocation 1:1 (48%); drowning 1:3 (28%); firearm or explosive in males 1:3 (27%) and in females 1:40 (2.5%); and jumping from a height in males 1:3 (26%) and in females 1:6 (15%).[549]

Among the population: odds of DSM anorexia nervosa are 1:300 (0.3%) among young women; odds of DSM bulimia nervosa are 1:100 (1%) among young women and 1:1000 (0.1%) among young men; and odds of binge eating depending on definition and population are 1:100–1:20 (1–4.5%).[550]

There are no clear reference standards for diagnosis of age-associated memory impairment, mild cognitive impairment or dementia, even at autopsy.[165]

In the general population, odds of dementia >50y are 1:10 (9%); odds of mild cognitive impairment >60y are 1:5 (17%); odds of memory problems ≥65y are 1:2 (25–50%); and odds of subjective memory problems aged 65–74y are 2:3 (43%), aged 70–85y are 1:1 (52%), and aged >85y are 7:1 (88%). For dementia or for mild cognitive impairment, subjective memory problems has LR+ 3, LR– 0.7.[551]

Among people >65y living at home in Ireland: for diagnosis of dementia (assessed by GMS-AGECAT, which showed good concordance with GMS-III), clock-ing drawing test subjective score <6/10 had LR+ 3, LR– 0.3.[552] Among people in the community in Edinburgh aged ≥75y for dementia using CAMCOG as reference standard: the Mini-Mental State Examination <21[553] had LR+ 40, LR– 0.2; and the Abbreviated Mental Test[554] had LR+ 8, LR– 0.3.[555]

Among community dwellers aged ≥65y, inability to do at least one activity of daily living with assistance (manage medication, use the phone, cope with a budget, and use transportation) had LR+ 3, LR– 0.1 for diagnosis of DSM-III dementia.[556]

Among the general population ≥64y in Finland, odds of documented dementia were 1:24 (4%); odds of undocumented dementia were 1:19 (5%); and for DSM-IV dementia general practitioner diagnosis had LR+ 120, LR– 0.5.[557]

Among consecutive elderly people in the United States diagnosed in life then at necropsy, results were as follows: with no cognitive impairment in life, necropsy odds of Alzheimer's disease were 2:3 (38%), infarct 1:3 (23%), Lewy body disease 1:30 (3%); with mild cognitive impairment in life, necropsy odds of Alzheimer's disease were 1:1 (54%), infarct 1:2 (33%), Lewy body disease 1:16 (6%); with Alzheimer's disease in life, necropsy odds of Alzheimer's disease were 7:1 (88%), infarct 2:3 (40%), and Lewy body disease 1:5 (17%).[164]

Among people >70y in England and Wales at death: for diagnosis of dementia (latest AGECAT organicity rating ≥O3), postmortem neuropathology features of

Alzheimer's or vascular disease had LR+ 1.7, LR– 0.5; for postmortem neuropathology features of Alzheimer's or vascular disease, diagnosis of dementia (latest AGECAT organicity rating ≥O3) had LR+ 2, LR– 0.6.[558]

Clock drawing test did not differentiate in the community between people with mild cognitive impairment and normal controls.[559]

Among people with clinical diagnosis of dementia in UK primary care, median life expectancies related to age at diagnosis are: 6y aged 60–69y; 5y aged 70–79y; 3y aged 80–89y; and 2y aged ≥90y.[560]

Among home-dwelling Australians aged 50–74y with memory problems or aged ≥75y, for DSM-IV dementia, GPCOG (General Practitioner's Assessment of Cognition (GPCOG online[561]) had LR+ 6, LR– 0.2.[562]

Care of people with learning disabilities (RCGP curriculum 14)

Among adults in India or sub-Sahara, odds of illiteracy are 2:3 (39–40%) in males and 2:1 (63–64%).[208]

Health literacy is the degree to which individuals have the capacity to obtain, process, and understand basic health information and services needed to make appropriate health decisions. Given appropriate information literature, adults with intermediate health literacy have a 67% chance of being able to, for instance: determine what time to take prescription medicine, identify three substances that interact with a medicine, find the age range during which a child should receive a vaccination, or determine a healthy weight range for a person of specified height given a BMI chart. Among U.S. adults using English or Spanish, the odds of having intermediate health literacy were 1:1 (53%), the odds of a higher level were 1:7 (12%), and the odds of a lower level were 1:2 (36%).[563]

Among people with low educational attainment aged 55–64y in Australia invited for colorectal cancer screening: odds of making an informed choice were 1:2 (34%) with decision aid (paper booklet and DVD) and 1:7 (12%) without decision aid; odds of completing faecal occult blood testing were 3:2 (59%) with decision aid and 4:1 (79%) without decision aid.[564]

Among institutionalised adults and children with IQ < 50, odds of constipation (having a bowel movement less than three times a week or the necessity of using laxatives more than three times a week) were 2:1 (69%).[565]

Cardiovascular problems (RCGP curriculum 15.1)

Among patients on warfarin with INR >5: during the following month, none died; odds of vitamin K therapy were 1:11 (9%); odds of major haemorrhage were 1:100 (1%) with INR 5–9 and 1:10 (10%) with INR >9.[566]

Among the U.S. general adult population, odds of valvular disease by age were: 18–54y 1:200 (0.1–1.3%); 55–64y 1:50 (1–3%); 65–74y 1:11 (8–9%); and >75y 1:7 (12–15%).[567] Among emergency room patients in Switzerland, for valve lesion on echocardiogram, loudness ≤2/6 in patient <50y had NPV of 98%.[568]

Among patients discharged in Europe with diagnosis of heart failure: odds of normal left ventricular systolic function were in men 1:3 (22%) and in women 1:1 (45%); odds of readmission within 12w were 1:3 (24%); and odds of death by 12w were 1:7 (13%).[569]

Among U.S. primary care patients who had been assessed acutely for oedema, odds of investigation leading to diagnosis not revealed by history and examination were 1:6 (15%); odds of identifying physical cause were 1:2 (36%); and odds of improvement were 2:1 (64%).[480]

Among white patients discharged from U.S. hospitals with diagnosis of heart failure, odds of preserved left ventricular ejection fraction were 1:1 (47%) (increasing in older, obese women with atrial fibrillation and without valve lesions).[570]

Among people >45y in England, odds of definite or probably heart failure were 1:30 (3%).[571] Among people >45y in England, odds of left ventricular systolic dysfunction with left ventricular ejection fraction <40% were 1:60 (2%) overall; 1:9 (10%) in patients with hypertension, myocardial infarction, angina, or diabetes; 1:5 (16%) in patients on diuretics; and 1:2 (34%) in patients with prior diagnosis of heart failure.[572]

For heart failure due to left ventricular systolic dysfunction, atrial fibrillation, or valvular disease (but not diastolic dysfunction), N-terminal pro-brain natriuretic peptide >305 pg/mL (>36 pmol/L) had LR+ 3.4, LR– 0 in the general population; LR+ 1.8, LR– 0 in patients with hypertension, myocardial infarction, angina, or diabetes; LR+ 1.5, LR– 0.2 in patients on diuretics; and LR+ 1.2, LR– 0 in patients with prior diagnosis of heart failure.[572] NICE N-terminal pro-brain natriuretic peptide thresholds are: normal < 400 pg/mL (47 pmol/L); raised 400–2000 pg/mL (47–236 pmol/L); high > 2000 pg/mL (236 pmol/L).[59]

Among white patients discharged from hospital in United States with diagnosis of heart failure, odds of death at 1y were 1:2 (29–32%) and odds of death at 5y were 2:1 (65–68%).[570]

Among people >45y in England, odds of death at 5y were 1:2 (31%) if reduced left ventricular ejection fraction (<40%) without heart failure; 2:3 (38%) if heart failure with preserved left ventricular ejection fraction; and 1:1 (47%) if heart failure with reduced left ventricular ejection fraction (<40%).[573]

Treatment of heart failure with preserved ejection fraction improves morbidity but not mortality.[574]

Visit-to-visit variability of systolic blood pressure predicts stroke; drugs that bring about the greatest reduction in visit-to-visit variability (calcium antagonists and diuretics) are associated with the best stroke prevention.[575, 576, 577]

Among Australian known and suspected hypertensives and among normal advertisement recruits, doctor clinic blood pressure measurements were 9/7 mm Hg higher than staff clinic measurements; staff clinic measurements were 6/3 mm Hg higher than daytime ambulatory measurements and 10/5 mm Hg higher than 24-hour blood pressure measurements.[578]

Among primary care patients >35y (derivation group in Germany, validation group in Switzerland) with volunteered or elicited history of chest pain, initial odds of ischaemic heart disease were 1:7 (13%). A point was given for each of the following: man >55y or woman >65y; known vascular disease; patient assumes pain is cardiac or is 'very worried' about it; pain is worse during exercise; and pain is not reproducible by palpation. For IHD, score 3–5 had LR+ 5, LR– 0.2.[579]

Among patients presenting to primary care, ambulance, or emergency room with suggestion of acute myocardial infarction or acute coronary syndrome, the initial odds of acute myocardial infarction are 1:8 (12%) and of acute coronary syndrome are 1:3 (26%); for either, pain in right arm or shoulder has LR+ 2–4, LR– 0.8–0.9; sweating has LR+ 1–3, LR– 0.7–0.9; chest wall tenderness has LR+ 0.1–0.2, LR– 1.4–1.5; pain elsewhere, nausea, and vomiting are fairly non-discriminatory.[580]

Among patients admitted with chest discomfort who were asked 'How does it feel?', 'Can you show me where it is?', and 'Can you show me what it feels like?', for ischaemic heart disease: clenched fist to chest had LR+ 0.6, LR– 1; flat palm to chest had LR+ 1.2, LR– 0.9; touching left arm with right arm had LR+ 0.7, LR– 1.1; and pointing with one or two fingers had LR+ 0.1, LR– 50.[413]

Among patients aged 45–74y in England in 1989–91, odds of ischaemic heart disease were 1:13 (7%). Among patients aged 45–74y in England in the 1990s with entry for angina in the general practice record, odds of ischaemic heart disease on follow-up were 2:1 (70%).[581]

Among U.S. primary care patients who had been assessed acutely for chest pain, odds of investigation leading to diagnosis not revealed by history and examination were 1:15 (6%); odds of identifying physical cause were 1:9 (11%); and odds of improvement were 2:1 (65%).[480]

For ischaemic heart disease with >70% loss of luminal diameter on angiography, three questions were asked: 'If you go up a steep hill (or do whatever brings the pain on) on 10 separate occasions, on how many of these would you experience chest pain?' (positive answer is 10); 'If you have 10 episodes of pain in a row, how many occur sitting quietly?' (positive answer is 0 or 1); 'What is the usual duration of your chest pain?' (positive answer is five minutes or less). Zero positive responses had LR+ <0.1, one positive had LR+ 1.4, two positives had LR+ 3, and three positives had LR+ 4.[582]

Among men aged 45–69y in England, odds of 3.1–8 cm abdominal aortic aneurysm were 1:200 (0.6%); diagnosis within three examinations by general practitioner had LR+ 80, LR 0.2.[457]

Among people aged 55–74y in Scotland, odds of intermittent claudication diagnosed by World Health Organization questionnaire were 1:20 (4.5%); odds of major asymptomatic peripheral arterial disease diagnosed non-invasively were 1:12 (8%); and odds of moderate asymptomatic peripheral arterial disease were 1:5 (17%).[583]

For peripheral arterial disease, intermittent claudication has LR+ 3, LR– 1; bruit in any of iliac, femoral, or popliteal arteries has LR+ 6; LR– 0.4.[584]

Among general practice patients >15y in the Netherlands with possible arrhythmia, odds of a clinically significant arrhythmia on a single ECG were 1:10 (9%).[585]

Among general practice patients >18y in England with new palpitations, odds of a clinically significant arrhythmia on ambulatory ECG were 1:4 (19%); among those who complied with investigations, odds were 1:2 (32%).[586]

Among people >65y in England, for atrial fibrillation, radial pulse palpation by a trained nurse had LR+ 3–6, LR– <0.1.[587]

Among U.S. primary care patients who had been assessed acutely for dizziness, odds of investigation leading to diagnosis not revealed by history and examination were 1:10 (9%); odds of identifying physical cause were 1:4 (18%); and odds of improvement were 3:2 (59%).[480]

Among adults in the Framingham study who had syncope in the community, odds of various causes were: unknown 1:2 (37%); vasovagal 1:4 (21%); cardiac 1:9 (10%); orthostatic 1:10 (9%); medication 1:14 (7%); seizure 1:20 (5%); stroke or TIA 1:24 (4%); and other 1:12 (8%).[588]

Digestive problems (RCGP curriculum 15.2)

After presentation in primary care in England with dysphagia, odds of having no specific diagnosis by 90d were 4:1 (77% for men and 83% for women) and by 3y were 2:1 (61% for men and 66% for women);[527] and odds of having oesophageal cancer by 3y were 1:17 (6%) for men and 1:40 (2%) for women.[528]

In men ≥55y presenting to primary care with dysphagia coded on computer, initial odds of oesophageal cancer are ≥1:20 (≥5%).[501]

Among U.S. primary care patients who had been assessed acutely for abdominal pain, odds of investigation leading to diagnosis not revealed by history and examination were 1:8 (11%); odds of identifying physical cause were 1:9 (10%); and odds of improvement were 1:1 (44%).[480]

Among people aged 18–60y in the UK, in the previous 2w odds of indigestion/heartburn were 1:4 (18%) and of stomach/abdominal pain were 1:6 (15%).[479]

In primary care patients in Finland with dyspepsia, diagnoses with odds were: functional (including heartburn without oesophagitis) 1:1 (55%); oesophagitis 1:6 (15%); lactose intolerance 1:10 (9%); duodenal ulcer 1:10 (9%); gastric ulcer 1:25 (4%); erosive duodenitis 1:50 (2%); gallstones 1:50 (2%); and malignancy 1:50 (2%).[589]

Among patients in England referred for upper endoscopy, diagnoses with odds were: benign stricture, severe oesophagitis, and peptic ulcer 1:7 (13%); and malignancy 1:25 (4%). For malignancy, weight loss had LR+ 1.4, LR– 0.2; age >55y with any alarm feature had LR+ 1.4, LR– 0.2.[590]

For peptic ulcer, *Helicobacter pylori* positivity in blood or by carbon-13 urea breath test had LR+ 2, LR– 0.6.[591]

Among primary care patients and the general population of all ages in England, after apparently infectious intestinal disease, odds of continuing symptoms at 3w were: diarrhoea 1:3 (24%); vomiting 1:7 (13%); and abdominal pain 1:3 (28%).[592]

Odds of coeliac disease are 1:100 (1%) in general Western populations; 1:20 (3–6%) in type 1 diabetes; 1:12 (5–10%) in first-degree relatives of coeliacs; 1:8 (10–15%) in symptomatic iron deficiency anaemia; 1:20 (3–6%) in asymptomatic iron deficiency anaemia; and 1:50 (1–3%) in osteoporosis.[593]

For coeliac disease in adults, IgA anti-tissue transglutaminase antibodies have LR+ 38, LR– 0.1 and IgA anti-endomysial antibodies have LR+ 170, LR– 0.1.[594]

Among U.S. primary care patients who had been assessed acutely for constipation, odds of investigation leading to diagnosis not revealed by history and examination were nil (0%); odds of identifying physical cause were nil (0%); and odds of improvement were 1:2 (33%).[480]

After presentation in primary care in England with rectal bleeding, odds of having no specific diagnosis by 90d were 4:1 (83% for men and 85% for women) and by 3y were 4:1 (78% for men and women).[527]

Among all patients >45y presenting to primary care in England with new rectal bleeding, odds of colorectal cancer were 1:17 (6%) and odds of polyp were 1:20 (5%).[595]

In English general practice, initial odds of colorectal cancer over the next 12m in patients with rectal bleeding rose from <1:100 (<1%) in men and woman at 45y to 1:10 (9%) in men at 85y and 1:20 (5%) in woman at 85y; with change in bowel habit rose from <1:100 (<1%) in men and women at 50y to 1:12 (8%) in men and 1:25 (4%) in women at 85y; and with anaemia rose from about 1:100 (1%) at 50y to 1:30 (3%) at 85y in men and from 1:1000 (0.01%) to 1:50 (2%) in women at 85y; the presence of a second of these features approximately doubled odds conferred by the presence of the first feature.[596]

After presentation in primary care in England >40y, odds of having colorectal cancer were: diarrhoea presenting once 1:100 (0.9%), presenting twice 1:150 (1.5%); rectal bleeding presenting once 1:40 (2.4%), presenting twice 1:14 (7%); and abdominal pain presenting once 1:100 (1%), presenting twice 1:30 (3%).[314]

Odds for colorectal cancer >34y were: rectal bleeding with change in bowel habit 1:10 (9%); rectal bleeding without perianal symptoms 1:9 (11%); dark blood 1:9 (10%); and bright blood 1:24 (4%).[597]

In ulcerative colitis, odds of cancer are 1:50 (2%) after 10y, 1:12 (8%) after 20y, and 1:4 (18%) after 30y; rates are higher in the United States and the UK, lower in Scandinavia and other countries.[598]

In English open-access clinics in patients referred with rectal bleeding, initial odds of colorectal cancer were <50y 1:100 (1%); 50–69y 1:20 (5%); and ≥70y 1:12 (8%).[599]

Among patients in general practice in England, for colorectal cancer, rectal bleeding had LR+ 10; loss of weight had LR+ 5; abdominal pain had LR+ 5; diarrhoea had LR+ 4; constipation had LR+ 2; faecal occult blood had LR+ 31; blood sugar >10 mmol/L had LR+ 3; Hb <90 g/L had LR+ 27 in men, 43 in women; Hb <90–99 had LR+ 17 in men, 12 in women; Hb <100–109 had LR+ 7; Hb 110–119 had LR+ 3.5; and Hb 120–129 had LR+ 2.5.[449]

In patients ≥75y presenting to primary care with new rectal bleeding or rectal bleeding computer code, initial odds of colorectal cancer were ≥1:20 (≥5%).[501]

Among patients in primary care with iron deficiency anaemia, odds of colorectal cancer are ≥1:20 (≥5%): in men ≥60y with Hb <120 g/L; in women ≥70y with Hb <110 g/L; and in women ≥60y with Hb <90 g/L.[501]

Among UK indigenous primary care patients, odds of anaemia (Hb <120 g/dL in women, Hb <130 g/dL in men) were: women 18–40y 1:8 (12%), women ≥65y 1:6 (14%), men ≥65y 1:4 (20%), menorrhagia/polymenorrhoea 1:4 (20%), tiredness 1:5 (17%), shortness of breath 1:4 (20%), palpitations 1:5 (18%), pale conjunctivae 1:3 (24%), angular stomatitis 1:3 (24%), weight loss 1:2 (32%), and subnormal dietary intake 1:3 (23%).[600]

Among adult patients in tertiary hospital setting, for Hb <90 g/L, LRs for conjunctival pallor LRs were: present LR+ 4, borderline LR+ 2, and absent LR+ 0.6.[601]

Among laboratory samples in England from primary care showing new microcytic anaemia without haemoglobinopathy with Hb <120 g/L in men >20y and Hb <110 g/L in women >50y, diagnoses with odds were: none 2:3 (39%); gastrointestinal benign disease 1:3 (35%); gastrointestinal malignancy 1:8 (11%); other malignancy 1:20 (5%); and other disease 1:9 (10%).[602]

Among patients in Sweden with raised aminotransferase (42–300 u/L) for >6m, normal alkaline phosphatase and no symptoms, referred to hospital and biopsied, odds were as follows: steatosis 2:3 (40%); unexplained hepatitis 1:3 (24%); hepatitis C 1:5 (15%); and presumed alcohol 1:12 (8%).[603]

Drug and alcohol problems (RCGP curriculum 15.3)

For drinking that is risky (>4 drinks/occasion or >14 drinks/w for man, >1 drink/occasion or >7 drinks /w for woman), harmful (causing physical or psychological harm), or hazardous (with risk of adverse consequences), AUDIT-C (first three questions of Alcohol Use Disorders Identification Test)[604] ≥8 has LR+ 12, LR− 0.6.[605]

For alcohol abuse or dependence (defined variously), CAGE[606] (Have you ever felt you should Cut down on your drinking? Have people Annoyed you by criticizing your drinking? Have you ever felt bad or Guilty about your drinking? Have you ever had a drink first thing in the morning to steady your nerves or to get rid of a hangover—an Eye opener?) has the following approximate LRs: score 0 LR+ 0.2; score 1 LR+ 1; score 2 LR+ 4; score 3 LR+ >13; and score 4 LR+ >100.[607]

For ascites, LRs are as follows: symptom of increased girth LR+ 4, LR− 0.2; symptom of recent weight gain LR+ 3, LR− 0.4; symptom of ankle swelling LR+ 3, LR− 0.1; sign of peripheral oedema LR+ 4, LR− 0.2; fluid wave LR+ 5, LR− 0.6; and shifting dullness LR+ 2, LR− 0.4.[608]

Among primary care patients in the Canary Islands prescribed benzodiazepine for more than one month without alcohol or other substance abuse, for prescribed benzodiazepine dependency using reference standard of Composite International

Diagnostic Interview conducted by psychiatrist: self-assessment of at least possible dependency had LR+ 2, LR– 0.2; Severity of Dependence Scale with threshold of ≥7 had LR+ 16, LR– 0.02.[609] Odds of dependence assessed by Severity of Dependence Scale with threshold of ≥7 were 1:1 (47%).[610] A modified Severity of Dependence Scale (which can be downloaded from www.darmipc.net[428]) is as follows. These questions are about your use of the medication … In the last month: (1) Did you think your use of this medication was out of control? (2) Did the prospect of missing this medication make you anxious or worried? (3) Did you worry about your use of this medication? (4) Did you wish to stop this medication? (5) How difficult would you find it to stop or go without this medication? Score for Q1–4: 'never'/'almost never' = 0; 'sometimes' = 1; 'often' = 2'; 'always'/almost always' = 3; score for Q5: 'not difficult' = 0; 'quite difficult' = 1; 'very difficult' = 2; 'impossible' = 3.

Among UK general practice patients prescribed methadone or buprenorphine, annualised odds of death: on treatment were 1:60 (1.7%) during weeks 1–2, 1:80 (1.3%) during weeks 3–4, 1:170 (0.6%) after 4w; off treatment, 1:20 (5%) during weeks 1–2, 1:24 (4%) during weeks 3–4, 1:100 (1%) after 4w.[611]

Among injecting drug users in one Scottish general practice followed up for 6–25y: odds of stopping injecting for ≥5y were 2:3 (42%); odds of death within 25y of first injecting were all-cause 1:2 (35%), HIV 1:5 (16%), overdose/suicide 1:8 (11%), liver 1:25 (4%), and alcohol 1:60 (2%).[612]

ENT and facial problems (RCGP curriculum 15.4)

In the general population in the United States: odds of ≥5 episodes of apnoea/hypopnoea per hour of sleep were 1:3 (24%) in men and 1:10 (9%) in women; odds of sleep apnoea syndrome (≥5 episodes of apnoea/hypopnoea per hour of sleep plus daytime hypersomnolence) were 1:25 (4%) in men and 1:50 (2%) in women.[613]

Among Italian primary care patients with hypertension (without relevant pulmonary disease, neurological disease, or insomnia), odds of obstructive sleep apnoea were 1:25 (4%); in those with BMI ≥30 kg/m2, odds were 1:9 (10%); positive predictive value of Epworth Sleepiness Scale score ≥11[614] was 97%. All patients diagnosed in this study accepted and continued with continuous positive airway pressure treatment, and blood pressure was significantly improved.[615]

Conversational speech is at 45–60 dB. Hearing loss thresholds generally are: 25 dB mild, 40 dB moderate, and 60 dB severe.[616]

Among the population 55–99y in Australia, odds of hearing loss were >25 dB 2:3 (39%), >40 dB 1:7 (13%), and >60 dB 1:50 (2%). For hearing loss, asking 'Do you feel you have a hearing loss?' had LR+ 2, LR– <0.3.[617]

For hearing loss >25 dB, reply to a closed question about hearing difficulty has LR+ 2, LR– 0.5. For hearing loss >40dB, reply to a closed question about hearing difficulty has LR+ 2.5, LR– 0.1. For hearing loss >30dB, whisper test has LR+ 6, LR– 0.03. (Rub contra-lateral tragus against external auditory canal and with lips two feet from ipsi-lateral ear outwith patient's field of vision whisper: three items identified out of six is a pass).[616]

Eye problems (RCGP curriculum 15.5)

Among children aged 6m–12y in primary care in England with infective conjunctivitis, odds of resolution without antibiotics 7d after consultation were 5:1 (83%).[618]

Metabolic problems (RCGP curriculum 15.6)

In the general population in China, odds of diabetes are 1:30 (3%) at 20–39y, 1:8 (12%) at 40–59y, and 1:4 (20%) at ≥60y; odds of impaired glucose tolerance are 1:8 (11%) and of impaired fasting glucose are 1:40 (2–3%).[619]

Among diabetics in 13 countries with sizeable Muslim populations in 2001–02, odds of fasting during Ramadan were 2:3 (43%) if type 1 and 4:1 (79%) if type 2.[620]

Odds of hypothyroidism in patients are 1:170 (0.6%) at 40–60y, 1:120 (0.8%) at >60y, and 1:50 (2%) in woman at 70–80y.[621]

Among people aged 18–60y in the UK, in the previous 2w odds of unintentional weight loss were 1:60 (2%).[479]

Among U.S. primary care patients who had been assessed acutely for weight loss, odds of investigation leading to diagnosis not revealed by history and examination were zero (0%), odds of identifying physical cause were 1:20 (5%), and odds of improvement were 2:3 (40%).[480]

Neurological problems (RCGP curriculum 15.7)

Among primary care patients in Oxfordshire with suspected transient ischaemic attack referred to a specialist clinic, odds of stroke during 7d were: 1:250 (0.4%) with ABCD score <5; 1:7 (12%) with score 5; and 1:3 (31%) with score 6. ABCD score was as follows: age ≥60y = 1; BP systolic >140 ± diastolic ≥90 = 1; clinical features: unilateral weakness = 2, speech disturbance without weakness = 1, duration of symptoms ≥60 minutes = 2, 10–59 minutes = 1.[622]

Among people aged 18–60y in the UK, in the previous 2w odds of headache were 2:3 (39%).[479]

Among the population, odds of tension headache are 2:3 (38%) and of migraine are 1:8 (6–17%).[402]

Among primary care patients in the United States and Canada presenting with new headache, initial diagnostic odds were: tension 1:3 (24%), vascular 1:7 (13%), and other 1:1 (48%); odds of meeting National Institutes of Health criteria for computerised tomographic scanning were 1:1 (46%); odds of follow-up appointment were 1:6 (15%).[623]

For migraine, score 1 for each of: pulsating, untreated duration 4–72h, ever unilateral, nausea, and disabling: for definite or possible migraine, score 4–5 has LR+ 24, score 3 has LR+ 4, and score 1–2 has LR+ 0.4; for definite migraine, score 4–5 has LR+ 6, score 3 has LR+ 1, and score 1–2 has LR+ 0.4.[402]

For migraine, features and LRs are: nausea LR+ 19, photophobia LR+ 6, phonophobia LR+ 5, precipitation by chocolate LR+ 5, precipitation by cheese LR+ 5, and exacerbation by physical activity LR+ 4.[407]

Among U.S. primary care patients who had been assessed acutely for headache, odds of investigation leading to diagnosis not revealed by history and examination were 1:20 (5%); odds of identifying physical cause were 1:9 (10%); and odds of improvement were 2:3 (38%).[480]

For giant cell arteritis, features with LRs are: jaw claudication LR+ 4; diplopia LR+ 3; temporal artery abnormality LR+ 4, LR– 0.5; and ESR <50 LR– 0.4.[624]

For brain tumour: new seizure had LR+ 96; motor loss had LR+ 21; confusion had LR+ 16; weakness had LR+ 11; headache had LR+ 7; memory loss had LR+ 3; and visual disorder had LR+ 3.[449]

In the world population: odds of someone having essential tremor are 1:240–1:24 (0.4–4%); odds of someone >60y having essential tremor are 1:100–1:20 (1–5%).[625]

Among the population, odds of Parkinson's disease are 1:100 (1%) >65y and 1:50 (2%) >85y. For Parkinson's disease, signs with LRs are: tremor LR+ 1.5, LR– 0.5; rigidity LR+ 3, LR– 0.4; glabellar tap LR+ 5, LR– 0.1; soft voice LR+ 4, LR– 0.3; altered speech LR+ 3, LR– 0.7; and poor heel-toe gait LR+ 3, LR– 0.3.[626]

Among patients >16y having a single fit: odds of a fit in the 12m after a fit-free interval of 6m were 1:6 (14%) with immediate treatment and 1:5 (18%) with delayed treatment; odds of a fit in the 12m after a fit-free interval of 12–24m were 1:12 (7–8%) with immediate treatment and 1:8 (10–12%) with delayed treatment.[627]

Among patients aged >1m having first fit or early epilepsy without progressive disease or known cause in whom patient and doctor were both in equipoise about starting anti-epileptics: odds of a 2y remission at 2y were 1:1 (52%) in those having deferred treatment and 3:2 (64%) in those treated immediately; odds of a 2y remission at 5y were 10:1 (90%) in those having deferred treatment and 12:1 (92%) in those treated immediately; odds of being on anti-epileptics after 5y were 2:3 (41%) in those having deferred treatment and 3:2 (60%) in those treated immediately; odds of injury/scalds during 5y were 1:30 (3%) in those having deferred treatment and 1:25 (4%) in those treated immediately; and odds of any adverse event during 5y were 1:3 (31%) in those having deferred treatment and 2:3 (39%) in those treated immediately.[628]

Among epileptics on anti-epileptic drugs without fit for 2y: odds of being seizure-free after 2y were 3:2 (59%) in those slowly withdrawn from treatment and 3:1 (78%) in those continuing treatment.[629]

Among pregnancies exposed to carbamazepine monotherapy in the first trimester, odds of major congenital malformation are 1:30 (3%).[630]

Among U.S. primary care patients who had been assessed acutely for numbness, odds of investigation leading to diagnosis not revealed by history and examination were 1:8 (12%); odds of identifying physical cause were 1:4 (19%); and odds of improvement were 1:1 (53%).[480]

Among patients with hand tingling or numbness in median nerve distribution, odds of carpal tunnel syndrome are 1:13 (7%). For carpal tunnel syndrome, features with LRs are: hypalgesia in median nerve territory LR+ 3, LR− 0.7; weak thumb abduction LR+ 2, LR− 0.5; and Katz hand diagram[631] classic or probable LR+ 2, LR− 0.5.[632, 633]

Patients presenting with dizziness or vertigo to primary care in Ireland were asked: 'When you get dizzy spells, do you just feel light-headed or do you see the world spin around you as if you had just got off a playground roundabout?' Those who saw the world spin were diagnosed with vertigo. Among those with vertigo, the initial odds were as follows: benign positional vertigo 2:3 (42%); acute vestibular neuronitis 2:3 (41%); and Ménière's disease 1:9 (10%). For benign positional vertigo, the Dix-Hallpike test (of which there are videos on the Internet) had a positive predictive value of 83% and negative predictive value of 52%.[634]

Respiratory problems (RCGP curriculum 15.8)

After presentation with sore throat, in placebo groups, odds of sore throat at 3d are 3:2 (60%); odds of fever at 3d are 1:6 (15%); and odds of symptoms at 7d are 1:4 (18%).[429]

Among U.S. primary care patients who had been assessed acutely for cough, odds of investigation leading to diagnosis not revealed by history and examination were 1:7 (13%); odds of identifying physical cause were 2:3 (40%); and odds of improvement were 4:1 (80%).[480]

In Dutch primary care, among patients presenting with cough, initial odds were: self-limiting respiratory illness/viral 3:1 (78%), cough 1:6 (14%), asthma 1:50 (2%), pneumonia 1:50 (2%), chronic obstructive pulmonary disease/emphysema/bronchiectasis 1:100 (1%), and whooping cough 1:250 (0.4%).[137]

In children <5y seen in primary care with cough in England, odds of recovery after consultation were 1:1 (50%) at 10d and 9:1 (90%) at 25d.[635]

Among adult patients in primary care in Europe with new or worsening cough or possible lower respiratory tract infection, odds of being prescribed antibiotic were: Belgium, Spain, Norway, Germany, Sweden, Finland, and Holland 1:2 (20–42%); UK 2:1 (52–70%); Poland, Hungary, and Slovakia 3:1 (71–87%); median time to recovery was 11d and to zero symptom score 15d; rate of recovery was unrelated to antibiotic use; and odds of subsequent admission to hospital were 1:100 (1%).[636]

In respiratory infections, odds of resistance to an antibiotic are 1:7 in patients who have not had a recent antibiotic, 1:3 in patients 2m after an antibiotic, and 1:5 in patients 12m after an antibiotic.[227]

Among asymptomatic adults recruited through newspaper advertisements in Finland with ≥20 pack years smoking history, odds of chronic obstructive pulmonary disease on pulmonary function tests using Global Initiative for Chronic Obstructive Lung Disease criteria[637] were 1:9 (11%).[486]

Among patients in Netherlands seeing general practitioners with persistent cough (>>2w) and no prior diagnosis of chronic lung disease, odds of chronic obstructive airways disease were 1:2 (29%) and of asthma were 1:13 (7%).[638]

For chronic obstructive pulmonary disease, features with LRs are: smoking pack years >40 LR+ 12; smoking pack years <20 LR+ 0.5; wheezing symptom LR+ 4, LR– 0.3; wheezing sign LR+ 4, LR– 0.3; reduced breath sounds LR+ 3, LR– 0.7; and maximum laryngeal height ≤4cm LR+ 4, LR– 0.7.[639]

Among U.S. primary care patients who had been assessed acutely for dyspnoea, odds of investigation leading to diagnosis not revealed by history and examination were 1:2 (30%), odds of identifying physical cause were 1:3 (24%), and odds of improvement were 2:3 (39%).[480]

In Dutch primary care among patients presenting with shortness of breath, initial odds were: self-limiting respiratory tract illness/viral 2:3 (43%), asthma 1:9 (10%), shortness of breath 1:11 (9%), heart failure 1:10 (9%), hyperventilation 1:12 (8%), chronic obstructive pulmonary disease/emphysema/bronchiectasis 1:24 (4%), pneumonia 1:30 (3%), ischaemic heart disease 1:50 (2%), and atrial fibrillation 1:100 (1%).

For influenza, most features studied have LRs in the range 0.7–1.3, which are not discriminating. Features with more discriminating LRs are: fever LR+ 1.8, LR– 0.4; cough LR– 0.4; nasal congestion LR– 0.5; immunised LR+ 0.6; combination of fever, cough, and acute onset LR+ 2, LR– 0.5; and rapid diagnostic test positive LR+ 5, LR– 0.1.[640]

For asthma, Swedish general practitioner initial diagnosis had LR+ 60, LR– 0.4.[641]

Among the adult population of the Netherlands, odds of asthma were 1:13 (7%).[642]

After presentation in primary care in England with haemoptysis, odds of having no specific diagnosis by 90d were 3:1 (76% in men and 74% in women) and by 3y were 2:3 (44% in men and 38% in women);[527] odds of having respiratory tract cancer by 3y were 1:12 (8%) for men and 1:22 (4%) for women.[528]

In men ≥55y and women ≥65y presenting to primary care with computer code of haemoptysis, odds of lung cancer are ≥1:20 (≥5%).[501]

Among patients >40y in primary care, odds of lung cancer were: haemoptysis 1:40 (2%), haemoptysis with dyspnoea or chest pain 1:20 (5%), thrombocytosis with loss of weight 1:16 (6%), haemoptysis with weight loss 1:10 (9%), haemoptysis with loss of appetite >1:9 (>10%), haemoptysis with thrombocytosis >1:9 (>10%), and haemoptysis presenting twice 1:5 (17%).[643]

For lung cancer, haemoptysis had LR+ 13; loss of weight had LR+ 6; loss of appetite had LR+ 5; dyspnoea had LR+ 4; chest wall pain had LR+ 3; fatigue had LR+ 2; cough had LR+ 2; thrombocytosis had LR+ 19; and abnormal spirometry had LR+ 14.[449]

For lung cancer diagnosed within the following year in primary care in England, CXR reported as abnormal with possible malignancy had sensitivity of 77%.[644]

Rheumatology and conditions of the musculoskeletal system (including trauma) (RCGP curriculum 15.9)

Osteoporosis is defined by World Health Organization as bone mass density more than 2.5 standard deviations below that of 20–40-year-olds.[645] Odds of osteoporosis in white women are 1:6 (15%) aged 50–59y, 1:4 (22%) aged 60–69y, 2:3 (39%) aged 70–79y, and 2:1 (70%) aged ≥80y.[646] For osteoporosis in women, score 1 for each of: >10y since menopause, daily calcium intake <1200 mg, kyphosis, BMI <25, and history of fracture. Scores giving odds of osteoporosis are: 0 gives 1:24 (4%); 1 gives 1:4 (3–33%); 2 gives 1:2 (7–42%); 3 gives 1:1 (21–85%); 4 gives 4:1 (73–95%); 50:1 (98%).[647] For osteoporosis in women, weight <50 kg had LR+ 7, <60 kg had LR+ 2–4, and >60 kg had LR+ 0.3;[648] 10y risk of fracture can be estimated using the World Health Organization Fracture Risk Assessment Tool.[649]

Among people aged 18–60y in the UK, in the previous 2w, odds of back pain were 1:2 (30%).[479]

In Dutch primary care patients presenting with low back pain without radiation, initial odds were: low back pain/mechanical problem 3:1 (76%), disc lesion 1:16 (6%), spinal deformity 1:30 (3%), and osteoarthritis 1:30 (3%).[137]

Among U.S. primary care patients who had been assessed acutely for back pain, odds of investigation leading to diagnosis not revealed by history and examination were 1:30 (3%); odds of identifying physical cause were 1:9 (10%); and odds of improvement were 3:2 (62%).[480]

Among patients >14y presenting to GPs, physiotherapists, or chiropracters in Australia with non-specific low back pain of <2w duration: median time to complete recovery (return to work, no disability, and no pain) was 59d and odds of complete recovery were 2:3 (39%) by 6w, 1:1 (57%) by 12w, and 3:1 (72%) by 1y. Among those who reduced their work commitment, odds of returning to pre-back pain work hours and duties were 3:1 (75%) by 6w, 4:1 (83%) by 12w, and 9:1 (90%) by 1y.[650]

Among the healthy population, odds of missing ankle reflex are: unilateral aged <60y 1:20 (5%); bilateral aged <60y 1:20 (5%); unilateral aged >60y 1:9 (10%); and bilateral aged >60y 1:2 (30%).[651]

Malignant cord compression diagnosis depends on symptoms and MRI, signs being too late and the level unpredictable. The paper does not report on whether the cancer was active or on the results of blood tests.[652]

Among adults in the Netherlands presenting to primary care with new non specific knee pain, odds of self-assessed recovery were 1:3 (25%) at 3m and 1:1 (44%) at 12m.[653]

Among U.S. patients referred by primary care physician, rheumatologist, or self to an orthopaedic surgeon on account of knee problem, the surgeon's clinical diagnoses with odds were: meniscal lesion 1:2 (31%); degenerative 1:3 (25%); patellofemoral syndrome 1:3 (25%); cruciate ligament lesion 1:11 (8%); collateral ligament lesion 1:26 (4%); and odds of surgery within 6m were 1:4 (21%).[654]

Among patients with torn anterior cruciate ligament, structured rehabilitation with either immediate or deferred reconstruction had same improvement (in symptoms, function, and quality of life assessed by Knee and Osteoarthritis Outcome Score).[655, 656]

For meniscal knee injuries, signs with LRs are: joint effusion LR+ 6, LR– 0.7; medial-lateral grind test[657] LR+ 5; LR– 0.4. For ligamentous knee injuries, Lachmann test[658] has LR+ 42, LR– 0.1.[659]

For rheumatoid arthritis, anticitrullinated peptide antibody has LR+ 13, LR– 0.5.[660]

Among people aged 18–60y in the UK, in the previous 2w odds of joint pain were 1:2 (31%).[479]

In the United States among non-cancer patients on chronic opioid prescriptions equivalent to morphine >100mg/d, annual odds of overdose were 1:55 (1.8%).[661]

Skin problems (RCGP curriculum 15.10)

For malignant melanoma: asymmetry has LR+ 2, LR– 0.6; border irregularity has LR+ 2, LR– 0.6; colour has LR+ 2, LR– 0.6; diameter >6 mm has LR+ 2, LR– 0.2; and enlargement has LR+ 11, LR– 0.2. Number of positive ABCDE findings: 0 has LR+ 0.1; 1 has LR+ 2; 2 has LR+ 3; 3 has LR+ 3; 4 has LR+ 8; and 5 has LR+ 100.[662]

Among moles excised in primary care in Australia, odds of invasive melanoma were 1:30 (3%) and of additional potentially malignant melanocytic lesions were 1:30 (3%).[663]

Among soft tissue sarcomata and non-visceral lipomata assessed by histopathologist in Sweden, odds of sarcoma:lipoma were: <5 cm 1:150; 5–10 cm 1:20; ≥10 cm 1:6; thigh 1:6; and subfascial 1:4.[664]

CHAPTER 6

Words that count

'Histories must be received, not taken.'

Bayliss R. Pain narratives. In: Greenhalgh T, Hurwitz B, editors.
Narrative Based Medicine: dialogue and discourse in clinical practice.
London: BMJ Books; 1998.

'. . . don't teach the patient how to simulate disease.'

Barbour A. *Caring for Patients: a critique of the medical model.*
Palo Alto, CA: Stanford University Press; 1997.

SOME DOCTORS ARE BORN COMMUNICATORS, BUT MOST OF US HAVE TO LEARN

As the patient talks, I notice that my shelf is sagging under the weight of books on consulting skills.[665, 30, 94, 666, 667, 176, 668, 1, 109] Through one wall, I hear easy laughter as a partner's patient starts their consultation and, through the other wall, social chit-chat as another partner's patient leaves. And I recall sitting in on a colleague's consultation that felt as natural as a natter over coffee at a parents and toddlers group. The gifted communicator doesn't need to analyse their skills; they can hear what's left unsaid and reassure with a light verbal touch.[125] Most general practitioners settle into a style and don't vary it greatly from one consultation to the next.[1] If the style's a good one, that's okay. But most of us need to work on the art or craft of consulting, and with practice we can improve.[125, 669, 670]

There are aspects of a patient's experience of illness that are important whatever their medical problem, and the minimal communication skills required for a consultation can be reduced to just a few. When the consultation is being observed, one way of studying these communication skills is by concentrating on the doctor rather than the patient, on the process rather than the content of the consultation. We listen to the patient in order to hear primarily what they say rather than what they mean.[34] Then we transfer our attention back to the doctor. That makes the discussion between teacher and learner briefer, so observation, learning, teaching, practising, and using skills in subsequent consultations can be done rapidly, and an underused skill can be quickly identified and immediately tried out. The learner does need to feel safe and to accept the usefulness of this approach. Innovations are likely to be adopted if they fit in with what we already do, are simple to adopt and adapt, and offer benefits that are immediately apparent.[276] I hope that applies here.

BETTER SKILLS MAKE FOR BETTER CONSULTATIONS

Patient-centred consulting is a way of enabling us to keep both functional and medical-model channels of communication open. The doctor elicits the patient's account of their experience of illness while retaining some influence over the structure of the encounter.[671]

The term 'patient-centred medicine' in its original sense included use of the medical model[4] and does so also in this book. The phrase 'patient-centred', however, is used in this chapter with a different emphasis: it refers to skills that address the patient's perspective as distinct from doctor-centred skills that serve the doctor's medical agenda.[1] Patient-centred and doctor-centred skills form not a dichotomy but a spectrum of complementary skills, all of which are needed whatever aspect of the patient's problem we're concentrating on. They're skills as precise as those for making an appendicectomy incision. Acquiring good consulting skills doesn't make someone a fantastic family doctor any more than holding a scalpel by the correct end makes someone a brilliant surgeon. But both increase the chance of a favourable outcome.

SKILLS CAN BE LEARNED

Medical students begin their careers showing an interest in the patient; they often end up asking lots of closed questions and ignoring cues in an effort to make the diagnosis. This isn't inevitable. Consulting skills training leads to improved interviewing skills and greater diagnostic efficiency without necessarily longer consultations,[672] although general practitioner consultations that work well are generally longer than those that don't.[1] Research into skill acquisition shows that an acceptable standard can be expected within 50 hours, by which time there'll be a degree of automation.[673] Further improvement will occur only with motivation, feedback,[673] and stretching beyond comfort levels.[674] Expertise takes 10 000 hours to acquire,[674] which equates to about 10 years for a full-time general practitioner. There's always scope for imaginative flexibility such as inviting patients with poor speech to type into the computer[675] and inviting those with poor hearing to use your stethoscope.[676] And patients appreciate having a doctor who's skilful, respectful and socially graced[677]—so there's plenty to fill a 30-year career.

The biomedical model separates the process of consulting from the outcome, thinking from doing, and the acquisition of knowledge from the exercising of it. In general practice consultations, all these things happen concurrently. When we listen to the patient and touch them, not only are we learning about them, but we're communicating something to them. This is best appreciated in the process of doing it. The learner needs to be prepared, for a time, to suspend disbelief and to take a certain amount on trust until they discover what it's like.[187]

THE CONSULTATION GRID

This chapter is based on a grid (*see* Table 6.1)[428] that deals with history, diagnosis and management but not examination. The grid is divided vertically into two main columns dealing with the history phase and management phase. It's divided horizontally into three layers dealing in turn with the overall aims of the consultation, the more detailed objectives, and the skills required to achieve these aims and objectives. The aim of the history is a differential diagnosis. The objectives of history-taking are answers to a list of questions relating to the patient's experience of illness: these are questions in the doctor's mind, whether spoken or not. The aim of management is salutogenesis,[678] which is making the patient feel better, as opposed to pathogenesis, which is making them feel iller. The objectives of management are safety, safety-netting, satisfaction, and self-confidence—primarily for the patient, although the doctor benefits correspondingly.

THE AIM OF THE HISTORY IS DIAGNOSIS

The purpose of the history is to enable us to make a diagnosis. We need to cast a wide net: many people worried by symptoms don't consult, and some not worried by

TABLE 6.1 Consultation grid

	History	*Management*
AIMS	Diagnosis of disease/illness	Salutogenesis
OBJECTIVES	Effects	Safety
	Emotions	Safety-netting
	Explanations	Satisfaction
	Expectations	Self-confidence
	Epitasis—'Why now?'	
	Enquiries	
	Enything else	
SKILLS	Body language	
Most patient-centred	Acknowledge	Acknowledge
	Reflect	Check
↕	Open question	Answer question
Most doctor-centred	Doctor-centred question	New information

symptoms do, so the symptom or even worry about the symptom can't be assumed to be the reason for consulting;[12] patients often don't mention something relevant, even though they think their doctor's not aware of it;[100] and with good communication skills, the outcome is better—patients' complaints, concerns, and perceptions are more fully elicited and our advice is better given, received, and followed.[669]

We're not trying to provide formal psychotherapy,[34] attribute symptoms to psychosocial causes, or necessarily extend our remit to psychosocial factors beyond the problem that the patient brings: somatisers who were encouraged by a research doctor to reveal important things about their lives felt no better, consulted as much, took as many drugs, and were off sick as much as controls.[679] Our standing as doctors rests on science: we should extend our activities beyond that with scepticism and humility.

It's necessary to use rules of thumb to help bridge the gap between the ideal and the achievable, but don't let this become the unexamined norm.[155] Don't defer being holistic until you become more experienced later in your career: play your beginner's tunes on your new violin as musically as you can from the start. And allow yourself to be absorbed in, and confident about, what you're doing: that's conducive to happiness.[71]

THE AIM OF MANAGEMENT IS SALUTOGENESIS, NOT PATHOGENESIS

The aim of management is salutogenesis, that is, making the patient feel better. It includes providing appropriate reassurance, support, and whatever medical treatment is indicated. It excludes sharing a potentially frightening differential diagnosis with the patient and imparting irrelevant, technical information, both of which are likely to be pathogenic. A positive approach by the doctor[517] and a definite diagnosis[680] are associated with greater amelioration of symptoms. Unrealistic optimism on the part of the patient can have good psychological and physical effects without subsequent harm.[681] Patients need guiding away from negative toward positive states—of subjective well-being, optimism, happiness, and self-determination.[682]

Wording of diagnosis matters. A diagnosis of osteoarthrosis implying irreversible degeneration, progressive pain, and inevitable loss of function is pathogenic. A diagnosis of strain suggesting the possibility of recovery is salutogenic. Words have the potential to heal or to harm. Where diagnosis is uncertain and treatment options limited, we have little more than words to offer. Using them well is important. The term 'functional symptoms' is less likely to offend patients than alternatives such as 'all in the mind', 'hysterical', 'psychosomatic', 'medically unexplained', 'depression-associated', and 'stress-related'.[174] For functional symptoms, it's helpful to talk about mechanism rather than cause, the 'how' rather than the 'why'. The patient can be reassured that there's no damage to whichever body part is involved and told positively that the problem is in the message between that body part and the brain—indeed that the brain is overvigilant, more sensitive, or excessively aware.[683]

Somatisers prefer a physical explanation that doesn't blame them and gives them something concrete to work with.[684]

A good consultation, without tests or prescriptions, is a form of treatment. This treatment can be thought of as a drug called 'doctor'.[182] Its active ingredients are expertise, personality, and—even after only a few minutes—our relationship with the patient. This drug does more good than an inappropriate prescription.[680] Medical expertise improves medical outcome and satisfaction. Interpersonal expertise also improves medical outcome—but not necessarily satisfaction.[685] The manner in which we express concern is a matter of judgment, personality, and context. I don't believe that it's always necessary or helpful for our communications to be imbued with feeling—certainly not sentimentality or the affectation of feeling.[686] For my part, perhaps attentiveness is the quality that I can bring honestly to one consultation after another, the drug I can offer the patient. I suggest to juniors that, in responding to distress, silence or sensitive words are more valuable than facial expressions of grief or shock. Facilitating a patient to recall and relive past painful experiences may be unhelpful and positively counterproductive.[173] The reflection of themself that the baby sees in the responsive mother's face[687] is a beneficent pretence.[191] So the doctor's acknowledgement of the patient's distress is refracted, muted, tempered—contained and containing. The doctor's manner will in turn be reflected in the patient's behaviour.[162] The high prevalence of personality disorder among patients[547, 152] means the onus is often on the doctor to sustain the relationship.

Examination is a form of communication. My father, a carpenter, learned about the timber he was working with by touching it, and we learn about patients in the same way. At the same time, we're communicating something to them. The majority of patients, if upset, would feel comforted by being touched by the doctor, their preferred site being the upper arm.[688] Sometimes I abandon the semi-automatic blood pressure monitor and use my stethoscope specifically so that the patient can get 20 seconds of uninterrupted bodily contact. Resting a hand on the shoulder while auscultating the chest is another form of physical contact that seems natural in context. Appropriate touching is healing.[689]

Reassuring talk, also, is therapeutic. When examining an ear, don't shout: 'There's enough wax to polish my desk!'; say quietly, 'Good, a normal amount of healthy wax'. The PR patter might go: Now, roll over and face the wall. Pull your knees up into your tummy. Good, that's right. Now, rest your head down on the pillow and breathe in and out to allow yourself to relax. Good. Now, I've got a glove on, and some jelly on the glove. You'll feel me pressing and sliding my finger in. This might be uncomfortable—that's natural. You might feel you're doing a poo, but you aren't—that's just my finger coming out. Good. That's done. I'll wipe away the jelly. Well done.' Toward the end of the procedure, when the patient is comfortable, take your time: the patient will remember mainly not the duration of the procedure but the pain at its most intense—which you can't eliminate—and the pain in the last few moments—which you can minimise.[690] Notice the language is all positive, reassuring, precise, and moderate and delivered in synchrony with the procedure.

How the diagnosis is expressed to the patient is important.[691, 692] A conversation is a process of creating a common language between the participants[3] and the same applies to a consultation. Patients describing angina often use words like 'heaviness' rather than 'pain'.[693, 694, 695] There's a mismatch between the language used by patients and that used by doctors, not only in the medical literature, but also in patient information leaflets.[696] What we learn, while taking the history, about the words patients use and the meanings they attach to them can guide our choice of words when discussing diagnosis and management.[109] Beware of replacing the patient's breathless, living account with a case history that's dead, unbreathing.[126]

Don't turn people into patients by giving everyday experiences medical labels.[97] Avoid causing iatrogenic disease[97] and wasting resources with inappropriate use of dangerous tests and powerful drugs: investigations are arranged and prescriptions written often not because the patient wants them, but because the doctor thinks the patient wants them,[697] so, rather than make assumptions, ask. Build on the helpful ideas they have, challenge the unhelpful ones, and avoid introducing new worrying notions needlessly. We can 'normalise', that is re-attribute a symptom to a less frightening, more everyday process:[698, 156] we might draw on our own medical knowledge or, better, on an explanation proffered by the patient.[156] We can offer general reassurance: this might reinforce the myth of medical infallibility[699] and be considered deceptive and paternalistic—which is ethically dubious[70]—but I think of it more as pastoral. And we can be grown-up, admit ignorance, and acknowledge that nothing's ever certain[699]—but this needs careful handling if it's not to come across as indifference. Which of these approaches we use on any particular occasion is a matter of judgment. Lastly, don't tell the patient what's going to happen next time they consult, especially if they're seeing someone other than yourself: you can't know, so don't solve your problem by creating a problem for someone else.

I've read of[173] and observed among my partners a different way of talking to the patient. The doctor outlines at some length and without interruption a medical account of the problem and a plan of action while the patient appears to listen without necessarily taking in all the detail. The doctor has a quiet confidence and gently undulating rhythm of speech and invites no particular response. The patient, freed from active participation, drifts into an apparent reverie, merely nodding in agreement. The medical details matter less than the underlying reassuring message, which probably bypasses consciousness as in hypnosis.

The general public wants to be involved in decisions about their health.[465] If there's a good match between what the patient wants and what they get in terms of information and participation, outcome is better; even when they don't anticipate wanting to participate, in retrospect they prefer having done so.[205] How do we negotiate this in practice? We might learn from the patient with a sore throat that they would like an antibiotic. If we don't comply, we can let them choose, instead, the formulation of paracetamol we prescribe. Serial attempts at cooperation—tempered where necessary with prompt and moderate confrontation then reconciliation—offer the best chance of a satisfactory outcome[335] for both doctor and patient. This cycle can be repeated in a consultation—and many times during a doctor-patient relationship.

If we think the patient has a lifestyle problem, it might help to know where they are in the cycle of change. Motivational interviewing[671]—guiding rather than directing, eliciting the patient's own motivation to change, listening, and encouraging 'change talk' from the patient—has small, durable, and statistically significant outcome benefits compared with treatment-as-usual.[700] If the patient is not ready for change, the matter can be left for another day. Dry leaves on a windy day just can't be swept up. Wait until the wind drops and try again.

THE OBJECTIVE OF THE HISTORY IS TO DISCOVER WHAT'S TROUBLING THE PATIENT

The objectives in history taking are to find out what's troubling the patient. If we let them talk initially without interruption, the history is slightly shorter—although the whole consultation becomes longer.[701] We shouldn't artificially limit the consultation to a single problem: revealing the range and nature of the symptoms and worries helps the patient feel understood and us to understand. If we're walking along a country road and hear a car approaching from behind, we might step onto the grass verge. It's easy then to step back into the path of a second car behind the first. The patient often has a second worry on the tail of the first: listen and look out for it.

THE OBJECTIVES OF MANAGEMENT ARE SAFETY, SAFETY-NETTING, SATISFACTION, AND SELF-CONFIDENCE

The patient should leave the room with an evidence-based medical management plan to reduce their risk of death and disease, including a safety net—what's likely to happen and what to do if it doesn't.[666] They should also feel satisfied with the consultation and more self-confident. Satisfied patients feel they've spent more time with their doctor, and longer consultations make doctors less stressed and more satisfied.[702]

SKILLS IN HISTORY-TAKING

The first skill to be used is body language. Go into the waiting room to welcome the patient. Face them directly, smile, and introduce yourself in a normal speaking voice.[125] Guide them to your consulting room, blending your deportment with theirs as you go, offer them a seat, sit down, mirror their posture, pay them full attention, and say the minimum—which might be nothing. Be interested, not interesting.[125] I've observed that all my partners—whatever their differences in style—give undivided attention at the start of the consultation.

SHOW YOU'RE LISTENING BY ACKNOWLEDGING

The verbal skills we use in the consultation form a spectrum from the most patient-centred to the most doctor-centred. Patient-centred and doctor-centred skills aren't mutually exclusive but complementary and which we use at any point in the consultation can be a matter of conscious choice. The first—and most patient-centred—skill is acknowledgement, saying 'Yes, uh-huh, I see'. This will encourage the patient to talk. We should listen and respond equally to what we hear, whether it's physical, social, or psychological.[173]

THEN REFLECT

Reflecting (or summarising, echoing) is the second most patient-centred skill. In my experience, this is the skill that's least understood and least used by students and junior doctors. In its simplest form, it's a repetition of the patient's last word or phrase in order to encourage the patient to carry on talking. It's not a challenge, confirmation, or question—and it's certainly not a leading question; it's neutral. It's not followed by an exclamation mark, a full stop or a question mark but by silence. It's particularly useful in responding to cues. Cues are puzzling verbal or non-verbal communications, sometimes incongruent and beyond the awareness of the patient. We should always notice and, in general, explore them.[173] Don't ignore cues while pursuing a series of closed questions.[672]

A more elaborate summary indicates to the patient that we're attending and allows them to confirm or correct our understanding.[669] A still more sophisticated form helps draw the history to a close: 'You've got a few problems and I'm wondering where to go from here'. An important detail here is the use of 'and' rather than 'but'. 'You've got a few problems BUT I'm wondering where to go from here' conveys to my ear rejection rather than acceptance. Be wary of putting your BUT in the face of an unhappy person.[703, 704] 'But' can, however, follow something negative: 'You don't know where to go from here, BUT I think we can come up with something'. A complementary skill that I've learned from one of my colleagues is saying 'no' assertively, calmly and confidently. It clears the way for finding areas of agreement— which are always larger than areas of disagreement—and moving on.

THEN ASK OPEN QUESTIONS

Questions, open or closed, interrupt the patient's train of thought and should be deferred. When we ask questions, we get answers:[182] we don't necessarily find out what the patient is trying to tell us or what we need to know. Symptoms that prompt the patient to consult and are volunteered may have more diagnostic value than those elicited by closed questioning.[705]

TABLE 6.2 Seven 'E' questions

Patient's experience	Examples of questions
Effects of the symptom	How is this affecting you?
Emotions surrounding it	How would you say you feel about this?
Explanations for it	What possible causes cross your mind?
Expectations of the consultation	Where did you think we might go with this?
Epitasis	What made you decide to make this appointment?
Enquiries	Is there anything you want to ask me?
Enything else	Is there anything else we need to think about just now?

When we do start questioning, we begin with patient-centred open questions. These might be of a general nature such as 'How have things been?' or more specific. A useful set of pegs is provided by seven 'E' questions (*see* Table 6.2) that I've derived from various sources.[671, 706, 94, 34] One of these questions might need clarification: epitasis is the main action in a drama leading to the climax[707]—this is what's precipitated the consultation. The 'E' questions form a checklist for distress equivalent to the checklist for, say, physical pain[708] or the features of a lump. They can be learned and recited by rote like questions in a foreign-language phrase book and, if not raised in every consultation, asked routinely when necessary. When it comes to the Clinical Skills Assessment, incidentally, you should use your own wording and, despite the artificiality of the occasion, ask these questions with conviction, showing an interest in the patient as a person.[709] If one of these questions doesn't draw a response from the patient, it can be repeated with or without variation. What we're looking for is any contribution by the patient. Once we have that, we can, if necessary, focus on detail.[97]

Leading questions should be avoided. Questions may be conveyed as statements or offers—'I'm wondering ...'. One advantage of the open question over the closed question is that it gives the doctor more time to think. A gap of three seconds after the patient has spoken serves the same purpose for both doctor and patient.[30]

You'll notice that questions are divided into open (including patient-centred) questions and doctor-centred (including closed) questions, and that the terminology is asymmetrical. The reason is that when I was developing these ideas, my colleagues and I had got bogged down trying to differentiate four types of question (open or closed and patient-centred or doctor-centred). We found that we could generally classify any question as either doctor-centred or open and further subdivision was unnecessary.

THEN ASK DOCTOR-CENTRED QUESTIONS

The doctor-centred question is the most doctor-centred skill: it's necessary but not sufficient for good consulting. I use it mainly to narrow the differential diagnosis and generally delay its use until the end of the history. I have, however, seen my colleagues use it effectively and efficiently earlier on but it's always part of a spectrum including patient-centred skills. The most common error I've observed among juniors is moving straight from acknowledging to closed questioning and never developing facility with open questions and, particularly, with reflections.

DIAGNOSIS

There are two aspects to diagnosis that are relevant here. One is the 'doctor bit'[710] in which the doctor gives their interpretation of the situation. The other is the 'story stuff',[711] in which the resolution, or dissolution, of the problem[34] comes from the patient.[712] The doctor should be patient-centred without making unwelcome intrusions on the patient's privacy and sensibilities; aware that the patient does not have a fixed pre-determined agenda to be discovered but is open to suggestions; neutral if possible without awkwardness; and, where not neutral, aware of bias.[34]

For biomechanical aspects of the problem, and for separating the biomechanical from the functional, the 'doctor bit' predominates; for functional aspects, the 'story stuff' predominates.

THERE ARE FOUR INTERWEAVING SKILLS IN THE MANAGEMENT PHASE

When we take a history, the flow of information is from patient to doctor. In management, the flow is in the opposite direction. The skills in the management phase are therefore mirror images of those in the history phase. There's another difference between history and management phases. In the history phase, we begin with the most patient-centred skill and end with the most doctor-centred. In the management phase, we begin with the most doctor-centred skill and interweave the others. I'll describe them in turn and then show how they fit together.

The first and most patient-centred skill is acknowledgement. Ideal management might simply involve nodding as the patient outlines their self-management plan. The patient says 'So, I'll take this antacid and come back if I'm not getting better' and the doctor says 'Yes, that's right'.

The second, third, and fourth management skills make sense only in combination. The second skill is checking, the third answering a patient's question, and the fourth providing new information. There are two types of checking: when the patient asks a question, we respond not with an immediate answer, but by checking what prompted their question and whether they have other questions—only then do we answer; also, after we volunteer new information, we check with the patient what they make of it.

These skills form little sequences. One sequence is a quickstep: patient asks question, doctor checks, patient clarifies, doctor replies. Another is a rather lumpen waltz: doctor gives information, doctor checks, patient replies. A third is a tango, a dance which doesn't require much movement: only one step need be taken before pausing, and you can rock gently or reverse at any time.

HISTORY-TAKING AND MANAGEMENT SKILLS CAN BE LEARNED BY ROTE

The skills described in this chapter—body language and four verbal skills—are useful only if recalled and enacted immediately in the commotion of the consultation. So they need to be learned. That learning will be enhanced by the following techniques: establish in your mind what you already know about consulting skills, add this new information in a meaningful way, try it out repeatedly in your head, your tutorials and your consultations, and use mnemonics.[713] To complement this dry learning, also remember that the consultation is a performance of great mental, physical and emotional intensity: create that sense of vitality as you learn and practise so that the consultation proper is no different from the rehearsal except that there happens to be a patient in the room.

A mnemonic for consultation skills is BLAck ROqCq, which refers to: Body Language, Acknowledgements, Reflections, Open questions, Closed questions.

HISTORHYME

Something more ridiculous—and therefore more memorable—is the poem I call the HistoRhyme. This refers to the four history taking skills: acknowledgement, reflection, open (or patient-centred) question and doctor-centred (or closed) question.

> When you take a history
> First say, 'YES, uh-huh, I see;'
> REFLECT; then question OPENly;
> And lastly ask DOCTORlyly.

The HistoRhyme can be abbreviated to 'YES REFLECT OPEN DOCTOR' and even recited in front of a mirror accompanied by an open gesture of the arms. The belief that people have different learning styles (visual, auditory, and kinaesthetic) doesn't enhance and may inhibit learning.[714] Use of distinct, bizarre images does improve recall.[715] If you're not usually physically demonstrative, the memory of yourself in a mirror with your arms wide apart saying 'Yes, uh-huh, I see . . . reflect!' might bring the words to mind. The crucial thing is that when your mind goes blank in a consultation— or in the Clinical Skills Assessment—you don't dry up or resort to a series of closed questions. Instead, you repeat the patient's last word and you wait three seconds.

MANAGEMODE

The poem I call the ManagemOde reminds you to follow each of the patient's questions and each of your statements with a checking question.

> When asked a question, first explore:
> 'What prompted that?' and 'Any more?'
> Having answered or said something new,
> Ask the patient, 'What's your view?'

The ManagemOde might run through your mind and rescue you at moments of panic. A shorter reminder would be: 'When asked, ask; having answered, ask.'

USE THE GRID IN LEARNING AND TEACHING

I use the grid when teaching. I ask medical students and junior doctors to make a mark against a skill each time they observe my using it. This keeps us both on our toes. With their permission I reciprocate. In general, in the history phase, marks should appear earliest and most plentifully against acknowledgements, and latest and most sparsely against doctor-centred questions. In the management phase, each question asked by the patient and each answer or new information given by the doctor should be followed by a checking question.

The first task I set medical students when they consult is to discover answers to the seven 'E' questions: this is within their capacity and usually shows that the patient-centred approach effectively and efficiently elicits information and builds rapport.

If a skill is never or rarely demonstrated, this can be identified from the marked grid: it can then be taught and practised immediately, either with the patient or through role-play—which for the stage-shy means simply saying the words or sounds, not acting. For effective learning, the doctor should observe themself on video, or recall a moment in one of their own consultations, identify the under-used skill, demonstrate it, practise it in role-play perhaps 10–20 times, then try it in their next consultation. If a skill whose phrasing has been approved by your trainer doesn't seem to work well initially, don't overcompensate: just try it again.[716]

If learner and teacher accept the validity of this approach, learning is likely to benefit. Feedback is specific, descriptive and challenging, and progress can be monitored by the learner. Of course, the grid shouldn't dominate: it's just one of many tools.[717]

IN PRACTICE, THE STRUCTURE OF THE CONSULTATION VARIES

The consultation has four components: history, examination, diagnosis, and management; these components can occur in any sequence and often overlap. History and diagnosis begin when we look at the patient's record before the consultation. Ideally, during the history, we elicit the questions the patient wants answered but we might well defer answering them until the management phase—at which time further questions might emerge. Examination starts as soon as we meet the patient. It's helpful to begin preparing the patient for formal examination in the middle of the history phase: this saves time, indicates that you know what you're about, and shows that you're taking the patient's problem seriously. And treatment, especially reassurance of a distressed patient, might well begin during the history, as long as you don't curtail disclosure. It's important, however, to be clear in your own mind what part of the consultation you're in and what you're trying to achieve at any one time. For instance, you can continue the history while examining a skin rash but not while palpating the abdomen. Be particularly wary of the computer.[718, 719] It's necessary for printing prescriptions and patient information leaflets but it mustn't be allowed to take over. You might find you've been reading the tourist guide all holiday and never seen the sights.

DON'T GET IN A MUDDLE: CONCENTRATE ON ONE THING AT A TIME

The consultation should form a coherent whole and its component parts intermingle. But be clear where your focus is at any one time. Before the patient comes in, study the notes and prepare your medical agenda. While fetching the patient and sitting down, establish rapport by mirroring and matching body language. During the early part of the history, give the patient's agenda your mental attention and use the HistoRhyme. During the examination, give the patient your physical attention while you think. If you need more time to think, wash your hands slowly. Give the computer attention while you find prescriptions and patient information leaflets. In the management phase, use the ManagemOde: here the focus changes frequently and you have to be nimble, just as in dancing the weight is transferred from foot to foot.

EXERCISE

Use a video or observer to record the consulting skills you use on the grid from this chapter. In the history phase, is there a spread of skills with many patient-centred skills at the start and a few doctor-centred skills toward the end? Is any skill too frequent or infrequent? In the management phase, before answering each of the patient's questions and after each new bit of information, did you ask an open checking question?

CHAPTER 7

Pattern design

'It is the large generalisation, limited by a happy particularity, which is the fruitful conception.'

Alfred North Whitehead. *Science and the Modern World.*
Cambridge: Cambridge University Press; 1946.

'... the notion of a disease is essentially abstract—an ideal model, a template against which the more untidy experiences of individual doctors and their patients can be tested and observed ...'

Marinker M. Sirens, stray dogs, and the narrative of Hilda Thomson.
In: Greenhalgh T, Hurwitz B, editors. *Narrative Based Medicine: dialogue and discourse in clinical practice.* London: BMJ Books; 1998.

Edinburgh's Royal Botanic Garden: grass underfoot, blackbird's song overhead, rustle of cherry tree leaf, rough bark, poetry on a plaque: *Aesculus hippocastanum.* I hesitate. *Hippos* is horse:[87] that's chestnut, not cherry. My tree book describes the chestnut leaf as palmate:[720] I'd call it digitate—there's no palm, and each finger is shaped like a cherry leaf. It's when you notice that the leaves cluster in fives and radiate that you say, 'Of course! It's a chestnut'.

The blackbird is identified by its musical song, bright orange beak, and black plumage. It also has characteristic movements by which ornithologists recognise it as it flashes across their field of vision: these movements are referred to as 'jizz'.[721] I suspect 'jizz' is a relative of 'gist', the word used by cognitive psychologists for a fuzzy trace encoded in memory alongside detail: most reasoning is thought to use not the detail but the 'gist'.[722]

PATTERNS

Bongard problems are collections of framed geometric shapes used to compare the performance of artificial intelligence with the functioning of the human brain.[106] Geometry, gist, jizz—they all depend on pattern recognition, which is one of the ways in which doctors make diagnoses. Pattern recognition is based on knowledge, experience, and skill acquired over decades: it's often exercised too rapidly for the clinician to be aware of it, let alone describe it to others. It's contrasted with hypothesis testing, the process that novices use predominantly, and that experts revert to occasionally when faced with an unusual problem.[723] But when we diagnose, we aren't using either pattern recognition or hypothesis testing alone: we're combining the two strategies. And we're not just recognising patterns but creating them: we're forming the elements of a messy consultation into a variety of shapes until we find one we're familiar with, one that we can make sense of. We then observe how the current instance resembles and differs from previous instances.[187] My guess is that expert diagnosticians are good at finding patterns and even better at creating them. If we settle for wondering at their intuition or marvelling at their clinical acumen, we won't learn from them. If we can find out how they do what they do, we might be better able to learn these skills ourselves, and to research and teach them.

In consultations, doctors experiment in a variety of ways: by exploring, by saying or doing something to see what happens, and by hypothesis testing.[187] Patients play an active part in this process. It's not easy to analyse because activities of different kinds are taking place cyclically over short periods of time. The doctor's obtaining information, reflecting on it, and deciding what further information to seek, often not quite knowing what they're looking for but trusting that they'll recognise it when they find it. This process is more readily appreciated when it's experienced than when it's conveyed in words. And it's an act of creation: the same patient consulting a different general practitioner will have a different consultation.

ISOLATED SYMPTOMS AND SIGNS

At medical school, from textbooks we learn symptoms and signs in isolation then in clusters. In the United States, an attempt has been made to draw up a curriculum of signs that hospital trainees should be familiar with.[724] These include rectal examination, eliciting ankle reflexes, and palpating and percussing the spleen. As postgraduates we discover, from experience and the evidence-based literature, that some of these traditional clinical features are relatively undiscriminating in the contexts in which we work. Rectal examination is useful.[530, 725] Ankle reflexes, however, are so often lost with normal ageing[651] that their absence doesn't predict pathology. And I can't remember an occasion during my 20 years as a general practitioner in the UK when my management hinged on palpating and percussing the spleen. Some signs are too rare or unpredictive for general practice use.[726]

Clinical features studied and reported in the literature may not be representative. They may have been selected for a variety of reasons—because they were common or rare, obvious or subtle, elicited with ease or with difficulty. They may be atypical in a variety of ways. So, the fact that many haven't proved to be particularly discriminating doesn't tell us that all isolated features have the same failing. However, as far as the limited evidence goes, it does seem that isolated signs and symptoms often have low discriminatory value.

CLUSTERS OF FEATURES

How about clusters of features? Traditionally we learn how groups of symptoms and signs form syndromes. The literature sometimes supports this approach and sometimes brings it into question. For instance, although the patient with irritable bowel syndrome might see a gastroenterologist and the patient with tension headache a neurologist, the two patients have more similarities than differences—as do their conditions.[91] Pain is 'an unpleasant sensory and emotional experience associated with actual or potential tissue damage, or described in terms of such damage'.[727] This definition says nothing about mechanism or site; instead it refers to the intimate interaction between psyche and soma. Psychosocial context plays a part in eliciting and maintaining what might be called pain behaviours. Attending to a patient's pain increases their pain rating. Recalled severity of past pain diminishes over time until pain recurs, at which time recalled pain severity rises again.[186] Juniors sometimes ask patients to rate their pain on a scale of 0 to 10. Such scoring has some uses[186] and may be a means by which the patient can communicate to the doctor their degree of distress. But it might lend a false objectivity to a subjective experience. A high rating doesn't indicate that the condition is more dangerous nor that we should necessarily respond with greater pharmaceutical intensity. The significance of pain and pain rating depends on context.

One way in which clustered features are appraised is by means of global, subjective impressions. These sometimes prove to be discriminating. In children with illness of less than five days' duration, the parent's feeling that 'this illness is different' and the doctor's feeling that 'something is wrong' have higher positive predictive values for serious infection than any other feature or combination of features.[497]

Research evidence, then, offers us new ways of weighting and grouping symptoms and signs. Decision aids help us to incorporate the research findings into practice with the aim of improving diagnosis and therefore clinical care. Such decision aids are available on paper[171, 456] and on the Web,[457, 458] and Chapter 5 in this book makes a contribution. To be useful in general practice, these tools sometimes need to occupy as yet uncharted territory somewhere between screening procedures[728] and diagnostic tests. What's wrong is often less important than whether something's wrong and how serious or urgent it is. Urinalysis is too insensitive to use as a screening test for diabetes;[729] on the other hand, it might be sensitive enough to identify diabetes as the cause of polyuria or weight loss, although I can find no literature to support or refute this. Chest radiography might do more harm than good when used to screen for lung cancer;[730] however, it might be helpful when occult cancer is clinically suspected—again, I can find no evidence one way or the other. Research, clinical practice, and service delivery might be better organised not by organ and specialty but by optimal diagnostic pathway.

DISCRIMINATING SYMPTOMS

A complementary approach is to look more closely at the individual clues—the symptoms, signs, and combinations—that we find helpful in practice but which are underrepresented in the literature.

Let's start with symptoms. We can divide them into two groups. Symptoms that prompt a consultation and are volunteered by the patient can be called iatrotropic. Symptoms that are elicited in response to questions can be called non-iatrotropic.[336]

One might suppose that iatrotropic symptoms are better pointers to the diagnosis than non-iatrotropic symptoms are. This notion has received little direct research but there are indications that it might be justified: experienced clinicians base their diagnoses on fewer items of information than novices do;[731] and the process of refining a clinical decision tool involves removal of redundant or confounding symptoms and signs.[410] Iatrotropic symptoms aren't necessarily stated bluntly at the start of the consultation. They might be slipped in as asides: 'While I'm here', for instance, might mean 'Why I'm here'.[109] Or they might be revealed by cues.[173] Cues are verbal or non-verbal communications, sometimes incongruent or beyond the awareness of the patient, that don't fit with what else is going on.[173] In cognitive behavioural therapy, the clinician might be particularly interested in beliefs or behaviours that arouse the patient's emotions.[732] We look for the underlying causes of ripples on the surface of the water.

An iatrotropic symptom—a symptom that prompts the patient to consult—is always important because it tells you about the patient. If it has a high positive likelihood ratio it also tells you about the patient's disease. Attempted suicide by hanging, strangulation, or suffocation has a high positive likelihood ratio for subsequent completed suicide.[549] I suspect that, in the context of breathlessness, tingling of the lips and hands would prove to have a high positive likelihood ratio for hyperventilation. 'Change of bowel habit' is a more powerful predictor of colorectal cancer than 'diarrhoea' or 'constipation'[313] but its discriminating value is still low. Curiously, occult blood has a higher positive predictive value than frank blood.[449] So, symptoms and signs in colorectal cancer are of limited discriminating value. This observation, while disheartening, is useful. It tells us that abdominal symptoms—compared with symptoms related to other systems—predict diagnostic uncertainty[109] and might well warrant repeated assessment.

Non-iatrotropic symptoms—those that are elicited by questioning—are most useful for excluding diagnoses. The symptom that's best for this is one with a low negative likelihood ratio. Being keen to stop smoking has a low negative likelihood ratio for successful cessation. Not being keen to stop smoking—the equivalent of a negative test result—means that the patient probably won't stop. We might intuit this: research confirms it.[486] For ascites, ankle swelling has a low negative likelihood ratio:[608] that means the absence of ankle swelling makes ascites unlikely—something we might be unsure about without empirical evidence.

DISCRIMINATING SIGNS

Now consider signs. Formal examination makes little positive contribution to diagnosis in primary care. Extensive examination—that is, beyond a single system—is associated with less confidence in diagnosis.[109] The role of formal examination in diagnosis is to exclude: mostly, we're looking for the absence of signs with a low negative likelihood ratio. Informal and global assessment of the patient, however, provides a lot of information. Rather like pattern recognition, it takes place quickly and often subliminally.[733]

One reaction to the unpredictability of clinical outcome in the context of a risk averse and litigious society is to measure and record vital signs. Junior doctors recommend this to their peers[734, 735] and guideline writers to the rest of us,[736] but it's unclear how useful measuring these vital signs is.[737]

Perhaps, rather than measurement of vital signs, it's their assessment that matters. In children, we begin this process before touching. Assessment of respiration means looking at the toddler sitting quietly on their parent's lap and deciding whether their chest is moving more effortfully than expected. Capillary refilling time might be a useful measure in certain situations, but relatively cool, blotchy skin in a hot child, while being less definable, is probably more helpful.[738] Whether or not the heart rate is normal depends—except in a rare condition such as supraventricular tachycardia—on what the child is doing: the number of beats per minute contributes little further. There's no table of normal values to refer to. We acquire our own internal nomogram through experience.

INCONGRUENCE

This example of the feverish child indicates the importance of incongruence: the mismatch between respiratory effort and level of physical activity or between heart rate and emotional upset; and the contrast between cool periphery and hot core.

A single symptom or sign is a melody. Add another and we get harmony, either consonance or dissonance. A musical ear will hear the difference.

Incongruence or inconsistency can make physical pathology less likely. There might be a mismatch between what the patient says and how they say it. The patient may follow one account of their symptoms with a contradictory account. Or they might show 'lack of commitment' to a symptom:[710] as soon as the doctor tries to explore it, they abandon it and move on to another. Some signs change when the patient is distracted: unilateral leg weakness can improve when attention is directed to the other leg;[683] and spontaneous use of an apparently painful limb is often more revealing than formal examination. Some generalisations, although not evidence-based, might be helpful. Physical pathology is unlikely to be the cause of symptoms that are multiple, in recognised functional clusters, biologically improbable, inconsistent, unaccompanied by signs, described incongruously, non-progressive, unaffected by biomechanical treatment, or not mentioned at follow-up consultations. The single most useful investigation here is the test of time.[317]

TIME COURSE

Time course is useful for diagnosis. Diseases vary in their natural history. Some are relentlessly progressive, some chronically fluctuating, and some self-limiting.[109, 411] Knowledge of the natural history improves diagnosis and safety-netting.[666] Of coughs in children in general practice, 10% last more than 25 days.[635] This time course contrasts with the time course of childhood meningococcal illness in which an acute onset is followed within hours by death. In acute feverish illness in children, the combination of a rapid onset and early consultation prompts us to consider meningococcal disease. If such a feverish child seems ill but not ill enough for immediate referral to hospital, we might review them half an hour or a couple of hours later: such safety-netting might improve the chances of timely diagnosis.

When someone's ill, they don't experience the illness in a series of disconnected temporal fragments. On the contrary, they're looking backward and forward in time, trying to make sense of what's happening and preparing for what might be going to happen. At each stage, they're weighing up the competing merits of succumbing to illness or attempting restitution.[640] This is an active process. How healthy they feel at any stage doesn't depend just on their physical condition. It depends on their mental state and whether they perceive themself to be on the road to recovery or not. Health is the process of adaptability, or even an aptitude for adaptability. In the case of most acute illnesses, the patient recovers, fully or partially. When and how much they recover is partly a function of the pathology and partly a matter of personal disposition, of choice. They might opt to remain ill, to become invalids.[739] They might make that decision and take the necessary action on their own or they might seek their doctor's help. The doctor can choose how to respond, and one option is collusion. Patient and doctor may have similar reasons not to confront a problem.[100] Examples of collusion might be prescribing of long-term benzodiazepines for the anxious, protein pump inhibitors for the obese dyspeptic,[740] and opiates for patients with chronic non-cancer pain.[546] But it's not always clear when we're colluding in a destructive process and when we're holding the person[331] pending restitution.

During an illness, the progression in time scale from days to weeks and then to months changes the diagnosis, not just in degree but in kind. For instance, acute pain, a symptom of disease, becomes chronic pain, a disease in itself. Whereas recall of acute pain is a matter of 'remembering', recall of chronic pain is more a matter of 'knowing'.[186] The pain becomes a daily companion or an integral part of the person. Any attempt to separate the pain from the patient will probably fail.

MAJOR ILLNESS

Minor illness can sometimes be adequately dealt with by diagnosis and treatment. Major illness or distress requires a different response. The experience has changed the person's life and changed the person.[741] For a time, it might overwhelm the patient or defy technology: it mustn't overwhelm or defy the doctor. Our fortitude, through our relationship with the patient, gives them strength.[332] Referral to another agency might signal our inability to cope with their problem or with the demands of the relationship. We respond with ourselves, partly involved and partly detached.[742] When involved, we react in a variety of ways: we may be dismayed by the patient's progressive debility rather than adaptability, indulge their sense of victimhood,[686] or admire the determination of the person living with disability.[743] With detachment, we look more objectively at the patient's condition and our reaction to it. To these two reactions, emotional and cognitive, we add a third, 'bodily empathy': hearing the patient's story as an account of them as a person, not as a catalogue of symptoms,[744] meeting their eyes with ours.[745]

The effects of severe illness on someone's life[741] are similar to the effects of other devastating experiences such as loss of a child.[746, 747] At times, one can't distinguish between the person who wants to die because of despair and the one who's going to die because of disease. When people do approach death, illness, pain, and ageing prepare the way.[745] The policy directive might say 'advance care planning' but where the journey starts and what route to follow aren't clear.[748, 749] The patient needs their doctor to travel with them.

That the chestnut leaf is not a cherry leaf becomes apparent only when we seek out the whole. So with our patients.

EXERCISE

During a consultation, look for a the crucial bit of information or combination of symptoms and signs that tips you toward a particular diagnosis or course of action, write it down, discuss it with a colleague, learn more about it, and teach it.

CHAPTER 8

Medical education

'Only level-headed people, then, will know themselves and be able to examine what they know and don't know; and be able to inspect others in the same way and see - when they know or think they know something - whether they do know it; or, more importantly, when they think they know something but actually don't. No-one else will be able do this.'

Plato. *Charmides*. (Translated by Jo Wright and Wilfrid Treasure)

'Teaching, in my estimation, is a vastly overrated function.'

Rogers CR. *Freedom to Learn: a view of what education might become.*
Columbus, OH: Charles E. Merrill Publishing Company; 1969.

The requirements for qualifying as a general practitioner are many and detailed. Fortunately, these are explicit, so it's possible systematically to set about satisfying them. This chapter addresses the following areas: the relationship between the behaviour of medical undergraduates and subsequent professional conduct; the demographic markers of success in the examination for Membership of the Royal College of General Practitioners; the criteria that have to be met by would-be general practitioners from medical school entry to passing MRCGP; and, finally, continuing professional development.

UNDERGRADUATE BEHAVIOUR AND PROFESSIONAL CONDUCT

Risk factors for a doctor's poor performance might become evident during the undergraduate years. In the United States, disciplinary action among practising physicians by medical boards was associated with previous unprofessional undergraduate behaviour.[750] In Canada, doctors in the bottom quartile of the undergraduate finals written paper were more likely to be assessed by their peers almost a decade later as demonstrating an unacceptable quality of care: the clinical component of the examination was of no additional predictive value.[751] Among UK graduates, male sex, early undergraduate examination failures, and lower social-class background were independent risk factors for later professional misconduct.[752]

Primary care physicians who hadn't been the subject of malpractice investigations differed from those who had: they had longer consultations, they were better at interacting with their patients, and they laughed more.[753] Whether misconduct will be exposed is largely a matter of chance. Complaints against doctors are common in total but they're rare in relation to the number of consultations we do[754] and they don't often progress to an advanced stage.[755]

Medicine is a stressful occupation, general practitioners, for example, having a higher rate of suicide than the general population.[756] The work is probably unusual in terms of the demands made and rewards offered.[328, 757, 758] Support is available for doctors in difficulties.[759, 760, 761, 762, 763, 764]

DEMOGRAPHIC MARKERS OF SUCCESS IN THE MRCGP

You're most likely to pass the MRCGP Applied Knowledge Test and Clinical Skills Assessment if you're a white, female, UK graduate at ST2 or ST3 level attempting the examination for the first time. You're least likely to pass if you're a black, male, European Economic Area graduate at ST1 level in the southwest UK re-sitting the examination.[476]

A small study in an English deanery suggested possible reasons why international medical graduates had lower pass rates than other candidates: they were less familiar with the English language, with the UK, and with the NHS; they had different attitudes to learning and related differently to patients and to their peers; and they perceived half-day release courses as relatively unhelpful and attended fewer of them.[765] The General Medical Council isn't allowed to test the language skills of doctors from the European Union seeking registration in the UK and are negotiating this with the UK government and European Commission.[766]

CURRICULA

The positive qualities required of medical school applicants are indicated by the contents of the United Kingdom Clinical Aptitude Test, which involves verbal, quantitative and abstract reasoning along with decision analysis. This test has good reliability but unknown validity: that means that a single candidate will get the same result if they re-sit but the result doesn't indicate how good they'll be as undergraduates or as doctors.[767] In the United States, medical school applicants are required to provide evidence of personal qualities as well as of academic achievements. However, compared with academic achievements, personal qualities predict later performance less reliably and are less attended to by admission committees.[74] Increasingly close attention, however, is being applied to fraud. Evidence of fraud is found in 5% of applicants to residences in the United States and is monitored by the UK Universities and Colleges Admissions Service.[768]

In selecting general practice specialty trainees, the following qualities are prioritised: empathy and sensitivity, communication skills, clinical expertise, problem solving, professional integrity, and coping with pressure.[188] Other qualities—important but harder to assess—are other personal attributes; organisational and administrative skills; managing others and team involvement; legal, ethical, and political awareness; and learning and personal development.[769]

The syllabus for general practice training can be subdivided into formal, informal, assessed, and hidden curricula.[770] The formal curriculum is defined by the Royal College of General Practitioners[771, 18] the assessed curriculum by MRCGP[475] and the e-portfolio. The informal curriculum can be thought of as those things mentioned over coffee, and the hidden curriculum as those things not spoken of but implied by behaviour.

Analysis of the assessed curriculum suggests that the trainee is expected to be knowledgeable, reflective, and able to perform.[772] The MRCGP is a highly researched and audited set of examinations assessing knowledge and performance. The e-portfolio is a tool to enable formative and summative assessment of both minimum and excellent achievement in the areas of knowledge, performance, and reflectiveness.[773] The informal and hidden curricula are, by their nature, not so easily analysed. They might be gleaned from institutional policies, resource allocation, actions rather than words, asides, and slang.[774]

Among competencies not formally assessed are emotional intelligence,[775] self-awareness, and the ability to form relationships.[333, 332] These competencies are aspects of, or related to, a quality that might be called humaneness, and are features of the system of thought called humanism. They're the values that prevent the erosion of professionalism by expediency; more positively, they're the values that inspire professionalism.[74] A weakness in these areas might hide in the lower right-hand pane of the Johari window, unknown both to the trainee and to others.[776] It's possible that, with the e-portfolio, medical training is following a societal trend toward public displays of what traditionally might have remained private,[686] and that records of reflection will reveal the presence or absence of humaneness in the trainee. But it's the trainer, the person with whom the trainee inevitably forms some sort of relationship, who's in the best position to notice a weakness in this area and to nurture this quality of humaneness. Ideally, the trainer is a role model, someone decent and responsible that the trainee can look up to,[777] a guide who can enable the trainee to achieve their potential through a relationship based on genuineness, acceptance, and understanding.[778]

THE CLINICAL SKILLS ASSESSMENT

Passing the MRCGP Clinical Skills Assessment depends on an appropriate level of knowledge, skills, and attitude, for which guidance is available elsewhere.[206] Feedback to, and about, unsuccessful candidates indicates a spread of failings scattered over a variety of criteria. However, the biggest single failing is in relation to management and an important reason for this is that the candidate runs out of time.[709]

The Clinical Skills Assessment is a stressful experience. Preparation for it includes years of work, mostly beyond the scope of this book. One determinant of success is examination technique. You need to have a formula that works reliably, whatever the clinical content and however anxious you're feeling on the day. Fortunately, the general practice consultation and the Clinical Skills Assessment are sufficiently similar that the skills required for one serve well for the other. Good habits need to be practised so that they become the default mode under stress. The skills described in Chapter 6 of this book include asking stock open questions. Might repetition reveal the formulaic nature of this technique? In the Clinical Skills Assessment, each consultation is observed by a different pair of examiners so they won't be aware of repetition, although they will be on the alert for things being said parrot-fashion without interest in the patient as a person. In general practice, approximately half of patients consult less than 10 times in 41 months,[220] which is about three times during the course of a trainee year. In March 2010, I found that 86% of the patients seen by our ST3 in a six-month period had seen him only once. So most patients will be exposed to few repetitions of the same set of questions—and it's reasonable to suppose that patients returning to see the same doctor are fairly satisfied with their consultations. It's probably sensible, therefore, to become confident with a small repertoire of questions: this is better than improvising and getting tongue-tied.

COMPETENCE

Self-assessment and external assessment of competence often don't correlate.[779] Incompetent people overrate their level of competence[779] both in absolute terms and relative to the competence they perceive in others. This can be ameliorated by improving their competence. Competent people slightly underestimate their own competence and assume other people are as competent as they.[780] This suggests that the poor trainee will think that they're better than they really are and that their trainer, better as a doctor than as an educator, might not realise that the trainee's confidence masks incompetence.

Teaching can be made more effective and efficient if the trainer identifies the trainee's needs before imparting wisdom. When trainees ask for advice about patients, one option is to use the following formula: ask them to commit themselves to a diagnosis or management plan and to identify any quandary; ask them what has brought them to that point; then teach them general principles, commend their achievements, and correct their errors. When learners sit in during consultations, they can be given specific observational tasks and quizzed afterwards.[83] New students, especially when they might spend only a few hours with you and then move on, can be invited to talk about something they're good at outwith medicine: recounting their success in other fields will build their confidence, inform their medical learning, and keep their thinking broad. Disproportionate emphasis on facts (as measured by the Applied Knowledge Test), performance (Clinical Skills Assessment), and written reflection (e-portfolio) risks overlooking or even promoting hidden incompetence in other areas such as humaneness. Indeed, we should beware privileging a few qualities at the expense of other undervalued or unrecognised ways of being a good doctor.[772]

Orthodoxy needs challenged. Experiential learning might seem self-evidently good but has unpredictable consequences.[781] Workplace-based assessment doesn't necessarily improve performance.[782] Audit and feedback have variable effect on professional practice from slight worsening to moderate improvement. They're more beneficial when baseline adherence to recommended practice is low and when feedback is delivered intensively.[783] Group learning has a positive impact on knowledge but small or negligible impact on clinical behaviour and patient outcome.[784] Rather than beginning continuing professional development from the physician's self-perceived needs, it might be better to begin with competencies required and work backward toward learning needs.[784] Testing and repeated recall enhance learning.[785] Professionals need formative assessment; they also need summative assessment not just of their static competence, but also of their ability to learn,[784, 786] not only of what decisions they make, but how they make them,[787] not merely of their ability to follow rules of thumb, but of their capacity for deeper, reflective practice.[155]

On the other hand, we must be wary of self-indulgence: we might like thinking about what we do and how we can do it better: the public just wants us to get it right.[784] In response to this, revalidation is being introduced in the UK within the next year or two and is likely to require the following areas to be covered: annual appraisal including a personal development plan agreed and reviewed; learning credits; feedback from colleagues and patients; and complaints, significant events, and audit.[788] For the doctor just starting in a new practice, Table 8.1 is a checklist of things to consider. It's based on the GMC appraisal framework[20] and the RCGP curriculum.[18]

EXERCISE

Identify from reflection, observation and discussion three items in the informal and hidden curricula that are not present in the formal and assessed curricula. Are they things to be proud of, things to pay more attention to, reflections of human weakness rather than saintliness, or troubling lapses from good practice?

TABLE 8.1 Induction checklist

When?	What?	Done?
Preceding weeks	I'm immunised.	
	I've GMC membership, insurance, driving licence.	
	I've read about the general practice consultation.	
Preceding days	I know where I need to be when and can get there.	
	I'm healthy and presentable.	
	I'm appropriately confident and motivated.	
	I've a local map for house calls.	
First consultation	I know what's expected of me and the supervision arrangements.	
	I have the necessary equipment.	
	I can stop patients seeing other patients' details on the computer.	
	I can read the patient record.	
	I can prescribe.	
	I read the prescriptions I'm signing.	
	I can record my consultations.	
	I check patient identity, contact details, and follow-up arrangements when arranging investigations.	
	I know how to get help for a medical emergency.	
	I know how to get help if I'm in danger.	
	I've turned off my mobile phone.	
First days	I can contact ambulance, hospital, etc.	
	I can communicate with colleagues personally and by other means as appropriate.	
	I'm respectful of patients and colleagues.	
	I tell my supervisor if I feel out of my depth.	
	I have a structure for the consultation.	
	I examine the part complained of.	
	I look up every drug I'm not familiar with.	
	I use guidelines.	
	I respond to prevention prompts.	
	I've access to patient information leaflets, support groups, local services, etc.	
	I keep a learning log.	

CHAPTER 9

Risk management

'Rule number four: the patient is the one with the disease.'

Samuel Shem. *The House of God*. London: Black Swan; 1985.

'... a medicine which regards the patient not only as an object but also as a subject continues to exist in general practice ... precisely because the patient refuses to be ill according to the best precepts of modern medical education.'

Marinker M. Sirens, stray dogs, and the narrative of
Hilda Thomson. In: Greenhalgh T, Hurwitz B, editors.
Narrative Based Medicine: dialogue and discourse in clinical practice.
London: BMJ Books; 1998.

INTRODUCTION

Risk management is the process of evaluating risk in order to maximise the probability of success and minimise the likelihood of failure.[789] In business, the outcomes are principally financial[199] and their management falls within the remit of managers and accountants. In medicine, the outcomes are human, and risk management is therefore the concern of doctors. This chapter deals with two types of risk, risk to the doctor of a complaint and to the patient of being harmed, particularly through diagnostic error. We probably don't enjoy dwelling on these uncomfortable topics and would rather avoid thinking about them. But these events, complaints and harm, tell us something useful about our day-to-day practice and are worth exploring.

PATIENT DISSATISFACTION

Countries differ in the quality of their healthcare systems: a recent international study of healthcare outcomes and the experiences of patients and physicians produced the following rankings: Netherlands came top followed by the UK, Australia, Germany, New Zealand, Canada, and, lastly, the United States. Primary care in the UK ranked low for certain aspects of patient-centredness: patients couldn't understand their doctors' explanations, they weren't informed about their care or treatment options, and they weren't involved in decisions or encouraged to ask questions.[303]

Some dissatisfied patients take action.[790] They may approach agencies without jurisdiction such as the media or democratic representatives, agencies with jurisdiction such as the General Medical Council, whose main role is to assess fitness to practice, or the relevant healthcare organisation that is in a position to resolve the matter or redress a wrong.[755] There are prescribed systems for responding to complaints in the UK[791] and principles to be followed include attention to both process and outcome, with, where possible and appropriate, restitution, compensation, and remediation.[792] In England, for the first time in 2009, a constitution was drawn up for the National Health Service and patients' rights formally defined.[793] Those who complain to the ombudsman in Scotland are often dissatisfied with the complaints process, saying that they were not listened to or that they didn't get an apology.[755] Taking legal action is sometimes a way of getting heard.[794]

MEASURING DISSATISFACTION

Ratings by patients of doctor communication skills don't tell us much about the doctor. The ratings vary randomly, or by patient, more than by doctor.[258] Satisfaction ratings depend on local expectations and the means by which the ratings are elicited: for instance, discussions in focus groups might magnify dissatisfaction in a way that one-to-one exit interviews don't.[217] Satisfaction ratings might be affected by the fact of being asked[795] or by the views of others.[796] Some patients relate to their doctor as children relate to their parent.[666] Anger is sometimes misdirected from the disease to the doctor.[162]

In experimental research unrelated to healthcare, it's found that the more severe the consequences of a mistake, the greater the tendency of complainants to assign responsibility to someone, and the harsher their judgments.[797] Complainants—and more so third-party observers—tend to attribute someone's action to personal disposition rather than to the situation.[798] And bad perceptions tend to outweigh good ones.[799]

HEALTH COMPLAINTS AND HEALTHCARE COMPLAINTS

So the literature on patient dissatisfaction suggests that measurement is unreliable, that complainants are likely to elide mechanism and magnitude of error, that they tend to blame the individual doctor rather than the situation, and that they want someone to hear their story and to apologise.

Imprecision, subjectivity, interpersonal dynamics, the wish to be heard, apology for error—these all sound like the consultation. They also remind me of a comment by Balint that patient interaction with the practice—in relation to appointments and repeat prescriptions, for instance—is a symptom to be examined.[329] Perhaps dissatisfaction is also a symptom to be examined.

We use the term 'complaint' in two ways, relating firstly to the patient's health and secondly to their healthcare. The patient returning with a continuing respiratory illness might attribute or misattribute their symptoms variously to the natural course of their disease, to the doctor's previous refusal of an antibiotic, to prescribed ibuprofen or to over-the-counter paracetamol, or to other factors. The doctor will have their own array of attributions and misattributions. Patient and doctor may or may not express their opinions; if they express them, they may or may not reach agreement; and in most cases, there's no arbiter. Whether the problem is with the patient's health or with their healthcare is often unknowable.

A colleague told me recently how her openly acknowledged delay in diagnosing a man's fatal colorectal cancer was followed by a continuing therapeutic relationship with the widow rather than a pathogenic litigious one. The maturity and humanity revealed here by both doctor and patient represent an ideal, rarely met in reality, and serve as an impressive and humbling model.

So the consultation is an important means by which we hear about patients' health and healthcare complaints. What other sources of feedback are there? Patient satisfaction questionnaires commonly reveal dissatisfaction with the doctor-patient relationship, the giving of information and the gatekeeper role.[218] Patients who give a rating just less than perfect are particularly worth paying attention to because, while being positive, they may have identified areas for improvement.[800]

Audits, significant event analyses, and complaints are other sources of information that would not necessarily come to the doctor's attention if not collected systematically. These forms of data collection and analysis do, however, have disadvantages. They consume considerable resources, cover small areas of our work, are sometimes anonymised, obscure specifics by generalising, or are too specific to enable general lessons to be learned; they also lack immediacy, so the damage has been done before we know there's a problem. In any case, reporting error is not an activity that of itself improves quality.[716]

So the purpose served by reporting and discussing results of surveys and audits at, say, practice meetings is not so much in the content as in the process. We proclaim and rehearse our common purpose as a team and our readiness to subject our work to scrutiny. We indicate our receptiveness to routine, non-competitive, cooperative, mutual appraisal[801] and foster that openness in the next generation of doctors.

Formal complaints and educational activities, therefore, are epiphenomena. They're not the means by which most learning and development take place. In our daily work, this process of development—largely internalised and unrecorded—takes the form of constant sensitivity, responsiveness, and adaptability[802] to the needs of the individual patient in their unique situation.

Patient feedback needn't be separated from normal doctor-patient communication: it's possible to incorporate it into the consultation. Dissatisfaction isn't an aberration, but part of a range of normal human responses.

MEDICAL ERROR

Diagnostic error is inevitable. Mistakes with actual or potential harm occur frequently.[467] There are many organisations involved in addressing medical mishap and risk to patients,[803, 804, 805, 806, 807, 808, 809, 810, 809, 811, 812] guidelines to reduce error,[813] and mechanisms for reporting patient safety incidents.[814] A lot of work has been done in developed countries and in secondary care, and a little in primary care.[815, 816] Attempts have been made to categorise medical error in various ways, one attempt resulting in 23 major patient safety topics classified under the headings of structure, process, and outcome.[817] When causes of error are analysed, it's often found that the fault is in the system rather than in an individual, and parallels are drawn with other risky activities such as aviation from which it's thought medicine might learn.[818]

Healthcare appears to be a stable and reliable system for making mistakes,[716] and this state of affairs, while extensively studied and discussed, has defied remediation.[817]

It's remarkable how transparent this is. No other profession publishes so much evidence of fault[6] and no professional exposes their actions to the scrutiny of their peers more than the general practitioner referring a patient to hospital.[329] The UK complainant has the power to study their medical record and hold the professional to account, and the litigant is expected by medical defence organisations to receive an explanation and, where appropriate, an apology.[819] The legal profession may have led in such standards of professional ethics,[820] but medicine has caught up.

What's the scale of medical mishap? This is hard to quantify because it depends what's being measured. There's a steep gradient from error with the potential for harm—which is frequent—through actual harm and dissatisfaction with or without harm, to complaint or litigation—a court case being rare. In one study, of 53 mistakes reported by family physicians of which 47% were fatal, only four led to litigation.[821] There's also a discrepancy between what I read in the literature about high levels of disgruntlement and what my colleagues and I see in our practice from day to day—predominantly courteous, grateful patients and happy doctors.

DIAGNOSTIC ERROR

Diagnostic skill grows as medical knowledge is acquired, the two intertwining. Students learn biomedical facts which they apply in a clinical context,[822] learning iteratively, or spirally, covering the same topics repeatedly and developing progressively greater proficiency.[770] To what extent diagnostic skills can be taught is unclear.[823] For instance, having students use certain abstractions, such as 'recurrent cystitis' rather than 'cystitis three times over the last year', to help them generalise from the specific doesn't lead to greater diagnostic accuracy.[824] The student incorporates isolated facts and information processing skills into cognitive networks. Junior doctors gradually bypass intermediate steps and link basic concepts with clinical correlates. General practitioners develop a greater range of networks[825] and then proceed to illness scripts, which comprise pigeonholed diagnoses along with causes and consequences. They set clinical presentations against these prototypes and, using detailed knowledge, rapidly and efficiently test a hypothesis by means of a relatively small number of relevant questions.[731] Like expert chess players,[826] experienced clinicians don't generally have a longer list of alternatives than novices—they just have a better list. Furthermore what makes them more successful is not decontextualised reasoning ability but greater knowledge: their differential diagnosis is better than the novice's.[827] Non-experts—and experts solving non-routine problems—use backward reasoning[828] and refer sometimes to a long-buried biomedical fact.[822] So, a diagnostic pathway might begin with a presenting complaint or self-label and proceed to spot diagnosis or pattern recognition. Then there might be a series of loops involving forward and backward reasoning involving thought or spoken questions perhaps supplemented by a formal clinical prediction rule. Finalising the diagnosis might depend on test of treatment or of time.[829]

Research volunteers think mistakenly that the probability of either of two things happening singly is less than the probability of both of them happening together.[830] For doctors, this might be reinforced by the way we learn clusters of symptoms and signs. As a result, we don't realise how common variants of normal are in the general population. When experimental participants estimate the chance of something happening at the end of a chain of events, they tend to overestimate, probably because they assume on some level that the outcome of the first few events is definite rather than only possible.[831] A chain of events requires only one weak link for the whole chain to break. If we think that multiple links are more likely to remain intact than any one of them alone, we'll underestimate the risk of adverse outcomes. I suspect that this contributes to an unrealistic expectation that management will proceed according to plan.

Lay research participants calculate and intuit base rates inaccurately, partly because they're influenced by irrelevant information,[832] and they attribute chance events to skill.[833] Except at very low probabilities, when they overestimate probability, they tend to underestimate the probability of single events.[834]

Retrospectively, experimental participants remember their judgment about an outcome to have been better than it was at the time. Even if they're aware of the effect that knowledge of the outcome has on their recollection, they're unable to eliminate it. This reduces the educational impact of surprise at an unforeseen outcome and lessens their ability to learn from reviewing past events.[835]

So when we diagnose, we draw on past experience and acquired knowledge, weigh probabilities, and use a sophisticated combination of rules of thumb and more formal reasoning. Given that we don't do this perfectly, how can we improve?

MANAGING THE DIAGNOSIS

We must exercise our intelligence. Intelligence is described as the ability to be flexible, seize opportunities, negotiate ambiguity and contradiction, weigh evidence, spot hidden similarities and differences, identify patterns contained by and containing the clinical vignette, reformulate, and innovate.[106] Add humanity and community and I think we have the requirements for a diagnostician. Doctors in training—and that's all of us—must not settle for current orthodoxy but work, continually and with others, to create and share with colleagues new models of practice.

We must maintain a system of general practice in which experienced senior doctors are doing the most important part of the work: seeing patients. The transition in UK hospitals toward a service led by consultants rather than by juniors will lead to better care for patients and training for doctors:[836] we should be wary of a reverse trend in general practice with increasing numbers of trainees substituting for experienced general practitioners.

The use of patterns and rules of thumb works a lot of the time but can lead to diagnostic bias: one disease springs to mind more readily than another; the presentation bears a superficial relationship to an otherwise unrelated disease; it's difficult to separate likelihood of a diagnosis from its seriousness; the latest information is given disproportionate weight; supportive evidence is sought and weighted more than conflicting evidence; small probabilities are overestimated and large probabilities underestimated; corroborative detail gives verisimilitude;[837] having thought of a diagnosis we don't revise it enough; and seriousness is elided with probability.[825]

The use of rules of thumb is probably evolutionarily adaptive and efficient.[838] It doesn't require much conscious thought so we can apply our minds to other things[107]—such as the patient's unique story. Eliminating rules of thumb might be difficult and carries the risk of unintended consequences.[838] However, rules of thumb shouldn't be used exclusively. Premature closure during diagnosis should be consciously avoided by internal prompts to lengthen the diagnostic process such as: 'The diagnosis is this: What doesn't fit? What might not fit?'.[82] Like the auctioneer, we point at the highest bidder while looking elsewhere for 'any advance'.

The example of colorectal cancer will illustrate both the strengths and weaknesses of this approach. A sufficiently low risk of cancer might require no further action. At the other extreme, a barn door case, red flags, patient expectations, or doctor uncertainty might prompt immediate referral. Intermediate risk is hard to handle and one option is to temporise, reflect, perhaps discuss with colleagues, and see the patient again. Colorectal cancer is thought to arise in polyps and have an annual progression rate of 58% from Duke A to B, 66% from B to C and 86% from C to D.[438] It's not known whether delay in cancer diagnosis worsens mortality[839, 151] and it's possible that review before referral will improve the balance of benefit against risk. For what range of probability of cancer might the strategy of watchful waiting apply? Research results and clinical assessment are subject to error, both human and statistical. And scoring systems tend to be overconfident, underestimating low risk and overestimating high risk.[410] So we should be wary of false precision. Odds between, say, 1:100 and 1:20 might constitute a grey area within which judgment is particularly required. Disagreement or tension between patient and doctor makes sensible management of risk harder.[302] We might mitigate this by taking particular care to elicit and take account of the patient's views.

This example of colorectal cancer gives an account of the diagnostic problem along with a solution that is at best provisional. And it still doesn't convey the messiness of clinical practice. Overt diagnostic dilemmas—recognised as such at the time—are probably outnumbered by missed or late diagnoses that creep up on us and are obvious only in retrospect.

We deal with a wide range of problems, from the life-threatening to the trivial. We often don't know at the time how likely we are to have made a wrong decision and, if so, the likelihood, severity, or time course of the possible sequelae; decisions of minor consequence are often distinguishable from those with life-and-death importance only after the event. It's likely that the majority of adverse outcomes arise from these many situations of low apparent risk rather than the few situations of high risk.[98] Beneath a superficial repetitiveness, many of the judgments we make are specific to a unique context, a particular patient, with their own combination of illnesses, and a single decision balancing estimated risks against anticipated benefits in a situation of compromise. General practice consultations have an objectively higher complexity density per hour than cardiology or psychiatry consultations.[341] So how are we to spot the warning signs of a bad outcome? How do we know that we risk curtailing the diagnostic process, the patient's feedback or the consultation? And what can we do about it? Here are some observations.

If the patient starts the consultation with a briefly worded request with which we can't comply, we're likely to express less empathy: this scenario heralds conflict.[840] If we get upset,[841] the patient is likely to get upset as well.[162] A checklist of options—'agree, disagree, counsel, or refer'—might avert confrontation. When patients request sickness certificates, doctors are concerned that questioning them about fitness to work might compromise their relationship.[842] Patients don't always see it that way, value the opportunity to get advice about work, and might be disappointed if they don't get that opportunity.[843] It's easy to overlook the examination—because we've examined the patient before, because a specialist has examined them or because we get caught up in talking. This is risky. Remember to examine the part complained of. Finally, if we're having difficulty ending a consultation, something's probably going wrong[1] and it might be a good idea to continue the consultation or arrange a follow-up appointment.

When there's no single best treatment for a condition,[25] patient decision aids[354, 844] may be useful. They increase the likelihood of an informed decision based on the patient's values,[356] although there isn't always an aid available that suits the clinical or cultural context.[25] Electronic diagnostic aids might simply assist or actually direct:[845] real-time directive clinical decision aids that make recommendations during the consultation improve clinical practice.[237, 846, 847] Patients might benefit from sources of information or help beyond what the doctor can personally provide.

Information about these agencies can be stored as favourites on the computer for rapid access during the consultation. Patients might exchange experiences with others on-line[848] or access an expert patient programme that may improve self-efficacy and well-being.[849] They can also be given the opportunity to report drug adverse events.[850]

SUMMARY

In this chapter, I've dealt with two areas of risk: patient dissatisfaction resulting in complaints against the doctor and diagnostic error resulting in harm to the patient. I've argued that both patient dissatisfaction and diagnostic error can be mitigated by a consultation broad enough to encompass concerns about healthcare as well as about health, and a diagnostic mind that is always open to change. To summarise, I suggest we keep the consulting room large and the complaints form small. Clients appreciate diligence, punctuality, experience, and mastery of subject.[851] Patients also want us to be good listeners.

EXERCISE

Think back to a recent consultation in which you felt particularly uneasy about the possibility of a missed diagnosis. Deliberately review your latest surgery to see if, on reflection, any of your diagnoses were too hasty or uncritical. How did these situations come about? What can you learn for the future?

References

1. Byrne PS, Long BEL. *Doctors Talking to Patients: a study of the verbal behaviour of general practitioners consulting in their surgeries.* Exeter: RCGP; 1976.
2. Heath I. The Mystery of General Practice. In: *Matters of Life and Death: key writings.* Oxford: Radcliffe Publishing; 2008.
3. Hudson RA. *Sociolinguistics.* Cambridge: Cambridge University Press; 1996.
4. Balint M. Repeat-Prescription Patients—are they an identifiable group? In: Balint M, editor. *Treatment or Diagnosis: a study of repeat prescriptions in general practice.* London: Tavistock Publications; 1970.
5. Sackett DL, Rosenberg WM, Gray JA, Haynes RB, Richardson WS. Evidence-based medicine: what it is and what it isn't. *BMJ.* 1996; **312**(7023): 71–2.
6. Cochrane AL. *Effectiveness and Efficiency: random reflections on health services.* London: RSM Press; 1999.
7. Snow CP. The two cultures. In: *The Two Cultures.* Cambridge: Cambridge University Press; 1993.
8. Snow CP. The two cultures: a second look (1963). In: *The Two Cultures.* Cambridge: Cambridge University Press; 1993.
9. Meza J, Passerman D. *Integrating Narrative Medicine and Evidence-based Medicine: the everyday social practice of healing.* Oxford: Radcliffe Publishing; 2011.
10. Kuhn TS. *The Structure of Scientific Revolutions.* 2nd ed. Chicago: University of Chicago Press; 1970.
11. Loftus S, Higgs J. Learning the language of clinical reasoning. In: Higgs J, Jones MA, Loftus S, Christensen N, editors. *Clinical reasoning in the health professions.* Philadelphia: Elsevier Health Sciences; 2008.
12. Hannay DR. *The Symptom Iceberg: a study of community health.* London: Routledge & Kegan Paul; 1979.
13. Last JM. The iceberg "completing the clinical picture" in general practice. *Lancet.* 1963; **282**(7297): 28–31.
14. Cavell S. *Must We Mean What We Say? a book of essays.* Cambridge: Cambridge University Press; 1969.
15. *RCGP Position Statement on Climate Change and Health.* RCGP; 2010. Available at: www.rcgp.org.uk/pdf/Position_Statement_Climate_Change_and_Health.pdf
16. *The Millennium Development Goals Report.* United Nations Department of Economic and Social Affairs; 2010. Available at: www.un.org/millenniumgoals/pdf/MDG%20Report%202010%20En%20r15%20-low%20res%2020100615%20-.pdf

17. *World Health Report 2008. Primary Health Care: now more than ever.* World Health Organisation; 2008. Available at: www.who.int/whr/2008/whr08_en.pdf

18. *RCGP GP Curriculum Statements (revised January 2010).* RCGP; 2010 [cited 2010 Sep 5]. Available at: www.rcgp-curriculum.org.uk/PDF/curr_1_Curriculum_Statement_Being_a_GP.pdf

19. *Royal College of General Practitioners—RCGP Curriculum Site: Competence framework.* [cited 2010 Oct 21]. Available at: www.rcgp-curriculum.org.uk/nmrcgp/wpba/competence_framework.aspx

20. *General Medical Council. Revalidation—GMP framework for appraisal and revalidation.* 2010 Oct 19 [cited 2010 Oct 27]. Available at: www.gmc-uk.org/doctors/revalidation/revalidation_gmp_framework.asp

21. Cruess R, Cruess S. Expectations and obligations: professionalism and medicine's social contract with society. *Perspectives in Biology and Medicine.* 2008; **51**(4): 579–99.

22. Fugelli P. James Mackenzie Lecture. Trust—in general practice. *BJGP.* 2001; **51**(468): 575–9.

23. Jutel A. *Self-Diagnosis: a discursive systematic review of the medical literature.* Journal of Participatory Medicine. 2010 Sep [cited 2010 Nov 8]. Available at: www.jopm.org/evidence/research/2010/09/15/self-diagnosis-a-discursive-systematic-review-of-the-medical-literature/

24. Grime J, Richardson JC, Ong BN. Perceptions of joint pain and feeling well in older people who reported being healthy: a qualitative study. *BJGP.* 2010; **60**: 597–603.

25. Higgs J, Jones MA. Clinical decision making and multiple problem spaces. In: Higgs J, Jones MA, Loftus S, Christensen N, editors. *Clinical reasoning in the health professions.* Philadelphia: Elsevier Health Sciences; 2008.

26. Marinker M. Journey to the interior: the search for academic general practice. *J R Coll Gen Pract.* 1987; **37**(302): 385–8.

27. Kennedy I. *The Unmasking of Medicine: a searching look at health care today.* London: Granada Publishing; 1983.

28. Helman C. Diseases versus illness in general practice. *BJGP.* 1981; **31**: 548–52.

29. Lukes S. *Power: a radical view.* London: Macmillan Press Ltd; 1974.

30. Silverman DJ, Kurtz SM, Draper J. *Skills for communicating with patients.* Oxford: Radcliffe Publishing; 2005.

31. Adler RH. Engel's biopsychosocial model is still relevant today. *Journal of Psychosomatic Research.* 2009; **67**(6): 607–11.

32. Engel GL. The need for a new medical model: a challenge for biomedicine. *Science.* 1977; **196**(4286): 129–36.

33. Marinker M. Sirens, stray dogs, and the narrative of Hilda Thomson. In: Greenhalgh T, Hurwitz B, editors. *Narrative Based Medicine: dialogue and discourse in clinical practice.* London: BMJ Books; 1998.

34. Launer J. *Narrative-Based Primary Care: a practical guide.* Oxford: Radcliffe Publishing; 2002.

35. Marinker M. Studies of contact behaviour in a general practice. I. An exposition of methods and a consideration of meanings. *J R Coll Gen Pract.* 1967; **14**(1): 59–66.

36. Okkes IM, Polderman GO, Fryer GE, Yamada T, Bujak M, Oskam SK, *et al.* The role of family practice in different health care systems: a comparison of reasons

for encounter, diagnoses, and interventions in primary care populations in the Netherlands, Japan, Poland, and the United States. *J Fam Pract.* 2002; **51**(1): 31–6.

37. Mathers N, Rowland S. General practice—a post-modern specialty? *BJGP.* 1997; **47**(416): 177–9.

38. Porter R. *Blood and Guts: a short history of medicine.* New York: Penguin Books; 2002.

39. Lawrence C. 'Definite and Material': coronary thrombosis and cardiologists in the 1920s. In: Rosenberg CE, Golden J, editors. *Framing Disease: studies in cultural history.* New Brunswick, New Jersey: Rutgers University Press; 1992.

40. Guidance for doctors completing Medical Certificates of Cause of Death in England and Wales. 2008 Sep [cited 2010 Dec 19]. Available at: http://nazshua.blog.com/files/2010/12/Death-Cert-1.pdf

41. Health Protection Agency. *List of notifiable diseases.* 2010 Apr [cited 2010 Dec 19]. Available at: www.hpa.org.uk/Topics/InfectiousDiseases/InfectionsAZ/NotificationsOfInfectiousDiseases/ListOfNotifiableDiseases/

42. Peitzman SJ. From Bright's disease to end-stage renal disease. In: Rosenberg CE, Golden J, editors. *Framing Disease: studies in cultural history.* New Brunswick, New Jersey: Rutgers University Press; 1992.

43. Department of Health. National Service Framework for Renal Services—*Part Two: chronic kidney disease, acute renal failure and end of life care.* 2005 Feb [cited 2010 Nov 29]. Available at: www.dh.gov.uk/en/Publicationsandstatistics/Publications/PublicationsPolicyAndGuidance/DH_4101902

44. Spence D. Bad medicine: chronic kidney disease. *BMJ.* 2010 6; **340**(jun16 1): c3188–c3188.

45. Launer J. Narrative and Mental Health in Primary Care. In: Greenhalgh T, Hurwitz B, editors. *Narrative Based Medicine: dialogue and discourse in clinical practice.* London: BMJ Books; 1998.

46. Dowrick C. *Beyond Depression: a new approach to understanding and management.* 2nd ed. Oxford: Oxford University Press; 2009.

47. Szasz TS. *The Myth of Mental Illness: foundations of a theory of personal conduct.* St Albans, Herts: Paladin; 1962.

48. Reed P. *The One.* Edinburgh: Crescent; 2003.

49. UJJAY. This is my story. *The Haven: hearing voices network.* 2010 Spring; **28**: 6–7.

50. Campbell P. Hearing my voice. *The Psychologist.* 2007; **20**(5): 198–9.

51. Boyle M. The problem with diagnosis. *The Psychologist.* 2007; **20**(5): 290–2.

52. Moncrieff J. Diagnosis and drug treatment. *The Psychologist.* 2007; **20**(5): 296–7.

53. Wykes T, Callard F. Diagnosis, diagnosis, diagnosis: towards DSM-5. *J Ment Health.* 2010; **19**(4): 301–4.

54. Stannus HS. Memorandum. Typescript. 1927 Feb 3; Bodleian Library of Commonwealth and African Studies at Rhodes House, Oxford.

55. Brumber JJ. From Psychiatric Syndrome to "Communicable" Disease: the case of anorexia nervosa. In: Rosenberg CE, Golden J, editors. *Framing Disease: studies in cultural history.* New Brunswick, New Jersey: Rutgers University Press; 1992.

56. Zimmerman M. Is underdiagnosis the main pitfall in diagnosing bipolar disorder? No. *BMJ.* 2010; **340**(Feb 22_1): c855.

57. MacNee W. 15.6 Chronic obstructive pulmonary disease. In: Warrell DA, Cox TM, Firth JD, Benz EJ, editors. *Oxford Textbook of Medicine*. Oxford: Oxford University Press; 2003.

58. *Definition, Diagnosis and Classification of Diabetes Mellitus and its Complications. Part 1: diagnosis and classification of diabetes mellitus*. Geneva: World Health Organization Department of Noncommunicable Disease Surveillance; 1999.

59. NICE. CG108 Chronic heart failure: quick reference guide. 2010 [cited 2010 Sep 21]. Available at: http://guidance.nice.org.uk/CG108/QuickRefGuide/pdf/English

60. *Preamble to the Constitution of the World Health Organization as adopted by the International Health Conference*. New York: World Health Organization; 1946 [cited 2010 Nov 6]. Available at: www.who.int/about/definition/en/print.html

61. Plant M, Robertson R, Miller P, Plant M. *Drug Nation: patterns, problems, panics and policies*. Oxford: Oxford University Press; 2011.

62. *Disability Living Allowance—medical examination: Directgov—Disabled people*. [cited 2010 Dec 14]. Available at: www.direct.gov.uk/en/DisabledPeople/FinancialSupport/DisabilityLivingAllowance/DG_10022605

63. *Incapacity Benefit—Personal Capability Assessment: Directgov—Disabled people*. [cited 2010 Dec 14]. Available at: www.direct.gov.uk/en/DisabledPeople/FinancialSupport/IncapacityBenefit/DG_10023130

64. *IPC Classification Code and International Standards*. 2007 Nov [cited 2010 Dec 14]. Available at: www.paralympic.org/export/sites/default/IPC/Reference_Documents/2008_2_Classification_Code6.pdf

65. *What is Classification?* 2010 [cited 2010 Dec 14]. Available at: www.uksportsassociation.org/athlete_classification/procedure.html

66. Gardner DSL, Hosking J, Metcalf BS, Jeffery AN, Voss LD, Wilkin TJ. Contribution of early weight gain to childhood overweight and metabolic health: a longitudinal study (EarlyBird 36). *Pediatrics*. 2009; **123**(1): e67–3.

67. Kessler DA. *The End of Overeating*. London: Penguin; 2009.

68. Westendorp RGJ, Kirkwood. The biology of ageing. In: Bond J, Peace S, Dittman-Kohli F, Westerhof G, editors. *Ageing in Society: European perspectives on gerontology*. London: SAGE; 2007.

69. Plato. *The Dialogues of Plato*. 3rd ed. London: Oxford University Press; 1931.

70. Gillon R. *Philosophical Medical Ethics*. Chichester: Wiley; 1986.

71. Haidt J. *The Happiness Hypothesis: putting ancient wisdom and philosophy to the test of modern science*. London: Arrow Books; 2006.

72. Tännsjö T. Moral dimensions. *BMJ*. 2005; **331**(7518): 689–91.

73. Macartney FJ. Diagnostic logic. In: Phillips CI, editor. *Logic in Medicine*. London: BMJ Publishing Group; 1995.

74. Cohen JJ. Viewpoint: linking professionalism to humanism: what it means, why it matters. *Academic Medicine*. 2007; **82**(11): 1029–32.

75. New Gold Foundation. [cited 2010 Dec 11]. Available at: www.humanism-in-medicine.org/index.php

76. Hope T, Hope S, Foster C. Turning a blind eye to crime: health professionals and the Sexual Offences Act 2003. *BJGP*. 2010; **60**: 64–5.

77. General Medical Council. Confidentiality. 2009 [cited 2010 Jun 21]. Available at: www.gmc-uk.org/guidance/ethical_guidance/confidentiality.asp

78. Bhandari S. A single-centre audit of junior doctors' diagnostic activity in medical admissions. *J R Coll Physicians Edinb*. 2009; **39**(4): 307–12.

79. Weed LL. Medical records that guide and teach. *N Engl J Med.* 1968; **278**(12): 652–7.

80. Scott B. *Health Record and Communication Practice Standards for Team Based Care Version 1.0.* NHS Health Records and Communication Practice Standards Group; 2004 [cited 2010 Dec 30]. Available at: www.isb.nhs.uk/about/leadership/healthrec_compractice.pdf

81. *Quality and Service Improvement Tools: SBAR—situation—background—assessment—recommendation.* [cited 2010 Dec 11]. Available at: www.institute.nhs.uk/quality_and_service_improvement_tools/quality_and_service_improvement_tools/sbar_-_situation_-_background_-_assessment_-_recommendation.html

82. Norman GR, Eva KW. Diagnostic error and clinical reasoning. *Med Educ.* 2010; **44**(1): 94–100.

83. Irby DM, Wilkerson L. Teaching when time is limited. *BMJ.* 2008; **336**(7640): 384–7.

84. Van Houdt S, De Lepeleire J. Does the use of care plans improve the quality of home care? *Qual Prim Care.* 2010; **18**(3): 161–72.

85. Iliffe S, Peacock S, Seecharan A, *et al.* Making a jigsaw puzzle in ten minutes: is case management feasible in general practice? *London J Primary Care* 2011; 1–9. Available at: www.londonjournalofprimarycare.org.uk/articles/4244872.pdf

86. Marcoen A, Coleman PG, O'Hanlon. Psychological Ageing. In: Bond J, Peace S, Dittman-Kohli F, Westerhof G, editors. *Ageing in Society: European perspectives on gerontology.* London: SAGE; 2007.

87. Soanes C, Stevenson A. *Oxford Dictionary of English.* 2nd ed. Oxford: Oxford University Press; 2006.

88. Pinker S. *The Stuff of Thought: language as a window into human nature.* London: Penguin Books; 2008.

89. The Way. In: *World Philosophies: an historical introduction.* Oxford: Blackwell; 1996.

90. Blumhagen D. Hyper-Tension: a folk illness with a medical name. *Cult Med Psychiatry.* 1980; **4**(3): 197–224.

91. Wessely S, White PD. There is only one functional somatic syndrome. *The British Journal of Psychiatry.* 2004; **185**(2): 95–6

92. Croft P. Aches and pains in primary care: stay positive but critical. *BJGP.* 2010; **60**(571): 79–80.

93. Launer J. *How not to be a doctor, and other essays.* London: Royal Society of Medicine Press; 2007.

94. Stewart M, Brown J, Weston W, McWhinney I, McWilliam C, Freeman T. *Patient-Centered Medicine: transforming the clinical method.* London: Sage Publications, Inc.; 1995.

95. Kay J. Obliquity: *Why our goals are best achieved indirectly.* London: Profile Books; 2010.

96. Loftus S, Smith M. A history of clinical reasoning research. In: Higgs J, Jones MA, Loftus S, Christensen N, editors. *Clinical reasoning in the health professions.* Philadelphia: Elsevier Health Sciences; 2008.

97. Barbour A. *Caring for Patients: a critique of the medical model.* Stanford, CA: Stanford University Press; 1997.

98. Rose G. Sick individuals and sick populations. *International Journal of Epidemiology.* 2001; **30**(3): 427–32.

99. Morris L, Cameron J, Brown C, Wyatt JC. Sharing summary care records: results from Scottish emergency care summary. *BMJ*. 2010; **341**(8): c4305.

100. Tuckett D, Boulton M, Olson C, Williams A. *Meetings Between Experts: an approach to sharing ideas in medical consultations*. London: Tavistock Publications; 1985.

101. Herxheimer A. Principles of clinical pharmacology and drug therapy. In: Warrell DA, Cox TM, Firth JD, Benz EJ, editors. *Oxford Textbook of Medicine*. Oxford: Oxford University Press; 2003.

102. Ellis CG. Making dysphoria a happy experience. *BMJ (Clin Res Ed)*. 1986; **293**(6542): 317–18.

103. Gerrard TJ, Riddell JD. Difficult patients: black holes and secrets. *BMJ*. 1988; **297**(6647): 530–2.

104. Marinker M. Peace. In: Balint M, editor. *Treatment or Diagnosis: a study of repeat prescriptions in general practice*. London: Tavistock Publications; 1970.

105. Hunt J. Disturbances. In: Balint M, editor. *Treatment or Diagnosis: a study of repeat prescriptions in general practice*. London: Tavistock Publications; 1970.

106. Hofstadter DH. *Gödel, Escher, Bach*. Harmondsworth, Middlesex: Penguin Books; 1980.

107. Whitehead AN. *An Introduction to Mathematics*. Oxford: OUP; 1911.

108. Kuenssberg EV. Recording of morbidity of families: F. Book. *J Coll Gen Pract*. 1964; **7**: 410–22.

109. Morrell DC. *The Art of General Practice*. Oxford: Oxford University Press; 1991.

110. Freeman G, Hughes J. *Continuity of Care and the Patient Experience: an inquiry into the quality of general practice in England*. London: The King's Fund; 2010.

111. Treasure W. The primary care electronic health record: who's righting the software? *BJGP*. 2011; **61**(583): 152–4.

112. Jordan K, Porcheret M, Croft P. Quality of morbidity coding in general practice computerized medical records: a systematic review. *Fam Pract*. 2004; **21**(4): 396–412.

113. Mant J, Murphy M, Rose P, Vessey M. The accuracy of general practitioner records of smoking and alcohol use: comparison with patient questionnaires. *J Public Health Med*. 2000; **22**(2): 198–201.

114. Al-Agilly S, Neville R, Robb H, Riddell S. Involving patients in checking the validity of the NHS shared record: a single practice pilot. *Inform Prim Care*. 2007; **15**(4): 217–20.

115. García Rodríguez LA, Ruigómez A. Case validation in research using large databases. *BJGP*. 2010; **60**(572): 160–1.

116. Smith GE, Cooper DL, Loveridge P, Chinemana F, Gerard E, Verlander N. A national syndromic surveillance system for England and Wales using calls to a telephone helpline. *European Surveillance*. 2006; **11**(12): pii–667.

117. Treasure W. Data, please (letter). *BMJ*. 2009; **339**(Aug 11_1): b3247.

118. *Flu Watch*. [cited 2010 Dec 5]. Available at: www.fluwatch.co.uk/

119. Greenhalgh T, Potts HWW, Wong G, Bark P, Swinglehurst D. Tensions and paradoxes in electronic patient record research: a systematic literature review using the meta-narrative method. *Milbank Q*. 2009; **87**(4): 729–88.

120. Hodge P. The White Paper: a framework for survival? (commentary on a letter). *BJGP*. 2010; **60**(579): 782.

121. *Homosexuality and Sexual Orientation Disturbance: Proposed Change in DSM-II, 6th Printing, page 44 position statement (retired)*. 1973 Nov [cited 2010 Nov 25]. Available at: www.psychiatryonline.com/DSMPDF/DSM-II_Homosexuality_Revision.pdf

122. Treasure W. An examination of the ways in which the primary care electronic patient record in one practice fails to meet national guidelines. Poster at RCGP Conference, Oct. 2010.

123. Greenhalgh T, Hurwitz B. Why Study Narrative? In: Greenhalgh T, Hurwitz B, editors. *Narrative Based Medicine: dialogue and discourse in clinical practice.* London: BMJ Books; 1998.

124. Donald A. The Words We Live In. In: Greenhalgh T, Hurwitz B, editors. *Narrative Based Medicine: dialogue and discourse in clinical practice.* London: BMJ Books; 1998.

125. Spence SJC. *The Purpose and Practice of Medicine: selections from the writings of Sir James Spence.* Oxford: Oxford University Press; 1960.

126. Elwyn G, Gwyn R. Stories We Hear and Stories We Tell … analysing talk in clinical practice. In: Greenhalgh T, Hurwitz B, editors. *Narrative Based Medicine: dialogue and discourse in clinical practice.* London: BMJ Books; 1998.

127. Goyal RK, Charon R, Lekas H, Fullilove MT, Devlin MJ, Falzon L, *et al.* 'A local habitation and a name': how narrative evidence-based medicine transforms the translational research paradigm. *J Eval Clin Pract.* 2008; **14**(5): 732–41.

128. Hayward M, Slade M. Getting better … who decides? *The Psychologist.* 2008; **21**(3): 198–200.

129. Brody H. Foreword. In: Greenhalgh T, Hurwitz B, editors. *Narrative Based Medicine: dialogue and discourse in clinical practice.* London: BMJ Books; 1998.

130. Macnaughton J. Anecdote in Clinical Practice. In: Greenhalgh T, Hurwitz B, editors. *Narrative Based Medicine: dialogue and discourse in clinical practice.* London: BMJ Books; 1998.

131. Dixon A. There's a lot of it about: clinical strategies in family practice. *J R Coll Gen Pract.* 1986; **36**(291): 468–71.

132. Hansen MP, Bjerrum L, Gahrn-Hansen B, Jarbol DE. Quality indicators for diagnosis and treatment of respiratory tract infections in general practice: a modified Delphi study. *Scandinavian Journal of Primary Health Care.* 2010; **28**(1): 411.

133. Jones R, Barraclough K, Dowrick C. When no diagnostic label is applied. *BMJ.* 2010; **340**(7759): c2683.

134. Levenstein JH, McCrackend EC, McWhinney IR, Stewart MA, Brown JB. The patient-centred clinical method. 1. A model for the doctor-patient interaction in family medicine. *Fam Pract.* 1986; **3**(1): 24–30.

135. Shepherd J, Blauw GJ, Murphy MB, Bollen EL, Buckley BM, Cobbe SM, *et al.* Pravastatin in elderly individuals at risk of vascular disease (PROSPER): a randomised controlled trial. *Lancet.* 2002; **360**(9346): 1623–30.

136. Hall PS, Lord SR, El-Laboudi A, Seymour MT. Non-cancer medications for patients with incurable cancer: time to stop and think? *BJGP.* 2010; **60**: 243–4.

137. Okkes IM, Oskam SK, Lamberts H. The probability of specific diagnoses for patients presenting with common symptoms to Dutch family physicians. *J Fam Pract.* 2002; **51**(1): 31–6.

138. McNally M, Curtain J, O'Brien KK, Dimitrov BD, Fahey T. Validity of British Thoracic Society guidance (the CRB-65 rule) for predicting the severity of pneumonia in general practice: systematic review and meta-analysis. *BJGP.* 2010; **60**(579): 423–33.

139. Lim WS, Baudouin SV, George RC, Hill AT, Jamieson C, Le Jeune I, *et al*. BTS guidelines for the management of community acquired pneumonia in adults: update 2009. *Thorax*. 2009; **64**(Suppl 3): iii1–55.
140. Freedman D. *Out-of-hours Reporting of Laboratory Results Requiring Urgent Clinical Action to Primary Care: advice to pathologists and those that work in laboratory medicine.* (Version number 3., G025). The Royal College of Pathologists; 2010 [cited 2010 Dec 26]. Available at: www.rcpath.org/resources/pdf/g025_outofhoursreporting_nov10.pdf
141. Nash CE, Mickan SM, Del Mar CB, Glasziou PP. Resting injured limbs delays recovery: a systematic review. *J Fam Pract*. 2004; **53**(9): 706–12.
142. Chamnan P, Simmons RK, Khaw KT, Wareham NJ, Griffin SJ. Estimating the population impact of screening strategies for identifying and treating people at high risk of cardiovascular disease: modelling study. *BMJ*. 2010; **340**(Apr 23_2): c1693.
143. Whitehead AN. *Science and the Modern World*. Cambridge: Cambridge University Press; 1946.
144. NICE. *CG069 Respiratory tract infections—antibiotic prescribing*. 2008 [cited 2010 Dec 11]. Available at: www.nice.org.uk/nicemedia/pdf/CG69FullGuideline.pdf
145. Morgenstern H. Uses of ecologic analysis in epidemiologic research. *Am J Public Health*. 1982; **72**(12): 1336–44.
146. Robinson WS. Ecological correlations and the behavior of individuals. *American Sociological Review*. 1950; **15**(3): 351–7.
147. Mallen CD, Peat G, Thomas E, Dunn K, Croft P. Prognostic factors for musculoskeletal pain in primary care: a systematic review. *BJGP*. 2007; **57**: 655–61.
148. Mayes R, Horwitz AV. DSM-III and the revolution in the classification of mental illness. *J Hist Behav Sci*. 2005; **41**(3): 249–67.
149. Albertsen PC, Hanley JA, Fine J. 20-year outcomes following conservative management of clinically localized prostate cancer. JAMA. 2005; **293**(17): 2095–101.
150. Nelson HD, Tyne K, Naik A, Bougatsos C, Chan BK, Humphrey L. Screening for breast cancer: an update for the U.S. Preventive Services Task Force. *Annals of Internal Medicine*. 2009; **151**(10): 727–37.
151. Neal RD. Do diagnostic delays in cancer matter? *Br J Cancer*. 2009; **101**(Suppl 2): S9–12.
152. Alwin N, Blackburn R, Davidson K, Hilton M, Logan C, Shine J. *Understanding Personality Disorder: a report by the British Psychological Society*. Leicester: The British Psychological Society; 2006 [cited 2010 Nov 25]. Available at: www.bps.org.uk/downloadfile.cfm?file_uuid=28ECFB5B-1143-DFD0-7E28-C7CDA21A3E7F&ext=pdf&restricted=true
153. Haynes RB, You JJ. The architecture of diagnostic research. In: Knottnerus JA, Buntinx F, editors. *The Evidence Base of Clinical Diagnosis: theory and methods of diagnostic research*. Oxford: John Wiley and Sons; 2009.
154. Robertson A. A good diagnosis. *JRCGP*. 1970; **19**: 311–14.
155. Silva SA, Charon R, Wyer PC. The marriage of evidence and narrative: scientific nurturance within clinical practice. *J Eval Clin Pract*. 2010 Nov 10 [cited 2010 Jan 7]. Available at: www.ncbi.nlm.nih.gov/pubmed/21062389
156. Dowrick CF, Ring A, Humphris GM, Salmon P. Normalisation of unexplained symptoms by general practitioners: a functional typology. *BJGP*. 2004; **54**(500): 165–70.

157. Kostopoulou O, Delaney BC, Munro CW. Diagnostic difficulty and error in primary care—a systematic review. *Fam Pract.* 2008; **25**(6): 400–13.

158. Boyd K, Murray SA. Recognising and managing key transitions in end of life care. *BMJ.* 2010; **341**(sep 16_2): c4863.

159. Gill TM, Gahbauer EAM, Han LM, Allore HG. Trajectories of Disability in the Last Year of Life. *N Engl J Med.* 2010; **362**(13): 1173–80.

160. Braithwaite RS, Concato J, Chang CC, Roberts MS, Justice AC. A framework for tailoring clinical guidelines to comorbidity at the point of care. *Arch Intern Med.* 2007; **167**(21): 2361–5.

161. Lee SJ, Lindquist K, Segal MR, Covinsky KE. Development and validation of a prognostic index for 4-year mortality in older adults. *JAMA.* 2006; **295**(7): 801–8.

162. Kübler-Ross E. *On Death and Dying.* London: Tavistock Publications; 1970.

163. Clark B. *Whose Life Is It Anyway?* London: Heinemann; 1978.

164. Schneider JA, Arvanitakis Z, Leurgans SE, Bennett DA. The neuropathology of probable Alzheimer's disease and mild cognitive impairment. *Ann Neurol.* 2009; **66**(2): 200–8.

165. Richards M, Brayne C. What do we mean by Alzheimer's disease? *BMJ.* 2010; **341**(oct 12_2): c4670.

166. Greaves I, Jolley D. National Dementia Strategy: well intentioned—but how well founded and how well directed? *BJGP.* 2010; **60**(572): 193–8.

167. Greaves I, Jolley D. National Dementia Strategy: well intentioned—but how well founded and how well directed? *BJGP.* 2010; **60**(572): 193–8.

168. Murray SA. Illness trajectories and palliative care. *BMJ.* 2005; **330**(7498): 1007–11.

169. Albertsson DM, Mellström D, Petersson C, Eggertsen R. Validation of a 4-item score predicting hip fracture and mortality risk among elderly women. *Ann Fam Med.* 2007; **5**(1): 48–56.

170. Bentall RP. Researching psychotic complaints. *The Psychologist.* 2007; **20**(5): 293–5.

171. Polmear A. *Evidence-Based Diagnosis in Primary Care.* Oxford: Elsevier Health Sciences; 2008.

172. Canguilhem G. *The Normal and the Pathological.* New York: Zone Books; 1991.

173. Meador CK. *Symptoms of Unknown Origin.* Nashville, TN: Vanderbilt University Press; 2005.

174. Stone J. What should we say to patients with symptoms unexplained by disease? The 'number needed to offend'. *BMJ.* 2002; **325**(7378): 1449–50.

175. Dowrick C, Katona C, Peveler R, Lloyd H. Somatic symptoms and depression: diagnostic confusion and clinical neglect. *BJGP.* 2005; **55**(520): 829–30.

176. Thistlethwaite J, Morris P. *The Patient-Doctor Consultation in Primary Care.* London: Royal College of General Practitioners; 2006.

177. Kanaan RAA, Wessely SC. The origins of factitious disorder. *Hist Human Sci.* 2010; **23**(2): 68–85.

178. Burton C. Beyond somatisation: a review of the understanding and treatment of medically unexplained physical symptoms (MUPS). *BJGP.* 2003; **53**: 231–9.

179. Firth J. Idiopathic oedema of women. In: Warrell DA, Cox TM, Firth JD, Benz EJ, editors. *Oxford textbook of medicine.* Oxford: Oxford University Press. 2003. [cited 2011 July 24]. Available at: http://ovidsp.uk.ovid.com/sp-3.4.1b/ovidweb.cgi?&S=NKLOPDHLEBHFDNNGFNBLECAGPEPPAA00&Link+Set=S.sh.37|3|sl_11297244

180. Mayou R, Farmer A. ABC of psychological medicine: functional somatic symptoms and syndromes. *BMJ*. 2002; **325**(7358): 265–8.

181. Goadsby PJ. Medically unexplained symptoms: (Letter 2 of 5). *J R Soc Med*. 2003; **96**(7): 368–b.

182. Balint M. *The Doctor, His Patient, and the Illness*. New York: International Universities Press; 1957.

183. Bland JM, Altman DG. Statistic notes: regression towards the mean. *BMJ*. 1994; **308**(6942): 1499.

184. Ryle G. *The Concept of Mind*. Harmondsworth, Middlesex: Hutchinson; 1949.

185. Carson A, Sharpe M. *Scottish Neurological Symptoms Study Final Report: executive summary*. Edinburgh: School of Molecular and Clinical Medicine, University of Edinburgh; 2005.

186. Eich, Brodkin IA, Reeves JL, Chawla AF. Questions Concerning Pain. In: Kahneman D, Diener E, Schwarz N, editors. *Well-Being: the foundations of hedonic psychology*. New York: Russell Sage Foundation; 2003.

187. Schön DA. *Educating the Reflective Practitioner: toward a new design for teaching and learning in the professions*. San Francisco: Jossey-Bass; 1987.

188. Irish B, Patterson F. Selecting general practice specialty trainees: where next? *BJGP*. 2010; **60**(580): 849–52.

189. Warburton N. *Thinking from A to Z*. London: Routledge; 2000.

190. Bonnett A. *How to Argue*. Harlow, Essex: Pearson Education; 2001.

191. Holmes J. Narrative in Psychotherapy. In: Greenhalgh T, Hurwitz B, editors. *Narrative Based Medicine: dialogue and discourse in clinical practice*. London: BMJ Books; 1998.

192. Wanless D. *Our Future Health Secured: a review of NHS funding and performance*. The King's Fund; 2007 [cited 2010 Nov 10]. Available at: www.kingsfund.org.uk/applications/site_search/?term=wanless+2007&searchreferer_id=0&searchreferer_url=%2Fapplications%2Fsite_search%2Findex.rm&submit.x=0&submit.y=0

193. Lakhani M, Baker M, Field S. *The Future Direction of General Practice: a roadmap*. Royal College of General Practitioners; 2008. Available at: www.rcgp.org.uk/pdf/CIRC_RCGP%20Roadmap%20Future%20General%20Practice%2013th%20Sept%202007.pdf

194. Beattie A. *False Economy: a surprising economic history of the world*. New York: Penguin Group USA; 2009.

195. Royal College of General Practitioners—Patients P3. [cited 2010 Aug 26]. Available at: www.rcgp.org.uk/college_locations/rcgp_scotland/about_us/patients_p3.aspx

196. NHS Direct. [cited 2010 Nov 22]. Available at: www.nhsdirect.nhs.uk/

197. NHS choices. [cited 2010 Nov 22]. Available at: www.nhs.uk/Pages/HomePage.aspx

198. Department of Health. *Walk-in centres and GP health centres*. [cited 2010 May 7]. Available at: www.dh.gov.uk/en/Healthcare/Primarycare/WalkincentresandGPhealthcentres/index.htm

199. Pollock AM, Leys C, Price D, Rowland D, Gnani S. *NHS plc: the privatisation of our health care*. London: Verso; 2006.

200. WONCA. *The European Definition of General Practice/Family Medicine—2005*. 2005 [cited 2010 Aug 14]. Available at: www.woncaeurope.org/definition%20GP-FM.htm

201. Heath I. Connections. In: *Matters of Life and Death: key writings*. Oxford: Radcliffe Publishing; 2008.

202. Kringos DS, Boerma WGW, Hutchinson A, van der Zee J, Groenewegen PP. The breadth of primary care: a systematic literature review of its core dimensions. *BMC Health Serv Res.* 2010; **10**: 65.

203. Scruton R. *The Uses of Pessimism.* Oxford: Atlantic Books; 2010.

204. Delamothe T. A comprehensive service. *BMJ.* 2008; **336**(7657): 1344–5.

205. Kiesler DJ, Auerbach SM. Optimal matches of patient preferences for information, decision-making and interpersonal behavior: evidence, models and interventions. *Patient Education and Counseling.* 2006; **61**(3): 319–41.

206. RCGP. Clinical Skills Assessment. RCGP Curriculum Home: MRCGP: CSA. [cited 2010 Nov 6]. Available at: www.rcgp-curriculum.org.uk/nmrcgp/csa.aspx

207. Sokol DK. How to think like an ethicist. *BMJ.* 2010; **340**(7761): c3256.

208. Sen AK. *Development as Freedom.* Oxford: Oxford University Press; 1999.

209. Schwartz B. *The Paradox of Choice: why more is less.* New York: HarperCollins; 2005.

210. Hunter DJ. *The Health Debate.* Bristol: The Policy Press; 2008.

211. Protheroe J, Bower P. Choosing, deciding, or participating: what do patients want in primary care? *BJGP.* 2008; **58**(554): 603–4.

212. McPherson A. More brickbats than bouquets? *BMJ.* 2010; **341**(Jul 28_2): c3977.

213. Mathers N, Mitchell C. Are the gates to be thrown open? *BJGP.* 2010; **60**(574): 317–18.

214. Abel-Smith B. Foreword. In: *The Division in British Medicine: a history of the separation of general practice from hospital care, 1911–68.* New York: Kogan Page; 1979.

215. Coulter A. Do patients want a choice and does it work? *BMJ.* 2010; **341**(Oct 14_2): c4989.

216. Thaler RH, Sunstein CR. *Nudge: improving decisions about health, wealth, and happiness.* London: Penguin Books; 2009.

217. Schneider H, Palmer N. Getting to the Truth? Researching user views of primary health care. *Health Policy Plan.* 2002; **17**(1): 32–41.

218. Crow R, Gage H, Hampson S, Hart J, Kimber A, Storey L, *et al.* The measurement of satisfaction with healthcare: implications for practice from a systematic review of the literature. *Health Technol Assess.* 2002; **6**(32): 1–244.

219. Honigsbaum F. *The Division in British Medicine: a history of the separation of general practice from hospital care, 1911–68.* New York: Kogan Page; 1979.

220. Neal RD, Heywood PL, Morley S, Clayden AD, Dowell AC. Frequency of patients' consulting in general practice and workload generated by frequent attenders: comparisons between practices. *BJGP.* 1998; **48**(426): 895–8.

221. Christensen CM, Grossman JH, Hwang J. *The Innovator's Prescription: a disruptive solution for health care.* New York: McGraw-Hill Professional; 2009.

222. Bellón J, Rodríguez-Bayón A, de Dios Luna J, Torres-González F. Successful GP intervention with frequent attenders in primary care: randomised controlled trial. *BJGP.* 2008; **58**(550): 324–30.

223. Imison C, Naylor C. *Referral Management: lessons for success.* The King's Fund; 2010 [cited 2010 Nov 11]. Available at: www.kingsfund.org.uk/publications

224. Richards M. *Extent and causes of international variations in drug usage: a report for the Secretary of State for Health by Professor Sir Mike Richards CBE.* Department of Health; 2010 [cited 2010 Aug 16]. Available at: www.dh.gov.uk/en/Publicationsandstatistics/Publications/PublicationsPolicyAndGuidance/DH_117962

225. Cumming J, Mays N, Daube J. How New Zealand has contained expenditure on drugs. *BMJ*. 2010; **340**(7758): c2441.
226. Dugdale L, Siegler M, Rubin D. Medical professionalism and the doctor-patient relationship. *Perspectives in Biology and Medicine*. 2008; **51**(4): 547–54.
227. Costelloe C, Metcalfe C, Lovering A, Mant D, Hay AD. Effect of antibiotic prescribing in primary care on antimicrobial resistance in individual patients: systematic review and meta-analysis. *BMJ*. 2010; **340**(May 18_2): c2096.
228. Smith J, Sibthorpe B. Divisions of general practice in Australia: how do they measure up in the international context? *Australia and New Zealand Health Policy*. 2007; **4**(1): 15.
229. Jackson C, Askew D. Is there a polyclinic alternative acceptable to general practice? the 'beacon' practice model. *BJGP*. 2008; **58**(555): 733.
230. White J. Stepping up primary care. *The Psychologist*. 2008; **21**(10): 844–7.
231. Delamothe T. Universality, equity, and quality of care. *BMJ*. 2008; **336**(7656): 1278–81.
232. Gillies JC, Mercer SW, Lyon A, Scott M, Watt GC. Distilling the essence of general practice: a learning journey in progress. *BJGP*. 2009; **59**(562): e167.
233. *Patient-Centred Primary Care in Canada: bring it on home*. The College of Familiy Physicians of Canada; 2009. Available at: www2.cfpc.ca/local/files/Communications/Health%20Policy/Bring%20it%20on%20Home%20FINAL%20ENGLISH.pdf
234. Foot C, Naylor C, Imison C. *The Quality of GP Diagnosis and Referral: an enquiry into the quality of general practice in England*. The King's Fund; 2010. Available at: www.kingsfund.org.uk/current_projects/gp_inquiry/dimensions_of_care/diagnosis_and.html
235. Darzi A. *Healthcare for London: a framework for action*. 2nd ed. Available at: www.healthcareforlondon.nhs.uk/assets/Publications/A-Framework-for-Action/aFrameworkForAction.pdf
236. Main C, Moxham T, Wyatt JC, Anderson R, Stein K. *Computerised decision support systems in order communication for diagnostic, screening or monitoring test ordering: systematic reviews of the effects and cost-effectiveness of systems*. Health Technology Assessment. 2010 [cited 2010 Oct 28]; **14**(48). Available at: www.hta.ac.uk/project/1786.asp?src=alr
237. Kawamoto K, Houlihan CA, Balas EA, Lobach DF. *Improving clinical practice using clinical decision support systems: a systematic review of trials to identify features critical to success*. *BMJ*. 2005; **330**(7494): 765.
238. Øvretveit J. *Does Improving Quality Save Money? A review of evidence of which improvements to quality reduce costs to health service providers*. The Health Foundation; 2009 [cited 2010 Nov 10]. Available at: www.health.org.uk/public/cms/75/76/313/572/Does%20improving%20quality%20save%20money.pdf?realName=1d2aAZ.pdf
239. Mangin D. Urinary tract infection in primary care. *BMJ*. 2010; **340**(Feb 05_1): c657.
240. *Map of Medicine*. [cited 2010 Nov 22]. Available at: www.mapofmedicine.com/
241. Laurant M, Harmsen M, Faber M, Wollersheim H, Sibbald B, Grol R. *Revision of Professional Roles and Quality Improvement: a review of the evidence*. The Health Foundation; 2010. Available at: www.health.org.uk/publications/revision-of-professional-roles-and-quality-improvement/

242. Ridsdale L. *Evidence-Based General Practice: a critical reader.* London: W.B. Saunders Company Ltd; 1995.

243. Angelmar R, Angelmar S, Kane L. Building strong condition brands. *Journal of Medical Marketing.* 2007; **7**: 341–51.

244. Kiran T, Hutchings A, Dhalla IA, Furlong C, Jacobson B. The association between quality of primary care, deprivation and cardiovascular outcomes: a cross-sectional study using data from the UK Quality and Outcomes Framework. *J Epidemiol Community Health.* 2010; **64**(10): 927–34.

245. Tudor Hart J. The inverse care law. *Lancet.* 1971; **297**(7696): 405–12.

246. Marmot M. *Fair Society, Healthy Lives (The Marmot Review).* London: University College London—Department of Epidemiology and Public Health; 2010 [cited 2010 Dec 5]. Available at: www.marmotreview.org/AssetLibrary/pdfs/Reports/ FairSocietyHealthyLives.pdf

247. *Ideas from Darzi: polyclinics.* The NHS Confederation; 2008. Available at: www. nhsconfed.org/Publications/Documents/Ideas%20from%20Darzi%20 Polyclinics.pdf

248. Illich I. *Limits to Medicine: medical nemesis: the expropriation of health.* Harmondsworth, Middlesex: Penguin Books; 1977.

249. Fotaki M, Boyd A, Smith L, McDonald R, Roland M, Sheaff R, *et al. Patient Choice and the Organisation and Delivery of Health Services: scoping review.* Manchester: National Co-ordinating Centre for NHS Service Delivery and Organisation R&D (NCCSDO); 2005.

250. Hirschman AO. *Exit, Voice, and Loyalty: responses to decline in firms, organizations, and states.* Cambridge, MA: Harvard University Press; 1970.

251. Department of Health. *Equity and Excellence: liberating the NHS.* [cited 2010 Aug 7]. Available at: www.dh.gov.uk/en/Publicationsandstatistics/Publications/ PublicationsPolicyAndGuidance/DH_117353

252. *Our Theory of Change: why we do what we do.* The Health Foundation; [cited 2010 Nov 9]. Available at: www.health.org.uk/media_manager/public/75/publications_ pdfs/Our%20Theory%20of%20Change.pdf

253. *Shine 2011.* [cited 2010 Nov 9]. Available at: www.health.org.uk/areas-of-work/ improvement-programmes/shine-eleven/projects/

254. Spurling GK, Mansfield PR, Montgomery BD, Lexchin J, Doust J, Othman N, *et al.* Information from pharmaceutical companies and the quality, quantity, and cost of physicians' prescribing: a systematic review. *PLoS Med.* 2010; **7**(10): e1000352.

255. Glasziou P. *Why Bother with Evidence-Based Practice?* Available at: www.cebm.net/ mod_product/design/presentations/introduction-to-ebm-2010-03.ppt

256. Mickan S, Burls A, Glasziou P. *Patterns of Leakage—the pipeline from research to practice.* 2010 Nov 1 [cited 2010 Nov 10]. Available at: www.evidence2010.com/posters

257. Stange KC, Ferrer RL. The paradox of primary care. *Ann Fam Med.* 2009; **7**(4): 293–9.

258. Salisbury C, Wallace M, Montgomery AA. Patients' experience and satisfaction in primary care: secondary analysis using multilevel modelling. *BMJ.* 2010; **341** (Oct 12_1): c5004.

259. Schwartz LM, Woloshin S, Welch HG. Using a drug facts box to communicate drug benefits and harms: two randomized trials. *Ann Intern Med.* 2009; **150**(8): 516–27.

260. Gigerenzer G, Wegwarth O, Feufel M. Misleading communication of risk. *BMJ*. 2010; **341**(Oct 12_2): c4830.

261. Gigerenzer G, Gaissmaier W, Kurz-Milcke E, Schwartz LM, Woloshin S. Helping doctors and patients make sense of health statistics. *Psychological Science in the Public Interest Archive*. 2007; **8**(2): 54–96.

262. Lawson N. *Machines, Markets and Morals: the new politics of a democratic NHS*. Compass; 2008 [cited 2010 Oct 10]. Available at: www.unison.org.uk/file/B3905.pdf

263. Bauman Z. *Alone Again: ethics after certainty*. London: Demos; 1994.

264. Budd J. Comorbidity or Complexity: a primary care persepective on dual diagnosis. In: Phillips P, McKeown O, Sandford T, editors. *Dual Diagnosis: practice in context*. Oxford: John Wiley and Sons; 2009.

265. *Declaration of Alma-Ata*. International Conference on Primary Health Care; 1978. Available at: www.who.int/publications/almaata_declaration_en.pdf

266. Satz D. *Why Some Things Should Not Be for Sale: the moral limits of markets*. Oxford: Oxford University Press; 2010.

267. Wilkinson R, Pickett K. *The Spirit Level: why equality is better for everyone*. London: Penguin; 2010.

268. *The NHS Atlas of Variation in Healthcare*. Right Care; 2010 [cited 2010 Nov 25]. Available at: www.rightcare.nhs.uk/atlas/qipp_nhsAtlas-LOW_261110c.pdf

269. Jones R. The White Paper: a framework for survival? *BJGP*. 2010; **60**(578): 635–6.

270. Sieghart P. Professional ethics—for whose benefit? *J Med Ethics*. 1982; **8**(1): 25–32.

271. Relman AS. The new medical-industrial complex. *N Engl J Med*. 1980; **303**(17): 963–70.

272. *Marketisation and the NHS*. Socialist Health Association; 2010 [cited 2010 Oct 28]. Available at: www.sochealth.co.uk/Policy/marketisation.html

273. *Kaiser Permanente*. [cited 2010 Nov 6]. Available at: www.kaiserpermanente.org/

274. Lechler R. More brickbats than bouquets? *BMJ*. 2010; **341**(Jul 28_2): c3977.

275. McNulty T, Ferlie E. *Reengineering Health Care: The Complexities of Organizational Transformation*. Oxford: Oxford University Press; 2002.

276. Greenhalgh T, Macfarlane F, Maskrey N. Getting a better grip on research: the organizational dimension. *InnovAiT*. 2010; **3**(2): 102–7.

277. Maynard A. Is doctors' self interest undermining the National Health Service. *BMJ*. 2007; **334**(7587): 234.

278. Adamson SC, Bachman JW. Pilot study of providing online care in a primary care setting. *Mayo Clinic Proceedings*. 2010; **85**(8): 704–10.

279. Slack WV. Mayo Clinic Proceedings. *Mayo Clinic Proceedings*. 2010: 701–3.

280. Stevens S. More brickbats than bouquets? *BMJ*. 2010; **341**(Jul 28_2): c3977.

281. Shekelle PG, Goldzweig CL, Maglione M, Towfigh A. *Costs and Benefits of Health Technology Information: an updated systematic review*. Southern California Evidence-based Practice Centre, RAND Corporation: The Health Foundation; 2009. Available at: www.health.org.uk/publications/costs-and-benefits-of-health-technology- information/

282. NHS Scotland. *Plan, Do, Study, Act (PDSA)*. [cited 2010 Nov 10]. Available at: www.clinicalgovernance.scot.nhs.uk/section2/pdsa.asp

283. Kruk ME, Porignon D, Rockers PC, Van Lerberghe W. The contribution of primary care to health and health systems in low- and middle-income countries: a critical review of major primary care initiatives. *Social Science & Medicine*. 2010; **70**(6): 904–11.

284. Macinko J, Starfield B, Shi L. The contribution of primary care systems to health outcomes within Organization for Economic Cooperation and Development (OECD) countries, 1970–98. *Health Serv Res.* 2003; **38**(3): 831–65.

285. Starfield B, Shi L, Macinko J. Contribution of primary care to health systems and health. *Milbank Q.* 2005; **83**(3): 457–502.

286. May C, Montori VM, Mair FS. We need minimally disruptive medicine. *BMJ.* 2009; **339**(Aug 11_2): b2803.

287. Paré G, Moqadem K, Pineau G, St-Hilaire C. Clinical effects of home telemonitoring in the context of diabetes, asthma, heart failure and hypertension: a systematic review. *J Med Internet Res.* 2010 [cited 2010 Jul 8]; **12**(2): Available at: www.jmir.org/2010/2/e21

288. McLean S, Chandler D, Nurmatov U, Liu J, Pagliari C, Car J, *et al.* Telehealthcare for asthma. *Cochrane Database Syst Rev.* 2010; 10: CD007717.

289. Anderson D, Rowell H. *Hospital Care at Home: supporting independent and healthy lives.* Healthcare at Home Ltd. and Dr Foster Intelligence; 2010.

290. Tan E, Yung A, Jameson M, Oakley A, Rademaker M. Successful triage of patients referred to a skin lesion clinic using teledermoscopy (IMAGE IT trial). *British Journal of Dermatology.* 2009; **162**(4): 803–11.

291. Car J, Black A, Anandan C, Cresswell K, Pagliari C, McKinstry B, *et al. The Impact of eHealth on the Quality and Safety of Healthcare: a systemic overview and synthesis of the literature.* Report for the NHS Connecting for Health Evaluation Programme. The University of Edinburgh and Imperial College London; 2008 [cited 2010 Aug 22]. Available at: www.haps.bham.ac.uk/publichealth/cfhep/documents/NHS_CFHEP_001_Final_Report.pdf

292. Proprietary Association of Great Britain. *Making the Case for the Self Care of Minor Ailments.* 2009 [cited 2010 Sep 2]. Available at: www.pagb.co.uk/information/PDFs/Minorailmentsresearch09.pdf

293. Bosch M, Faber M, Voerman G, Cruijsberg J, Grol R, Hulscher M, *et al. Patient Care Teams.* The Health Foundation; 2009. Available at: www.health.org.uk/publications/patient-care-quality-enhancing-interventions/

294. Mitchell G, Del Mar C, Francis D. Does primary medical practitioner involvement with a specialist team improve patient outcomes? A systematic review. *BJGP.* 2002; **52**(484). 934–9.

295. Thomas KB. The consultation and the therapeutic illusion. *BMJ.* 1978; **1**(6123): 1327–8.

296. Martyn C. Why medicine is overweight. *BMJ.* 2010; **340**(7758): 1219.

297. Gordon JE. *Structures: or why things don't fall down.* Harmondsworth, Middlesex: Penguin Books; 1978.

298. Evans AT. Much ado about (doing) nothing. *Annals of Internal Medicine.* 2009; **150**(4): 270–W: 53.

299. Kirch W, Schafii C. Misdiagnosis at a university hospital in 4 medical eras. *Medicine* (Baltimore). 1996; **75**(1): 29–40.

300. Winkens R, Dinant G. Evidence base of clinical diagnosis: rational, cost effective use of investigations in clinical practice. *BMJ.* 2002; **324**(7340): 783–5.

301. van Bokhoven MA, Koch H, van der Weijden T, Grol RPTM, Kester AD, Rinkens PELM, *et al.* Influence of watchful waiting on satisfaction and anxiety among patients seeking care for unexplained complaints. *Ann Fam Med.* 2009; **7**(2): 112–20.

302. Wilson T, Holt T, Greenhalgh T. Complexity and clinical care. *BMJ*. 2001; **323** (7314): 685–8.

303. The Commonwealth Fund. Mirror, mirror on the wall: how the performance of the U.S. health care system compares internationally. 2010. Available at: www.commonwealthfund.org/~/media/Files/Publications/Fund%20Report/2010/Jun/1400_Davis_Mirror_Mirror_on_the_wall_2010.pdf

304. Fleetcroft R, Parekh-Bhurke S, Howe A, Cookson R, Swift L, Steel N. The UK pay-for-performance programme in primary care: estimation of population mortality reduction. *BJGP*. 2010; **60**(578): 345–52.

305. Martin S, Smith PC, Dusheiko M, Gravelle H, Rice N. *Do Quality Improvements in Primary Care Reduce Secondary Care Costs? primary research into the impact of the Quality and Outcomes Framework on hospital costs and mortality.* The Health Foundation; 2010.

306. Welch HG, Schwartz LM, Woloshin S. Are increasing 5-year survival rates evidence of success against cancer? *JAMA*. 2000; **283**(22): 2975–8.

307. Kalager M, Zelen M, Langmark F, Adami H. Effect of screening mammography on breast-cancer mortality in Norway. *N Engl J Med*. 2010; **363**(13): 1203–10.

308. Atkin WS, Edwards R, Kralj-Hans I, Wooldrage K, Hart AR, Northover JM, *et al.* Once-only flexible sigmoidoscopy screening in prevention of colorectal cancer: a multicentre randomised controlled trial. *Lancet*. 2010; **375**(9726): 1624–33.

309. Djulbegovic M, Beyth RJ, Neuberger MM, Stoffs TL, Vieweg J, Djulbegovic B, *et al.* Screening for prostate cancer: systematic review and meta-analysis of randomised controlled trials. *BMJ*. 2010; **341**(Sep 14_1): c4543.

310. Rembold CM. Number needed to screen: development of a statistic for disease screening. *BMJ*. 1998; **317**(7154): 307–12.

311. Ekelund G, Manjer J, Zackrisson S. Population-based screening for colorectal cancer with faecal occult blood test—do we really have enough evidence? *Int J Colorectal Dis*. 2010 [cited 2010 Aug 31]. Available at: www.springerlink.com/index/10.1007/s00384-010-1027-1

312. Round A, Weller D. Screening and Early Diagnosis of Cancer. In: Hamilton W, Peters TJ, editors. *Cancer Diagnosis in Primary Care*. London: Elsevier Health Sciences; 2007.

313. Hamilton W, Peters TJ, editors. *Cancer Diagnosis in Primary Care*. London: Elsevier Health Sciences; 2007.

314. Hamilton W, Round A, Sharp D, Peters TJ. Clinical features of colorectal cancer before diagnosis: a population-based case-control study. *Br J Cancer*. 2005; **93**(4): 399–405.

315. Hamilton W, Sharp DJ, Peters TJ, Round AP. Clinical features of prostate cancer before diagnosis: a population-based, case-control study. *BJGP*. 2006; **56**(531): 756–62.

316. Hamilton W, Peters TJ, Bankhead C, Sharp D. Risk of ovarian cancer in women with symptoms in primary care: population based case-control study. *BMJ*. 2009; **339**(Aug 25_2): b2998.

317. Almond SC, Summerton N. Test of time. *BMJ*. 2009; **338**(Jun 15_1): b1878.

318. Summerton N. Diagnosis and general practice. *BJGP*. 2000; **50**(461): 995–1000.

319. Jones R, White P, Armstrong D, Ashworth M, Peters M. *Managing Acute Illness: an enquiry into the quality of general practice in England.* London: The King's Fund; 2010 [cited 2010 Nov 4]. Available at: www.kingsfund.org.uk/current_projects/gp_inquiry/dimensions_of_care/the_management_of.html

320. Elliott K, Stacey C. *Local Awareness and Early Diagnosis Initiatives 2009/2010: programme summary report.* NHS National Cancer Action Team; 2010. Available at: info.cancerresearchuk.org/prod_consump/groups/cr_common/@nre/@hea/documents/generalcontent/cr_046646.pdf

321. Souhami R. Are UK cancer cure rates worse than in most other European countries? *BJGP.* 2010; **60**(571): 81–2.

322. Beral V, Peto R. UK cancer survival statistics. *BMJ.* 2010; **341**(Aug 11_1): c4112.

323. Cohen JT, Neumann PJ, Weinstein MC. Does preventive care save money? Health economics and the presidential candidates. *N Engl J Med.* 2008; **358**(7): 661–3.

324. Stott NC, Davis RH. The exceptional potential in each primary care consultation. *J R Coll Gen Pract.* 1979; **29**(201): 201–5.

325. McKinlay JB, Marceau LD. A tale of 3 tails. *Am J Public Health.* 1999; **89**(3): 295–8.

326. Moynihan R. Who benefits from treating prehypertension? *BMJ.* 2010; **341**(Aug 24_2): c4442.

327. Barondess J. Toward reducing the prevalence of chronic disease: a life course perspective on health preservation. *Perspectives in Biology and Medicine.* 2008; **51**(4): 616.

328. Wilke G, Freeman S. *How to be a good enough GP: surviving and thriving in the new primary care organisations.* Oxford: Radcliffe Publishing; 2001.

329. Balint M. Introduction. In: Balint M, editor. *Treatment or Diagnosis: a study of repeat prescriptions in general practice.* London: Tavistock Publications; 1970.

330. Getz L, Sigurdsson JA, Hetlevik I. Is opportunistic disease prevention in the consultation ethically justifiable? *BMJ.* 2003; **327**(7413): 498–500.

331. Cocksedge S, May C. Pastoral relationships and holding work in primary care: affect, subjectivity and chronicity. *Chronic Illn.* 2005; **1**(2): 157–63.

332. Beach MC, Inui T. Relationship-centered care. A constructive reframing. *J Gen Intern Med.* 2006; **21**(S1): S3–8.

333. Tresolini CP, and the Pew-Fetzer Task Force. *Health Professions Education and Relationship-Centered Care.* San Francisco, CA: Pew Health Professions Commission; 1994 [cited 2010 Dec 4]. Available at: http://rccswmi.org/uploads/PewFetzerRCCreport.pdf

334. Oberg E, Frank E. Physicians' health practices strongly influence patient health practices. *J R Coll Physicians Edinb.* 2009; **39**(4): 290–1.

335. Axelrod R. *The evolution of cooperation.* New York: Basic Books; 1984.

336. Summerton N. *Patient-Centred Diagnosis.* Oxford: Radcliffe Publishing; 2007.

337. Yarnall K, Pollak K, Østbye T, Krause K, Michener J. Primary care: is there enough time for prevention? *Am J Public Health.* 2003; **93**(4): 635–41.

338. Willis J. *The Paradox of Progress.* Oxford: Radcliffe Publishing; 1995.

339. Hays R. *Teaching and Learning in Primary Care.* Oxford: Radcliffe Publishing; 2006.

340. Hayek FA. The use of knowledge in society. *American Economic Review.* 1945; **35**(4): 519–30.

341. Katerndahl DA, Wood R, Jaén CR. A method for estimating relative complexity of ambulatory care. *Ann Fam Med.* 2010; **8**(4): 341–7.

342. *Laws of the Game 2010/2011.* Fédération Internationale de Football Association; Available at: www.fifa.com/mm/document/affederation/generic/81/42/36/lawsofthegame_2010_11_e.pdf

343. Armstrong D. The rise of surveillance medicine. *Sociol Health and Illness.* 1995; **17**(3): 393–404.

344. Maskrey N, Underhill J, Hutchinson A, Shaughnessy A, Slawson D. Getting a better grip on research: a simple system that works. *InnovAiT.* 2009; **2**(12): 739–49.

345. Berwick DM. A transatlantic review of the NHS at 60. *BMJ.* 2008; **337** (Jul 17_1): a838.

346. Ezzati M, Vander Hoorn S, Lopez AD, Danaei G, Rodgers A, Mathers CD, *et al.* Comparative Quantification of Mortality and Burden of Disease Attributable to Selected Risk Factors. In: Lopez AD, Mathers CD, Ezzati M, Jamison DT, Murray CJL, editors. *Global Burden of Disease and Risk Factors.* New York: Oxford University Press; 2006 [cited 2010 Sep 5]. 241–68. Available at: www.ncbi.nlm.nih.gov/books/NBK11813/

347. Tsai SP, Lee ES, Hardy RJ. The effect of a reduction in leading causes of death: potential gains in life expectancy. *Am J Public Health.* 1978; **68**(10): 966–71.

348. *Scottish Online Appraisal Resource (SOAR)—for Scotland's GPs.* [cited 2010 Dec 7]. Available at: www.scottishappraisal.scot.nhs.uk/

349. Byberg L, Melhus H, Gedeborg R, Sundström J, Ahlbom A, Zethelius B, *et al.* Total mortality after changes in leisure time physical activity in 50-year-old men: 35-year follow-up of population based cohort. *Br J Sports Med.* 2009; **43**(7): 482.

350. Hooper L, Summerbell CD, Higgins JP, Thompson RL, Clements G, Capps N, *et al.* Reduced or modified dietary fat for preventing cardiovascular disease. *Cochrane Database Syst Rev.* 2001; **3**: CD002137.

351. Berrington de Gonzalez A, Hartge P, Cerhan JR, Flint AJ, Hannan L, MacInnis RJ, *et al.* Body-mass index and mortality among 1.46 million white adults. *N Engl J Med.* 2010; **363**(23): 2211–19.

352. Iversen L, Hannaford PC, Lee AJ, Elliott AM, Fielding S. Impact of lifestyle in middle-aged women on mortality: evidence from the Royal College of General Practitioners' Oral Contraception Study. *BJGP.* 2010; **60**: 563–9.

353. Ebrahim S, Beswick A, Burke M, Davey Smith G. Multiple risk factor interventions for primary prevention of coronary heart disease. *Cochrane Database Syst Rev.* 2006; **4**: CD001561.

354. *Patient Decision Aids.* Patient Decision Aids. Available at: http://decisionaid.ohri.ca/AZinvent.php

355. Mayo Clinic. *Shared Decision Making National Resource Center.* Shared Decisions. [cited 2010 Nov 2]. Available at: http://shareddecisions.mayoclinic.org/

356. O'Connor AM, Bennett CL, Stacey D, Barry M, Col NF, Eden KB, *et al.* Decision aids for people facing health treatment or screening decisions. *Cochrane Database Syst Rev.* 2009; **3**: CD001431.

357. Haynes RB, McDonald HP, Garg AX. Helping patients follow prescribed treatment: clinical applications. *JAMA.* 2002; **288**(22): 2880–3.

358. McLaren L, McIntyre L, Kirkpatrick S. Rose's population strategy of prevention need not increase social inequalities in health. *Int J Epidemiol.* 2010; **39**(2): 372–7.

359. Shaw K, Gennat H, O'Rourke P, Del Mar C. Exercise for overweight or obesity. *Cochrane Database Syst Rev.* 2006; **4**: CD003817.

360. Cummings KM, Hyland A. Impact of nicotine replacement therapy on smoking behavior. *Ann Rev Public Health.* 2005; **26**: 583–99.

361. Fiore MC, Novotny TE, Pierce JP, Giovino GA, Hatziandreu EJ, Newcomb PA, *et al.* Methods used to quit smoking in the United States. Do cessation programs help? *JAMA.* 1990; **263**(20): 2760–5.

362. Russell LB, Suh D, Safford MA. Time requirements for diabetes self-management: too much for many? *J Fam Pract.* 2005; **54**(1): 52–6.

363. MacDonald B, Cockerell O, Sander J, Shorvon S. The incidence and lifetime prevalence of neurological disorders in a prospective community-based study in the UK. *Brain.* 2000; **123**(4): 665–76.

364. McDonald HP, Garg AX, Haynes RB. Interventions to enhance patient adherence to medication prescriptions: scientific review. *JAMA.* 2002; **288**(22): 2868–79.

365. Irving G. Goodbye to gobbledegook: an introduction to basic statistics in primary care. *InnovAiT.* 2009; **2**(6): 372–83.

366. Greenhalgh T. *How to Read a Paper: the basics of evidence-based medicine.* 3rd ed. Blackwell; 2006.

367. Slawson DC, Shaughnessy AF, Bennett JH. Becoming a medical information master: feeling good about not knowing everything. *J Fam Pract.* 1994; **38**(5): 505–13.

368. Schulz KF, Altman DG, Moher D, for the CONSORT Group. CONSORT 2010 Statement: updated guidelines for reporting parallel group randomised trials. *BMJ.* 2010; **340**(3): c332.

369. Bossuyt PM, Reitsma JB, Bruns DE, Gatsonis CA, Glasziou PP, Irwig LM, *et al.* Towards complete and accurate reporting of studies of diagnostic accuracy: the STARD initiative. *BMJ.* 2003; **326**(7379): 41–4.

370. Montori VM, Jaeschke R, Schünemann HJ, Bhandari M, Brozek JL, Devereaux PJ, *et al.* Users' guide to detecting misleading claims in clinical research reports. *BMJ.* 2004; **329**(7474): 1093–6.

371. Gould SJ. The Median isn't the Message. In: Greenhalgh T, Hurwitz B, editors. *Narrative Based Medicine: dialogue and discourse in clinical practice.* BMJ Books; 1998.

372. Chan A. Access to clinical trial data: results and protocols go hand in hand. *BMJ.* 2011; **342**(7789): 117–18.

373. NHS Evidence. *Evidence in Health and Social Care.* [cited 2010 Nov 9]. Available at: www.evidence.nhs.uk/default.aspx

374. *Scottish Intercollegiate Guidelines Network (SIGN).* [cited 2010 Nov 27]. Available at: www.sign.ac.uk/

375. Godlee F, Delamothe T, Smith J. Continuous publication. *BMJ.* 2008; **336**(7659): 1450.

376. Rees M, Wells F. Falling research in the NHS. *BMJ.* 2010; **340**: c2375.

377. *National Institute for Health Research, Research Design Service South East, Research or clinical audit project?* [cited 2010 Jan 2]. Available at: www.rds-se.nihr.ac.uk/resources/res_clin_audit.htm

378. Marinker M. Personal paper: writing prescriptions is easy. *BMJ.* 1997; **314**(7082): 747–8.

379. Treasure W. N of 1 trials. Placebos should be abandoned. (Letter). *BMJ.* 1996; **313**(Aug 17_7054): 427–8.

380. Goldacre B. *Bad science.* London: Fourth Estate; 2009.

381. Chamberlain P. Independence of nutritional information? *BMJ.* 2010; **340** (Mar 22_1): c1438.

382. Carlowe J. Ghostwritten articles overstated benefits of HRT. *BMJ.* 2010; **341** (Sep 07_1): c4894.

383. Skrabanek P, McCormick JS. *Follies and Fallacies in Medicine.* Glasgow: Tarragon Press; 1989.

384. Drazen JM, Leeuw PWD, Laine C, Mulrow C, DeAngelis CD, Frizelle FA, *et al.* Towards more uniform conflict disclosures. *BMJ.* 2010; **340**(Jun 30_3): c3239.

385. Delaney B, Moxham J, Lechler R. Academic health sciences centres: an opportunity to improve services, teaching, and research. *BJGP.* 2010; **60**(579): 719–20.

386. Maskrey N, Greenhalgh T. Getting a better grip on research: the fate of those who ignore history. *InnovAiT.* 2009; **10**(2): 619–25.

387. Darnton R. The Library: three Jeremiads. *The New York Review of Books.* 2010 Nov 23;

388. McPherson K. Screening for breast cancer—balancing the debate. *BMJ.* 2010; **340**(Jun 24_1): c3106.

389. Moher D, Liberati A, Tetzlaff J, Altman DG. Preferred reporting items for systematic reviews and meta-analyses: the PRISMA statement. *BMJ.* 2009; **339**(Jul 21_1): b2535.

390. von Elm E, Altman DG, Egger M, Pocock SJ, Gøtzsche PC, Vandenbroucke JP. Strengthening the Reporting of Observational Studies in Epidemiology (STROBE) statement: guidelines for reporting observational studies. *BMJ.* 2007; **335**(7624): 806–8.

391. Bossuyt PM, Reitsma JB, Bruns DE, Gatsonis CA, Glasziou PP, Irwig LM, *et al.* Towards complete and accurate reporting of studies of diagnostic accuracy: the STARD initiative. *Clin. Chem. Lab. Med.* 2003; **41**(1): 68–73.

392. Stroup DF, Berlin JA, Morton SC, Olkin I, Williamson GD, Rennie D, *et al.* Meta-analysis of observational studies in epidemiology: a proposal for reporting. Meta-analysis of Observational Studies in Epidemiology (MOOSE) group. *JAMA.* 2000; **283**(15): 2008–12.

393. *Article Requirements.* British Medical Journal. [cited 2010 Nov 12]. Available at: http://resources.bmj.com/bmj/authors/article-submission/article-requirements

394. Glasziou P, Meats E, Heneghan C, Shepperd S. What is missing from descriptions of treatment in trials and reviews? *BMJ.* 2008; **336**(7659): 1472–4.

395. de Silva V, Hanwella R. Why are we copyrighting science? *BMJ.* 2010; **341** (Sep 16_1): c4738.

396. Playing the numbers game. *Drug and Therapeutics Bulletin.* 2011; **49**(1): 1.

397. Greenhalgh T. Narrative Based Medicine in an Evidence Based World. In: Greenhalgh T, Hurwitz B, editors. *Narrative Based Medicine: dialogue and discourse in clinical practice.* London: BMJ Books; 1998.

398. Eddy DM. Probabilistic reasoning in clinical medicine: problems and opportunities. In: Kahneman D, Tversky A, editors. *Judgment under Uncertainty: heuristics and biases.* New York: Cambridge University Press; 1982.

399. Tversky A, Kahneman D. Belief in the law of small numbers. In: Kahneman D, Slovic P, Tversky A, editors. *Judgment under Uncertainty: heuristics and biases.* New York: Cambridge University Press; 1982.

400. Greenland S. Medical Statistics a Half Century after Bradford Hill, 1965: sometimes a blessing, often a curse. Or, is statistics the sick man of science dragging public health down with it? A presentation at the London School of Hygiene and Tropical Medicine, Apr 14 2010.

401. Harris M, Taylor G. *Medical statistics made easy.* Bloxham, Oxon: Informa Health Care; 2004.

402. Simel DL. Make the diagnosis: does this patient with headaches have a migraine or need neuroimaging?. In: Simel DL, Rennie D, editors. *The Rational Clinical*

Examination: evidence-based clinical diagnosis. New York: McGraw-Hill; 2009 [cited 2010 Jul 16]. Available at: www.jamaevidence.com/content/3494120

403. *CEBM.* [cited 2010 Nov 16]. Available at: www.cebm.net/index.aspx?o=1000

404. Senn S. Bayesian, likelihood, and frequentist approaches to statistics: a comparison of methods. *Applied Clinical Trials.* 2003 Aug: 35–8.

405. Senn S. *Dicing with Death: chance, risk, and health.* Cambridge: Cambridge University Press; 2003.

406. Quinn J, Cremin J. *The Definitive Guide: A–Z of betting.* Newbury, Berkshire: Raceform; 2008.

407. Smetana GW. The diagnostic value of historical features in primary headache syndromes: a comprehensive review. *Arch Intern Med.* 2000; **160**(18): 2729–37.

408. Thompson IM, Ankerst DP, Chi C, Lucia MS, Goodman PJ, Crowley JJ, *et al.* Operating characteristics of prostate-specific antigen in men with an initial PSA level of 3.0 ng/ml or lower. *JAMA.* 2005; **294**(1): 66–70.

409. Kavanagh AM, Giles GG, Mitchell H, Cawson JN. The sensitivity, specificity, and positive predictive value of screening mammography and symptomatic status. *J Med Screen.* 2000; **7**(2): 105–10.

410. Spiegelhalter DJ. Statistical methodology for evaluating gastrointestinal symptoms. *Clin Gastroenterol.* 1985; **14**(3): 489–515.

411. Del Mar C, Doust J, Glasziou P. *Clinical Thinking: evidence, communication and decision making.* Oxford: Blackwell; 2008.

412. Elton R. Likelihood ratios. Personal communication. 24 Oct 2010.

413. Marcus G, Cohen J, Varosy P, Vessey J, Rose E, Massie B, *et al.* The utility of gestures in patients with chest discomfort. *The American Journal of Medicine.* 2007; **120**(1): 83–9.

414. Wang K, Harnden A, Thomson A. Foreign body inhalation in children. *BMJ.* 2010; **341**(Aug 18_3): c3924.

415. Kiyan G, Gocmen B, Tugtepe H, Karakoc F, Dagli E, Dagli TE. Foreign body aspiration in children: the value of diagnostic criteria. *International Journal of Pediatric Otorhinolaryngology.* 2009; **73**(7): 963–7.

416. Treasure W. Likelihood ratios would help prevent misinterpretation of data (rapid response). *BMJ.* 2010 Sep 20 [cited 2010 Sep 21]. Available at: www.bmj. com/content/341/bmj.c3924/reply#bmj_el_241910?sid=d79bcb43-149b-4881-8575-f7909bb2f68e

417. Jenkins R, Smeeton N, Marinker M, Shepherd M. A study of the classification of mental ill-health in general practice. *Psychol Med.* 1985; **15**(2): 403–9.

418. Siriwardena AN. Why do GPs prescribe psychotropic drugs when they would rather provide alternative psychological interventions? *BJGP.* 2010; **60**(573): 241–2.

419. NHS Employers and the General Practitioners Committee. *Quality and Outcomes Framework guidance for GMS contract 2009/10.* 2009 Mar. Available at: www. nhsemployers.org/Aboutus/Publications/Documents/QOF_Guidance_2009_final. pdf

420. Whooley MA, Avins AL, Miranda J, Browner WS. Case-finding instruments for depression: two questions are as good as many. *Journal of General Internal Medicine.* 1997; **12**(7): 439–5.

421. Wyke S, Hunt K, Ford G. Gender differences in consulting a general practitioner for common symptoms of minor illness. *Soc Sci Med.* 1998; **46**(7): 901–6.

422 Mitchell AJ, Rao S, Vaze A. International comparison of clinicians' ability to identify depression in primary care: meta-analysis and meta-regression of predictors. *BJGP* 2011; **61**(583): 72–80.

423. Bergus GR, Hartz AJ, Noyes R, Ward MM, James PA, Vaughn T, *et al.* The limited effect of screening for depressive symptoms with the PHQ-9 in rural family practices. *J Rural Health.* 2005; **21**(4): 303–9.

424. Barbui C, Butler R, Cipriani A, Geddes J, Hatcher S. Depression in adults: drug and physical treatments. *Clinical Evidence.* Available at: http://clinicalevidence.bmj.com/ceweb/conditions/meh/1003/1003_I1.jsp

425. *Antidepressant drug adherence.* Bandolier. Available at: www.medicine.ox.ac.uk/bandolier/band84/b84-3.html

426. Fournier JC, DeRubeis RJ, Hollon SD, Dimidjian S, Amsterdam JD, Shelton RC, *et al.* Antidepressant Drug Effects and Depression Severity: A Patient-Level Meta-analysis. *JAMA.* 2010; **303**(1): 47–53.

427. *Hamilton Depression Rating Scale.* Available at: http://healthnet.umassmed.edu/mhealth/HAMD.pdf

428. Treasure W. *Diagnosis and Risk Management in Primary Care.* [cited 2011 Jan 15]. Available at: www.darmipc.net/

429. Spinks A, Glasziou P, Del Mar C. *Antibiotics for sore throat.* Cochrane Database of Systematic Reviews. 2006 [cited 2010 Aug 14]; (4). Available at: http://onlinelibrary.wiley.com/o/cochrane/clsysrev/articles/CD000023/pdf_fs.html

430. Ashworth M, Latinovic R, Charlton J, Cox K, Rowlands G, Gulliford M. Why has antibiotic prescribing for respiratory illness declined in primary care? a longitudinal study using the General Practice Research Database. *J Public Health* (Oxf). 2004; **26**(3): 268–74.

431. Kenealy T. *Sore throat.* Clinical Evidence. [cited 2010 Aug 23]. Available at: http://clinicalevidence.bmj.com/ceweb/conditions/rda/1509/1509.jsp

432. Wark P. *Bronchitis (acute).* Clinical Evidence. [cited 2010 Aug 23]. Available at: http://clinicalevidence.bmj.com/ceweb/conditions/rda/1508/1508.jsp

433. Woo WWK, Man S, Lam PKW, Rainer TH. Randomized double-blind trial comparing oral paracetamol and oral nonsteroidal antiinflammatory drugs for treating pain after musculoskeletal injury. *Ann Emerg Med.* 2005; **46**(4): 352–61.

434. WHO. *The Top 10 Causes of Death.* [cited 2010 Apr 29]. Available at: www.who.int/mediacentre/factsheets/fs310/en/index.html

435. Hamilton W, Lancashire R, Sharp D, Peters TJ, Cheng K, Marshall T. The risk of colorectal cancer with symptoms at different ages and between the sexes: a case-control study. *BMC Med.* 2009; **7**: 17.

436. Hamilton W. Cancer diagnosis in primary care. *BJGP.* 2010; **60**(571): 121–8.

437. Hamilton W, Sharp D. Diagnosis of colorectal cancer in primary care: the evidence base for guidelines. *Family Practice.* 2004; **21**(1): 99–106.

438. Tappenden P, Chilcott J, Eggington S, Sakai H, Karnon J, Patnick J. Option appraisal of population-based colorectal cancer screening programmes in England. *Gut.* 2007; **56**(5): 677–84.

439. Burt RW. Colorectal cancer screening. *Curr. Opin. Gastroenterol.* 2010; **26**(5): 466–70.

440. *Scottish Bowel Screening Programme.* [cited 2010 Sep 6]. Available at: www.bowelscreening.scot.nhs.uk/

441. Information Services Division, NHS National Services Scotland. *Scottish Bowel Screening Programme: key performance indicators concise report: May 2010 data submission.* 2010 [cited 2009 Sep 5]. Available at: www.isdscotland.scot.nhs.uk/Health-Topics/Cancer/Bowel-Screening/KPI_Report.pdf

442. Braithwaite RS, Fiellin D, Justice AC. The payoff time: a flexible framework to help clinicians decide when patients with comorbid disease are not likely to benefit from practice guidelines. *Med Care.* 2009; **47**(6): 610–17.

443. Romagnuolo J, Enns R, Ponich T, Springer J, Armstrong D, Barkun AN. Canadian credentialing guidelines for colonoscopy. *Can J Gastroenterol.* 2008; **22**(1): 17–22.

444. Colford L. Scottish Bowel Screening Programme. E-mail. 2010 Sep 16.

445. Hewitson P, Glasziou PP, Irwig L, Towler B, Watson E. Screening for colorectal cancer using the faecal occult blood test, Hemoccult. *Cochrane Database of Systematic Reviews.* 2007; **1**: Art No.: CD001216.

446. Ginsberg G, Lim S, Lauer J, Johns B, Sepulveda C. Prevention, screening and treatment of colorectal cancer: a global and regional generalized cost effectiveness analysis. *Cost Effectiveness and Resource Allocation.* 2010; **8**(1): 2.

447. Steele RJC, Kostourou I, McClements P, Watling C, Libby G, Weller D, *et al.* Effect of repeated invitations on uptake of colorectal cancer screening using faecal occult blood testing: analysis of prevalence and incidence screening. *BMJ.* 2010; **341**: c5531.

448. *Colorectal cancer.* Information Services Division, NHS National Services Scotland. Available at: www.isdscotland.org/Health-Topics/Cancer/Cancer-Statistics/Colorectal/#colorectal

449. Hamilton W The CAPER studies: five case-control studies aimed at identifying and quantifying the risk of cancer in symptomatic primary care patients. *Br J Cancer.* 2009; **101**(S2): S80–6.

450. Barton MB, Elmore JG, Fletcher SW. Breast symptoms among women enrolled in a health maintenance organization: frequency, evaluation, and outcome. *Ann Intern Med.* 1999; **130**(8): 651–7.

451. Bobo JK, Lee NC, Thames SF. Findings from 752,081 clinical breast examinations reported to a national screening program from 1995 through 1998. *J Natl Cancer Inst.* 2000; **92**(12): 971–6.

452. Wathne B, Holst E, Hovelius B. Vaginal discharge—comparison of clinical, laboratory and microbiological findings. *Acta Obstet Gynecol Scand.* 1994; **73**: 802–8.

453. Anderson MR, Klink K, Cohrssen A. Evaluation of vaginal complaints. *JAMA.* 2004; **291**(11): 1368–79.

454. Schwiertz A, Taras D, Rusch K, Rusch V. Throwing the dice for the diagnosis of vaginal complaints? *Annals of Clinical Microbiology and Antimicrobials.* 2006; **5**(1): 4.

455. Knottnerus JA, Muris JW. Assessment of the accuracy of diagnostic tests: the cross-sectional study. In: Knottnerus JA, Buntinx F, editors. *The Evidence Base of Clinical Diagnosis: theory and methods of diagnostic research.* New York: John Wiley and Sons; 2009.

456. Simel DL, Rennie D, Keitz SA. *The Rational Clinical Examination: evidence-based clinical diagnosis.* New York: McGraw-Hill; 2009.

457. *Essential Evidence Plus.* [cited 2010 Oct 18]. Available at: www.essentialevidenceplus.com/index.cfm

458. *JAMAevidence.* [cited 2010 Oct 5]. Available at: www.jamaevidence.com/

459. Langewitz W, Denz M, Keller A, Kiss A, Ruttimann S, Wossmer B. Spontaneous talking time at start of consultation in outpatient clinic: cohort study. *BMJ*. 2002; **325**(7366): 682–3.

460. Svab I, Katic M, Cuk C. [The time used by the patient when he/she talks without interruptions]. *Atencion Primaria/Sociedad Española De Medicina De Familia Y Comunitaria*. 1993; **11**(4): 175–7.

461. Thomas KB. Temporarily dependent patient in general practice. *BMJ*. 1974; **1**(5908): 625–6.

462. Deber RB, Kraetschmer N, Irvine J. What role do patients wish to play in treatment decision making? *Archives of Internal Medicine*. 1996; **156**(13): 1414–20.

463. Coulter A. *Engaging Patients in their Healthcare: how is the UK doing relative to other countries?* Picker Institute Europe; 2006. Available at: www.pickereurope.org/Filestore/PIE_reports/project_reports/Six_country_study_with_ISBN_web.pdf

464. Weiner S, Schwartz A, Weaver F, Goldberg J, Yudkovsky R, Sharma G, *et al*. Contextual errors and failures in individualizing patient care. *Annals of Internal Medicine*. 2010; **153**(2): 69–75.

465. O'Connor A, Stacey D. *Should patient decision aids (PtDAs) be introduced in the health care system*. Copenhagen: WHO Regional Office for Europe (Health Evidence Network); 2005 [cited 2010 May 2]. Available at: www.euro.who.int/__data/assets/pdf_file/0011/74666/E87791.pdf

466. Cramer JA, Mattson RH, Prevey ML, Scheyer RD, Ouellette VL. How often is medication taken as prescribed? A novel assessment technique. *JAMA*. 1989; **261**(22): 3273–7.

467. Wetzels R, Wolters R, van Weel C, Wensing M. Mix of methods is needed to identify adverse events in general practice: a prospective observational study. *BMC Family Practice*. 2008; **9**(1): 35.

468. Cox SJ, Holden JD. Presentation and outcome of clinical poor performance in one health district over a five-year period: 2002–2007. *BJGP*. 2009; **59**(562): 344–8.

469. National Clinical Assessment Service. *Use of NHS exclusion and suspension from work amongst doctors and dentists in 2009/10*. National Patient Safety Agency; [cited 2010 Nov 18]. Available at: www.ncas.npsa.nhs.uk/publications/statistics/

470. Khan N, Harrison S, Rose P. Validity of diagnostic coding within the General Practice Research Database: a systematic review. *BJGP*. 2010; **60**(572): e128–36.

471. Schoen C, Osborn R, Squires D, Doty MM, Pierson R, Applebaum S. *How Health Insurance Design Affects Access to Care and Costs, by Income, in Eleven Countries*. Health Affairs Web First. 2010 Nov 18 [cited 2010 Nov 25]. Available at: http://content.healthaffairs.org/cgi/content/full/hlthaff.2010.0862?ijkey=Ho5XaxzsdWHVE&keytype=ref&siteid=healthaff

472. Shojania KG, Sampson M, Ansari MT, Ji J, Doucette S, Moher D. How quickly do systematic reviews go out of date? A survival analysis. *Ann Intern Med*. 2007; **147**(4): 224–33.

473. Thuline HC. Color-vision defects in American school children. *JAMA*. 1964; **188**: 514–18.

474. Reiss MJ, Labowitz DA, Forman S, Wormser GP. Impact of color blindness on recognition of blood in body fluids. *Arch Intern Med*. 2001; **161**(3): 461–5.

475. *MRCGP*. Available at: www.rcgp-curriculum.org.uk/nmrcgp.aspx

476. *MRCGP: Statistics 2009. Second annual report on the results of the MRCGP AKT and CSA assessments.* RCGP; 2010 [cited 2010 Jul 2]. Available at: www.rcgp-curriculum. org.uk/PDF/MRCGP%20Statistics%202009%20Annual%20Report%20v%20 040710.pdf

477. Houben PHH, Winkens RAG, van der Weijden T, Vossen RCR, Naus AJM, Grol RPT. Reasons for ordering laboratory tests and relationship with frequency of abnormal results. *Scan J Prim Health Care.* 2010; **28**(1): 18–23.

478. Koch H, van Bokhoven MA, ter Riet G, van Alphen-Jager JT, van der Weijden T, Dinant G, *et al.* Ordering blood tests for patients with unexplained fatigue in general practice: what does it yield? Results of the VAMPIRE trial. *BJGP.* 2009; **59**(561): 93–100.

479. McAteer A, Elliott AM, Hannaford PC. Ascertaining the size of the symptom iceberg in a UK-wide community-based survey. *BJGP.* 2011 [cited 2011 Jan 9]. Available at: www.ingentaconnect.com/content/rcgp/bjgp/2011/00000061/00000582/art00001

480. Kroenke K, Mangelsdorff A. Common symptoms in ambulatory care: incidence, evaluation, therapy, and outcome. *Am J Med.* 1989; **86**: 262–66.

481. *Mortality Statistics Cause: review by the Registrar General on deaths by cause, sex and age, in England and Wales, 2005.* London: Office for National Statistics; 2006 [cited 2010 Jun 23]. Available at: www.statistics.gov.uk/downloads/theme_health/Dh2_32/ DH2_No32_2005.pdf

482. DCPP 3. *The Burden of Disease and Mortality by Condition: Data, Methods, and Results for 2001.* [cited 2010 Jun 22]. Available at: www.dcp2.org/pubs/GBD/3/Table/3.B1

483. de Oliveira C, Watt R, Hamer M. Toothbrushing, inflammation, and risk of cardiovascular disease: results from Scottish Health Survey. *BMJ.* 2010, **340**(May27_1): c2451.

484. Oberg M, Jaakkola MS, Woodward A, Peruga A, Prüss-Ustün A. Worldwide burden of disease from exposure to second-hand smoke: a retrospective analysis of data from 192 countries. *Lancet.* 2011; **377**(9760): 139–46.

485. Simpson CR, Hippisley-Cox J, Sheikh A. Trends in the epidemiology of smoking recorded in UK general practice. *BJGP.* 2010; **60**(572): e121–7.

486. Toljamo T, Kaukonen M, Nieminen P, Kinnula V. Early detection of COPD combined with individualized counselling for smoking cessation: a two-year prospective study. *Scan J Prim Health Care.* 2010; **28**(1): 41–6.

487. Stead LF, Perera R, Bullen C, Mant D, Lancaster T. Nicotine replacement therapy for smoking cessation. *Cochrane Database Syst Rev.* 2008; **1**: CD000146.

488. Doll R, Peto R, Boreham J, Sutherland I. Mortality in relation to smoking: 50 years' observations on male British doctors. *BMJ.* 2004; **328**(7455): 1519.

489. Bonneux LG, Huisman CC, de Beer JA. Mortality in 272 European regions, 2002–2004. An update. *Eur J Epidemiol.* 2010; **25**(2): 77–85.

490. *Drug Misuse Declared: findings from the 2009/10 British Crime Survey England and Wales.* London: Home Office; 2010 [cited 2010 Dec 12]. Available at: www.homeoffice. gov.uk/publications/science-research-statistics/research-statistics/crime-research/ hosb1310/hosb1310?view=Binary

491. Pilger D, Khakban A, Heukelbach J, Feldmeier H. Self-diagnosis of active head lice infestation by individuals from an impoverished community: high sensitivity and specificity. *Rev Inst Med Trop Sao Paulo.* 2008; **50**(2): 121–2.

492. Stevens J, Cai J, Pamuk ER, Williamson DF, Thun MJ, Wood JL. The effect of age on the association between body-mass index and mortality. *N Engl J Med.* 1998; **338**(1): 1–7.

493. Bobrow BJ, Spaite DW, Berg RA, Stolz U, Sanders AB, Kern KB, *et al.* Chest compression-only CPR by lay rescuers and survival from out-of-hospital cardiac arrest. *JAMA.* 2010; **304**(13): 1447–54.

494. Bird SM, Harris J. Time to move to presumed consent for organ donation. *BMJ.* 2010; **340**(7754): 1010–12.

495. Williamson HA. Lymphadenopathy in a family practice: a descriptive study of 249 cases. *J Fam Pract.* 1985; **20**(5): 449–52.

496. Dube SR, Anda RF, Felitti VJ, Chapman DP, Williamson DF, Giles WH. Childhood abuse, household dysfunction, and the risk of attempted suicide throughout the life span: findings from the adverse childhood experiences study. *JAMA.* 2001; **286**(24): 3089–96.

497. Van den Bruel A, Aertgeerts B, Bruyninckx R, Aerts M, Buntinx F. Signs and symptoms for diagnosis of serious infections in children: a prospective study in primary care. *BJGP.* 2007; **57**(540): 538–46.

498. Gorelick MH, Shaw KN, Murphy KO. Validity and reliability of clinical signs in the diagnosis of dehydration in children. *Pediatrics.* 1997; **99**(5): e6.

499. Orr PH, Nicolle LE, Duckworth H, Brunka J, Kennedy J, Murray D, *et al.* Febrile urinary infection in the institutionalized elderly. *Am J Med.* 1996; **100**(1): 71–7.

500. Jordan RE, Hawker JI. Influenza in elderly people in care homes. *BMJ.* 2006; **333**(7581): 1229–30.

501. Shapley M, Mansell G, Jordan JL, Jordan KP. Positive predictive values of ≥5% in primary care for cancer: systematic review. *BJGP.* 2010; **60**(578): e366–77.

502. Eberl MM, Phillips RL, Lamberts H, Okkes I, Mahoney MC. Characterizing breast symptoms in family practice. *Ann Fam Med.* 2008; **6**(6): 528–33.

503. Bachmann LM, ter Riet G, Clark TJ, Gupta JK, Khan KS. Probability analysis for diagnosis of endometrial hyperplasia and cancer in postmenopausal bleeding: an approach for a rational diagnostic workup. *Acta Obstet Gynecol Scand.* 2003; **82**(6): 564–9.

504. Bastian LA, Smith C, Nanda K. Is this woman perimenopausal? *JAMA.* 2003; **289**(7): 895–902.

505. Wise LA1, Krieger N, Zierler S, Harlow BL. Lifetime socioeconomic position in relation to onset of perimenopause. *Journal of Epidemiology.* 2002; **56**(11): 851–60.

506. Strote J, Chen G. Patient self assessment of pregnancy status in the emergency department. *Emergency Medicine Journal.* 2006; **23**(7): 554–7.

507. Conde-Agudelo A, Rosas-Bermudez A, Kafury-Goeta AC. Birth spacing and risk of adverse perinatal outcomes: a meta-analysis. *JAMA.* 2006; **295**(15): 1809–23.

508. Love ER, Bhattacharya S, Smith NC, Bhattacharya S. Effect of interpregnancy interval on outcomes of pregnancy after miscarriage: retrospective analysis of hospital episode statistics in Scotland. *BMJ.* 2010; **341**(Aug 05_2): c3967.

509. Wieringa-De Waard M, Bonsel GJ, Ankum WM, Vos J, Bindels PJ. Threatened miscarriage in general practice: diagnostic value of history taking and physical examination. *BJGP.* 2002; **52**: 825–9.

510. Cahill DJ, Wardle PG. Management of infertility. *BMJ.* 2002; **325**(7354): 28–32.

511. Gnoth C, Godehardt D, Godehardt E, Frank-Herrmann P, Freundl G. Time to preg-nancy: results of the German prospective study and impact on the management of infertility. *Hum. Reprod.* 2003; **18**(9): 1959–66.

512. Gnoth C, Godehardt E, Frank-Herrmann P, Friol K, Tigges J, Freundl G. Definition and prevalence of subfertility and infertility. *Hum. Reprod.* 2005; **20**(5): 1144–7.

513. Dunson DB, Colombo B, Baird DD. Reproductive epidemiology: changes with age in the level and duration of fertility in the menstrual cycle. *Hum. Reprod.* 2002; **17**(5): 1399–403.

514. Mayrand M, Duarte-Franco E, Rodrigues I, Walter SD, Hanley J, Ferenczy A, *et al.* Human papillomavirus DNA versus Papanicolaou screening tests for cervical can-cer. *N Engl J Med.* 2007; **357**(16): 1579–88.

515. Bent S, Nallamothu BK, Simel DL, Fihn SD, Saint S. Does this woman have an acute uncomplicated urinary tract infection? *JAMA.* 2002; **287**(20): 2701–10.

516. Little P, Rumsby K, Jones R, Warner G, Moore M, Lowes JA, *et al.* Validating the pre-diction of lower urinary tract infection in primary care: sensitivity and specificity of urinary dipsticks and clinical scores in women. *BJGP.* 2010; **60**: 495–500.

517. Little P, Merriman R, Turner S, Rumsby K, Warner G, Lowes JA, *et al.* Presentation, pattern, and natural course of severe symptoms, and role of antibiotics and antibiotic resistance among patients presenting with suspected uncomplicated urinary tract infection in primary care: observational study. *BMJ.* 2010; **340**(Feb 05_1): b5633.

518. Little P, Moore MV, Turner S, Rumsby K, Warner G, Lowes JA, *et al.* Effectiveness of five different approaches in management of urinary tract infection: randomised controlled trial. *BMJ.* 2010; **340**(Feb 05_1): c199.

519. Vellinga A, Cormican M, Hanahoe B, Murphy AW. Predictive value of antimicrobial susceptibility from previous urinary tract infection in the treatment of re-infection. *BJGP.* 2010; **60**(576): 511–13.

520. Portis AJ, Sundaram CP. Diagnosis and initial management of kidney stones. *Am Fam Physician.* 2001; **63**(7): 1329–38.

521. Eskelinen M, Ikonen J, Lipponen P. Usefulness of history-taking, physical examina-tion and diagnostic scoring in acute renal colic. *Eur Urol.* 1998; **34**(6): 467–73.

522. Hemmelgarn BR, Manns BJ, Lloyd A, James MT, Klarenbach S, Quinn RR, *et al.* Relation between kidney function, proteinuria, and adverse outcomes. *JAMA.* 2010; **303**(5): 423–9.

523. Cooper BA, Branley P, Bulfone L, Collins JF, Craig JC, Fraenkel MB, *et al.* A rand-omized, controlled trial of early versus late initiation of dialysis. *N Engl J Med.* 2010; **363**(7): 609–19.

524. Lipsky BA, Inui TS, Plorde JJ, Berger RE. Is the clean-catch midstream void proce-dure necessary for obtaining urine culture specimens from men? *Am J Med.* 1984; **76**(2): 257–62.

525. Hiatt R, Ordonez J. Dipstick urinalysis screening, asymptomatic microhema-turia, and subsequent urological cancers in a population-based sample. *Cancer Epidemiology, Biomarkers & Prevention.* 1994; **3**: 439–43.

526. Ritchie CD, Bevan EA, Collier SJ. Importance of occult haematuria found at screen-ing. *BMJ (Clinical research ed.).* 1986; **292**(6521): 681–3.

527. Jones R, Charlton J, Latinovic R, Gulliford MC. Alarm symptoms and identification of non-cancer diagnoses in primary care: cohort study. *BMJ.* 2009; **339**(Aug13_2): b3094.

528. Jones R, Latinovic R, Charlton J, Gulliford MC. Alarm symptoms in early diagnosis of cancer in primary care: cohort study using the General Practice Research Database. *BMJ*. 2007; **334**(7602): 1040.

529. Bruyninckx R., Buntinx F., Aertgeerts B., van Casteren V. The diagnostic value of macroscopic haematuria for the diagnosis of urological cancer in general practice. *BJGP*. 2003; **53**(486): 31–5.

530. Hoogendam A, Buntinx F, de Vet HC. The diagnostic value of digital rectal examination in primary care screening for prostate cancer: a meta-analysis. *Fam Pract*. 1999; **16**(6): 621–6.

531. Feldman HA, Goldstein I, Hatzichristou DG, Krane RJ, McKinlay JB. Impotence and its medical and psychosocial correlates: results of the Massachusetts Male Aging Study. *J Urol*. 1994; **151**(1): 54–61.

532. Serretti A, Chiesa A. Treatment-emergent sexual dysfunction related to antidepressants. *Journal of Clinical Psychopharmacology*. 2009; **29**(3): 259–66.

533. Speckens AE, Hengeveld MW, Lycklama ÀNijeholt GA, van Hemert AM, Hawton KE. Discrimination between psychogenic and organic erectile dysfunction. *Journal of Psychosomatic Research*. 1993; **37**(2): 135–45.

534. van den Berk GEL, Frissen PHJ, Regez RM, Rietra PJGM. Evaluation of the Rapid Immunoassay Determine HIV 1/2 for detection of antibodies to Human Immunodeficiency Virus types 1 and 2. *J Clin Microbiol*. 2003; **41**(8): 3868–9.

535. Seagroatt V, Goldacre MJ. Hospital mortality league tables: influence of place of death. *BMJ*. 2004; **328**(7450): 1235–6.

536. Zimmerman M, Ruggero CJ, Chelminski I, Young D. Is bipolar disorder overdiagnosed? *J Clin Psychiatry*. 2008; **69**(6): 935–40.

537. Sartorius N, Ustün TB, Lecrubier Y, Wittchen HU. Depression comorbid with anxiety: results from the WHO study on psychological disorders in primary health care. *Br J Psychiatry Suppl*. 1996; **30**: 38–43.

538. Bjelland I, Dahl AA, Haug TT, Neckelmann D. The validity of the Hospital Anxiety and Depression Scale: an updated literature review. *Journal of Psychosomatic Research*. 2002; **52**(2): 69–77.

539. Arroll B, Goodyear-Smith F, Kerse N, Fishman T, Gunn J. Effect of the addition of a "help" question to two screening questions on specificity for diagnosis of depression in general practice: diagnostic validity study. *BMJ*. 2005; **331**(7521): 884.

540. Rinaldi P, Mecocci P, Benedetti C, Ercolani S, Bregnocchi M, Menculini G, et al. Validation of the five-item geriatric depression scale in elderly subjects in three different settings. *Journal of the American Geriatrics Society*. 2003; **51**(5): 694–8.

541. Shakespeare J, Blake F, Garcia J. A qualitative study of the acceptability of routine screening of postnatal women using the Edinburgh Postnatal Depression Scale. *BJGP*. 2003; **53**(493): 614–19.

542. Harris B, Huckle P, Thomas R, Johns S, Fung H. The use of rating scales to identify post-natal depression. *Br J Psychiatry*. 1989; **154**: 813–17.

543. *Edinburgh Postnatal Depression Scale*. Available at: www.fresno.ucsf.edu/pediatrics/downloads/edinburghscale.pdf

544. Furukawa TA, Cipriani A, Barbui C, Geddes JR. Long-term treatment of depression with antidepressants: a systematic narrative review. *Can J Psychiatry*. 2007; **52**(9): 545–52.

545. Elliott AM, Smith BH, Hannaford PC, Smith WC, Chambers WA. The course of chronic pain in the community: results of a four-year follow-up study. *Pain*. 2002; **99**(1–2): 299–307.

546. Stein C, Reinecke H, Sorgatz H. Opioid use in chronic noncancer pain: guidelines revisited. *Curr Opin Anaesthesiol*. 2010; **23**(5): 598–601.

547. Moran P, Jenkins R, Tylee A, Blizard R, Mann A. The prevalence of personality disorder among UK primary care attenders. *Acta Psychiatr Scand*. 2000; **102**(1): 52–7.

548. Chen EYH, Hui CLM, Lam MML, Chiu CPY, Law CW, Chung DWS, *et al*. Maintenance treatment with quetiapine versus discontinuation after one year of treatment in patients with remitted first episode psychosis: randomised controlled trial. *BMJ*. 2010; **341**(Aug 19_1): c4024.

549. Runeson B, Tidemalm D, Dahlin M, Lichtenstein P, Langstrom N. Method of attempted suicide as predictor of subsequent successful suicide: national long term cohort study. *BMJ*. 2010; **341**(Jul 13_1): c3222.

550. Hoek HW, van Hoeken D. Review of the prevalence and incidence of eating disorders. *International Journal of Eating Disorders*. 2003; **34**(4): 383–96.

551. Iliffe S, Pealing L. Subjective memory problems. *BMJ*. 2010; **340**: c1425.

552. Kirby M, Denihan A, Bruce I, Coakley D, Lawlor BA. The clock drawing test in primary care: sensitivity in dementia detection and specificity against normal and depressed elderly. *Int J Geriatr Psychiatry*. 2001; **16**(10): 935–40.

553. *Mini-Mental State Examination*. Available at: www.patient.co.uk/doctor/Mini-Mental-State-Examination-%28MMSE%29.htm

554. *Abbreviated Mental Test (AMT)*. Available at: www.patient.co.uk/doctor/Abbreviated-Mental-Test-%28AMT%29.htm

555. MacKenzie D, Copp P, Shaw R, Goodwin G. Brief cognitive screening of the elderly: a comparison of the Mini-Mental State Examination (MMSE), Abbreviated Mental Test (AMT) and Mental Status Questionnaire (MSQ). *Psychological Medicine*. 1996; **26**(2): 427–30.

556. Barberger-Gateau P, Commenges D, Gagnon M, Letenneur L, Sauvel C, Dartigues JF. Instrumental activities of daily living as a screening tool for cognitive impairment and dementia in elderly community dwellers. *J Am Geriatr Soc*. 1992; **40**(11): 1129–34.

557. Löppönen M, Räihä I, Isoaho R, Vahlberg T, Kivelä S. Diagnosing cognitive impairment and dementia in primary health care—a more active approach is needed. *Age and Ageing*. 2003; **32**(6): 606–12.

558. Neuropathology Group of the MRC Cognitive Function and Ageing Study. Pathological correlates of late-onset dementia in a multicentre, community-based population in England and Wales. *Lancet*. 2001; **357**(9251): 169–75.

559. Ehreke L, Luppa M, Luck T, Wiese B, Weyerer S, Eifflaender-Gorfer S, *et al*. Is the clock drawing test appropriate for screening for mild cognitive impairment?—results of the German study on Ageing, Cognition and Dementia in Primary Care Patients (AgeCoDe). *Dement Geriatr Cogn Disord*. 2009; **28**(4): 365–72.

560. Rait G, Walters K, Bottomley C, Petersen I, Iliffe S, Nazareth I. Survival of people with clinical diagnosis of dementia in primary care: cohort study. *BMJ*. 2010; **341**(Aug 05_2): c3584.

561. *GPCOG Dementia test*. [cited 2010 Oct 19]. Available at: www.gpcog.com.au/prep.php

562. Brodaty H, Kemp NM, Low L. Characteristics of the GPCOG, a screening tool for cognitive impairment. *International Journal of Geriatric Psychiatry.* 2004; **19**(9): 870–4.

563. *The Health Literacy of America's Adults: results from the 2003 National Assessment of Adult Literacy.* U.S. Depratment of Education, Institute of Education Sciences, National Center for Education Statistics; [cited 2011 Jan 31]. Available at: http://nces.ed.gov/pubs2006/2006483.pdf

564. Smith SK, Trevena L, Simpson JM, Barratt A, Nutbeam D, McCaffery KJ. A decision aid to support informed choices about bowel cancer screening among adults with low education: randomised controlled trial. *BMJ.* 2010; **341**: c5370.

565. Böhmer CJ, Taminiau JA, Klinkenberg-Knol EC, Meuwissen SG. The prevalence of constipation in institutionalized people with intellectual disability. *J Intellect Disabil Res.* 2001; **45**(Pt 3): 212–18.

566. Garcia DA, Regan S, Crowther M, Hylek EM. The risk of hemorrhage among patients with warfarin-associated coagulopathy. *Journal of the American College of Cardiology.* 2006; **47**(4): 804–8.

567. Nkomo VT, Gardin JM, Skelton TN, Gottdiener JS, Scott CG, Enriquez-Sarano M. Burden of valvular heart diseases: a population-based study. *Lancet.* 2006; **368**(9540): 1005–11.

568. Reichlin S, Dieterle T, Camli C, Leimenstoll B, Schoenenberger RA, Martina B. Initial clinical evaluation of cardiac systolic murmurs in the ED by noncardiologists. *Am J Emerg Med.* 2004; **22**(2): 71–5.

569. Cleland JGF, Swedberg K, Follath F, Komajda M, Cohen-Solal A, Aguilar JC, *et al.* The EuroHeart Failure survey programm - a survey on the quality of care among patients with heart failure in Europe. *European Heart Journal.* 2003; **24**(5): 442–63.

570. Owan TE, Hodge DO, Herges RM, Jacobsen SJ, Roger VL, Redfield MM. Trends in prevalence and outcome of heart failure with preserved ejection fraction. *N Engl J Med.* 2006; **355**(3): 251–9.

571. Davies M, Hobbs F, Davis R, Kenkre J, Roalfe A, Hare R, *et al.* Prevalence of left-ventricular systolic dysfunction and heart failure in the Echocardiographic Heart of England Screening study: a population based study. *Lancet.* 2001; **358**(9280): 439–4.

572. Hobbs FDR. Reliability of N-terminal pro-brain natriuretic peptide assay in diagnosis of heart failure: cohort study in representative and high risk community populations. *BMJ.* 2002; **324**(7352): 1498.

573. Hobbs FDR, Roalfe AK, Davis RC, Davies MK, Hare R. Prognosis of all-cause heart failure and borderline left ventricular systolic dysfunction: five-year mortality follow-up of the Echocardiographic Heart of England Screening Study (ECHOES). *European Heart Journal.* 2007; **28**(9): 1128–34.

574. British Heart Foundation. *Diastolic heart failure.* 2010 [cited 2010 May 4]. Available at: www.bhf.org.uk/idoc.ashx?docid=bc1f0d09-4b77-49cf-aff2-151b2a91ed10&version=-1

575. Carlberg B, Lindholm LH. Stroke and blood-pressure variation: new permutations on an old theme. *Lancet.* 2010; **375**(9718): 867–9.

576. Rothwell PM, Howard SC, Dolan E, O'Brien E, Dobson JE, Dahlöf B, *et al.* Prognostic significance of visit-to-visit variability, maximum systolic blood pressure, and episodic hypertension. *Lancet.* 2010; **375**(9718): 895–905.

577. Webb AJS, Fischer U, Mehta Z, Rothwell PM. Effects of antihypertensive-drug class on interindividual variation in blood pressure and risk of stroke: a systematic review and meta-analysis. *Lancet.* 2010; **375**(9718): 906–15.

578. Head GA, Mihailidou AS, Duggan KA, Beilin LJ, Berry N, Brown MA, *et al*. Definition of ambulatory blood pressure targets for diagnosis and treatment of hypertension in relation to clinic blood pressure: prospective cohort study. *BMJ*. 2010; **340**: c1104.

579. Bösner S, Haasenritter J, Becker A, Karatolios K, Vaucher P, Gencer B, *et al*. Ruling out coronary artery disease in primary care: development and validation of a simple prediction rule. *CMAJ*. 2010; **182**(12): 1295–300.

580. Bruyninckx R, Aertgeerts B, Bruyninckx P, Buntinx F. Signs and symptoms in diagnosing acute myocardial infarction and acute coronary syndrome: a diagnostic meta-analysis. *BJGP*. 2008; **58**(547): 105–11.

581. Gill D, Mayou R, Dawes M, Mant D. Presentation, management and course of angina and suspected angina in primary care. *Journal of Psychosomatic Research*. 1999; **46**(4): 349–58.

582. Cooke RA, Smeeton N, Chambers JB. Comparative study of chest pain characteristics in patients with normal and abnormal coronary angiograms. *Heart*. 1997; **78**(2): 142–6.

583. Fowkes FG, Housley E, Cawood EH, Macintyre CC, Ruckley CV, Prescott RJ. Edinburgh Artery Study: prevalence of asymptomatic and symptomatic peripheral arterial disease in the general population. *Int J Epidemiol*. 1991; **20**(2): 384–92.

584. Khan NA, Rahim SA, Anand SS, Simel DL, Panju A. Does the clinical examination predict lower extremity peripheral arterial disease? *JAMA*. 2006; **295**(5): 536–46.

585. Zwietering PJ, Knottnerus JA, Rinkens PE, Kleijne MA, Gorgels AP. Arrhythmias in general practice: diagnostic value of patient characteristics, medical history and symptoms. *Fam Pract*. 1998; **15**(4): 343–53.

586. Summerton N, Mann S, Rigby A, Petkar S, Dhawan J. New-onset palpitations in general practice: assessing the discriminant value of items within the clinical history. *Fam Pract*. 2001; **18**(4): 383–92.

587. Sudlow M, Rodgers H, Kenny RA, Thomson R. Identification of patients with atrial fibrillation in general practice: a study of screening methods. *BMJ*. 1998; **317**(7154): 327–8.

588. Soteriades E, Evans J, Larson M, Chen M, Chen L, Benjamin E, *et al*. Incidence and prognosis of syncope. *Journal of Medicine*. September 19, 2002; **347**(12): 878–5.

589. Heikkinen M, Pikkarainen P, Takala J, Räsänen H, Julkunen R. Etiology of dyspepsia: four hundred unselected consecutive patients in general practice. *Scand J Gastroenterol*. 1995; **30**(6): 519–23.

590. Kapoor N, Bassi A, Sturgess R, Bodger K. Predictive value of alarm features in a rapid access upper gastrointestinal cancer service. *Gut*. 2005; **54**(1): 40–5.

591. Weijnen CF, Numans ME, de Wit NJ, Smout AJPM, Moons KGM, Verheij TJM, *et al*. Testing for *Helicobacter pylori* in dyspeptic patients suspected of peptic ulcer disease in primary care: cross sectional study. *BMJ*. 2001; **323**(7304): 71–5.

592. Cumberland P, Sethi D, Roderick PJ, Wheeler JG, Cowden JM, Roberts JA, *et al*. The infectious intestinal disease study of England: a prospective evaluation of symptoms and health care use after an acute episode. *Epidemiol Infect*. 2003; **130**(3): 453–60.

593. Jones R, Sleet S. Coeliac disease. *BMJ*. 2009; **338**(Feb 19_1): a3058.

594. van der Windt DAWM, Jellema P, Mulder CJ, Kneepkens CMF, van der Horst HE. Diagnostic testing for celiac disease among patients with abdominal symptoms: a systematic review. *JAMA*. 2010; **303**(17): 1738–46.

595. du Toit J, Hamilton W, Barraclough K. Risk in primary care of colorectal cancer from new onset rectal bleeding: 10 year prospective study. *BMJ.* 2006; **333**(7558): 69–70.

596. Lawrenson R, Logie J, Marks C. Risk of colorectal cancer in general practice patients presenting with rectal bleeding, change in bowel habit or anaemia. *J Cancer Care.* 2006; **15**(3): 267–71.

597. Ellis BG, Thompson MR. Factors identifying higher risk rectal bleeding in general practice. *BJGP.* 2005; **55**(521): 949–55.

598. Eaden JA, Abrams KR, Mayberry JF. The risk of colorectal cancer in ulcerative colitis: a meta-analysis. *Gut.* 2001; **48**(4): 526–35.

599. Robertson R, Campbell C, Weller DP, Elton R, Mant D, Primrose J, *et al.* Predicting colorectal cancer risk in patients with rectal bleeding. *BJGP.* 2006; **56**(531): 763–7.

600. Challand GS, Michaeloudis A, Watfa RR, Coles SJ, Macklin JL. Distribution of haemoglobin in patients presenting to their general practitioner, and its correlation with serum ferritin. *Ann Clin Biochem.* 1990; **27**(Pt 1): 15–20.

601. Sheth TN, Choudhry NK, Bowes M, Detsky AS. The relation of conjunctival pallor to the presence of anemia. *J Gen Intern Med.* 1997; **12**(2): 102–6.

602. Yates JM, Logan ECM, Stewart RM. Iron deficiency anaemia in general practice: clinical outcomes over three years and factors influencing diagnostic investigations. *Postgraduate Medical Journal.* 2004; **80**: 405–10.

603. Mathiesen UL, Franzén LE, Frydén A, Foberg U, Bodemar G. The clinical significance of slightly to moderately increased liver transaminase values in asymptomatic patients. *Scandinavian Journal of Gastroenterology.* 1999; **34**(1): 85–91.

604. *Alcohol Use Disorders Identification Test (AUDIT).* Patient UK; [cited 2011 Jan 21]. Available at: www.patient.co.uk/doctor/Alcohol-Use-Disorders-Identification-Test-%28AUDIT%29.htm

605. Simel DL, Yancy WS. Update: alcohol abuse. In: Simel DL, Rennie D, editors. *The Rational Clinical Examination: evidence-based clinical diagnosis.* New York: McGraw-Hill; 2009 [cited 2010 Jul 16]. Available at: www.jamaevidence.com/resource/523

606. *CAGE Questionnaire.* Patient UK [cited 2010 Oct 25]. Available at: www.patient.co.uk/doctor/CAGE-Questionnaire.htm

607. Kitchens JM. Original article: does this patient have an alcohol problem? In: Simel D, Rennie D, editors. *The Rational Clinical Examination: evidence-based clinical diagnosis.* New York: McGraw-Hill; 2009 [cited 2010 Oct 25]. Available at: www.jamaevidence.com/content/3475115

608. Simel DL, Hatala R, Edelman D. Update: ascites. In: Simel DL, Rennie D, editors. *The Rational Clinical Examination: evidence-based clinical diagnosis.* New York: McGraw-Hill; 2009 [cited 2010 Oct 25]. Available at: www.jamaevidence.com/content/3475877

609. De Las Cuevas C, Sanz EJ, De La Fuente JA, Padilla J, Berenguer JC. The Severity of Dependence Scale (SDS) as screening test for benzodiazepine dependence: SDS validation study. *Addiction.* 2000; **95**(2): 245–50.

610. de las Cuevas C, Sanz E, de la Fuente J. Benzodiazepines: more "behavioural" addiction than dependence. *Psychopharmacology.* 2003; **167**(3): 297–303.

611. Cornish R, Macleod J, Strang J, Vickerman P, Hickman M. Risk of death during and after opiate substitution treatment in primary care: prospective observational study in UK General Practice Research Database. *BMJ.* 2010; **341**: c5475.

612. Kimber J, Copeland L, Hickman M, Macleod J, McKenzie J, De Angelis D, *et al.* Survival and cessation in injecting drug users: prospective observational study of outcomes and effect of opiate substitution treatment. *BMJ.* 2010; **341**(Jul 01_1): c3172.

613. Young T, Palta M, Dempsey J, Skatrud J, Weber S, Badr S. The occurrence of sleep-disordered breathing among middle-aged adults. *N Engl J Med.* 1993; **328**(17): 1230–5.

614. *Epworth Sleepiness Scale. British Snoring & Sleep Apnoea Association;* [cited 2010 Oct 25]. Available at: www.britishsnoring.co.uk/sleep_apnoea/epworth_sleepiness_scale.php

615. Di Guardo A, Profeta G, Crisafulli C, Sidoti G, Zammataro M, Paolini I, *et al.* Obstructive sleep apnoea in patients with obesity and hypertension. *BJGP.* 2010; **60**(574): 325–8.

616. Bagai A, Thavendiranathan P, Detsky AS. Does this patient have hearing impairment? *JAMA.* 2006; **295**(4): 416–28.

617. Sindhusake D, Mitchell P, Smith W, Golding M, Newall P, Hartley D, *et al.* Validation of self-reported hearing loss: the Blue Mountains Hearing Study. *Int. J. Epidemiol.* 2001; **30**(6): 1371–8.

618. Rose PW, Harnden A, Brueggemann AB, Perera R, Sheikh A, Crook D, *et al.* Chloramphenicol treatment for acute infective conjunctivitis in children in primary care: a randomised double-blind placebo-controlled trial. *Lancet.* 2005; **366**(9479): 37–43.

619. Yang W, Lu J, Weng J, Jia W, Ji L, Xiao J, *et al.* Prevalence of diabetes among men and women in China. *N Engl J Med.* 2010; **362**(12): 1090–101.

620. Salti I, Bénard E, Detournay B, Bianchi-Biscay M, Le Brigand C, Voinet C, *et al.* A population-based study of diabetes and its characteristics during the fasting month of ramadan in 13 countries: results of the epidemiology of diabetes and ramadan 1422/2001 (EPIDIAR) study. *Diabetes Care.* 2004; **27**(10): 2306–11.

621. Helfand M, Redfern CC. Screening for thyroid disease: an update. *Annals of Internal Medicine.* 1998; **129**(2): 144–58.

622. Rothwell P, Giles M, Flossmann E, Lovelock C, Redgrave J, Warlow C, *et al.* A simple score (ABCD) to identify individuals at high early risk of stroke after transient ischaemic attack. *Lancet.* 2005; **366**(9479): 29–36.

623. Becker L, Iverson DC, Reed FM, Calonge N, Miller RS, Freeman WL. Patients with new headache in primary care: a report from ASPN. *J Fam Pract.* 1988; **27**(1): 41–7.

624. Smetana GW, Shmerling RH. Does this patient have temporal arteritis? *JAMA.* 2002; **287**(1): 92–101.

625. Louis ED, Ottman R, Hauser WA. How common is the most common adult movement disorder? estimates of the prevalence of essential tremor throughout the world. *Mov Disord.* 1998; **13**(1): 5–10.

626. Rao G, Fisch L, Srinivasan S, D'Amico F, Okada T, Eaton C, *et al.* Does this patient have Parkinson Disease?. In: Simel DL, Rennie D, editors. *The Rational Clinical Examination: evidence-based clinical diagnosis.* New York: McGraw-Hill; 2009 [cited 2010 Jun 17]. Available at: www.jamaevidence.com/content/3485159

627. Bonnett LJ, Tudur-Smith C, Williamson PR, Marson AG. Risk of recurrence after a first seizure and implications for driving: further analysis of the Multicentre study of early epilepsy and single seizures. *BMJ*. 2010; **341**: c6477.

628. Marson A, Jacoby A, Johnson A, Kim L, Gamble C, Chadwick D. Immediate versus deferred antiepileptic drug treatment for early epilepsy and single seizures: a randomised controlled trial. *Lancet*. 2005; **365**(9476): 2007–13.

629. Medical Research Council Antiepileptic Drug Withdrawal Study Group, Bessant P, Chadwick D, Eaton B, Taylor J, Holland A, *et al*. Randomised study of antiepileptic drug withdrawal in patients in remission. *Lancet*. 1991; **337**(8751): 1175–80.

630. Jentink J, Dolk H, Loane MA, Morris JK, Wellesley D, Garne E, *et al*. Intrauterine exposure to carbamazepine and specific congenital malformations: systematic review and case-control study. *BMJ*. 2010; **341**: c6581.

631. *Katz hand symptom diagram*. [cited 2010 Oct 25]. Available at: www.carpal-tunnel-symptoms.com/hand-symptom-diagram.html

632. D'Arcy CA, McGee S. Original Article: does this patient have carpal tunnel syndrome? In: Simel DL, Rennie D, editors. *The Rational Clinical Examination: evidence-based clinical diagnosis*. New York: McGraw-Hill; 2009 [cited 2011 Jan 22]. Available at: www.jamaevidence.com/content/3474226

633. Simel DL, Bedlack R. Update: carpal tunnel syndrome. In: Simel DL, Rennie D, editors. *The Rational Clinical Examination: evidence-based clinical diagnosis*. New York: McGraw-Hill; 2009 [cited 2010 Jul 17]. Available at: www.jamaevidence.com/abstract/3474286

634. Hanley K, O' Dowd T. Symptoms of vertigo in general practice: a prospective study of diagnosis. *BJGP*. 2002; **52**(483): 809–12.

635. Hay AD, Wilson A, Fahey T, Peters TJ. The duration of acute cough in pre-school children presenting to primary care: a prospective cohort study. *Fam Pract*. 2003; **20**(6): 696–705.

636. Butler CC, Hood K, Verheij T, Little P, Melbye H, Nuttall J, *et al*. Variation in antibiotic prescribing and its impact on recovery in patients with acute cough in primary care: prospective study in 13 countries. *BMJ*. 2009; **338**(Jun 23_2): b2242.

637. *GOLD—The Global initiative for chronic Obstructive Lung Disease*. [cited 2011 Jan 22]. Available at: www.goldcopd.org/

638. Broekhuizen BD, Sachs AP, Hoes AW, Moons KG, van den Berg JW, Dalinghaus WH, *et al*. Undetected chronic obstructive pulmonary disease and asthma in people over 50 years with persistent cough. *BJGP*. 2010; **60**: 489–94.

639. Simel DL, Keitz S. Update: airflow limitation. In: Simel DL, Rennie D, editors. *The Rational Clinical Examination: evidence-based clinical diagnosis*. New York: McGraw-Hill; 2009 [cited 2010 Jul 17]. Available at: www.jamaevidence.com/abstract/3477922

640. Call S, Vollenweider M, Hornung C, Simel DL, Mckinney W. Original Article: does this patient have influenza? In: Simel DL, Rennie D, editors. *The Rational Clinical Examination: evidence-based clinical diagnosis*. New York: McGraw-Hill; 2009 [cited 2010 Jun 17]. Available at: www.jamaevidence.com/content/3481909

641. Montnemery P, Hansson L, Lanke J, Lindholm L, Nyberg P, Lofdahl C, *et al*. Accuracy of a first diagnosis of asthma in primary health care. *Fam Pract*. 2002; **19**(4): 365–8.

642. van Schayck CP, van der Heijden FMMA, van den Boom G, Tirimanna PRS, van Herwaarden CLA. Underdiagnosis of asthma: is the doctor or the patient to blame? The DIMCA project. *Thorax.* 2000; **55**(7): 562–5.

643. Hamilton W, Peters TJ, Round A, Sharp D. What are the clinical features of lung cancer before the diagnosis is made? A population based case-control study. *Thorax.* 2005; **60**(12): 1059–65.

644. Stapley S, Sharp D, Hamilton W. Negative chest X-rays in primary care patients with lung cancer. *BJGP.* 2006; **56**: 570–3.

645. Green AD, Colón-Emeric CS, Bastian L, Drake MT, Lyles KW. Original article: does this patient have osteoporosis? In: Simel DL, Rennie D, editors. *The Rational Clinical Examination: evidence-based clinical diagnosis.* New York: McGraw-Hill; 2009 [cited 2011 Jan 22]. Available at: www.jamaevidence.com/content/3484613

646. Colón-Emeric CS, Simel DL, Lyles KW. Make the diagnosis: osteoporosis. In: Simel DL, Rennie D, editors. *The Rational Clinical Examination: evidence-based clinical diagnosis.* New York: McGraw-Hill; 2009 [cited 2011 Jan 22]. Available at: www.jamaevidence.com/abstract/3484589

647. Colón-Emeric CS, Simel DL, Lyles KW. Update: osteoporosis. In: Simel DL, Rennie D, editors. *The Rational Clinical Examination: evidence-based clinical diagnosis.* New York: McGraw-Hill; 2009 [cited 2010 Jun 17]. Available at: www.jamaevidence.com/abstract/3484715

648. Green AD, Colón-Emeric CS, Bastian L, Lyles KW. Original article: does this patient have osteoporosis?. In: Simel DL, Rennie D, editors. *The Rational Clinical Examination: evidence-based clinical diagnosis.* New York: McGraw-Hill; 2009 [cited 2010 Jun 17]. Available at: www.jamaevidence.com/content/3484605

649. *FRAX.* [cited 2011 Jan 24]. Available at: www.shef.ac.uk/FRAX/

650. Henschke N, Maher CG, Refshauge KM, Herbert RD, Cumming RG, Bleasel J, *et al.* Prognosis in patients with recent onset low back pain in Australian primary care: inception cohort study. *BMJ.* 2008; **337**(Jul 07_1): a171.

651. Stern B, Deyo RA, Rainville J, Bedlack RS. Update: low back pain. In: Simel DL, Rennie D, editors. *The Rational Clinical Examination: evidence-based clinical diagnosis.* New York: McGraw-Hill; 2009 [cited 2010 Jun 17]. Available at: http://jamaevidence.com/abstract/3476058

652. Levack P, Graham J, Collie D, Grant R, Kidd J, Kunkler I, *et al.* Don't wait for a sensory level—listen to the symptoms: a prospective audit of the delays in diagnosis of malignant cord compression. *Clin Oncol (R Coll Radiol).* 2002; **14**(6): 472–80.

653. van der Waal JM, Bot SDM, Terwee CB, van der Windt DAWM, Scholten RJPM, Bouter LM, *et al.* Course and prognosis of knee complaints in general practice. *Arthritis Rheum.* 2005; **53**(6): 920–30.

654. Solmon DH, Avorn J, Warsi A, Brown CH, Martin S, Martin TL, *et al.* Which patients with knee problems are likely to benefit from nonarthroplasty surgery? development of a clinical prediction rule. *Arch Intern Med.* 2004; **164**(5): 509–13.

655. *Knee and Osteoarthritis Outcome Score (KOOS), English version LK1.0.* Available at: www.biomedcentral.com/content/supplementary/1471-2474-7-38-S1.pdf

656. Frobell R, Roos E, Roos H, Ranstam J, Lohmander L. A Randomized trial of treatment for acute anterior cruciate ligament tears. *N Engl J Med.* 2010; **363**(4): 331.

657. *Medial Lateral Grind Test.* 2009 [cited 2011 Jan 22]. Available at: www.youtube.com/watch?v=VyPYakQD0gI

658. *Lachman Test.* 2008. Available at www.youtube.com/watch?v=_5WyoDY31Fc&feature=youtube_gdata_player

659. Solomon DH, Simel DL, Bates DW, Katz JN, Schaffer JL. Original article: does this patient have a torn meniscus or ligament of the knee? In: Simel DL, Rennie D, editors. *The Rational Clinical Examination: evidence-based clinical diagnosis.* New York: McGraw-Hill; 2009 [cited 2010 Jun 17]. Available at: www.jamaevidence.com/abstract/3482053

660. Whiting PF, Smidt N, Sterne JA, Harbord R, Burton A, Burke M, *et al.* Systematic review: accuracy of anti–citrullinated peptide antibodies for diagnosing rheumatoid arthritis. *Annals of Internal Medicine.* 2010; **152**(7): 456–64.

661. Dunn KM, Saunders KW, Rutter CM, Banta-Green CJ, Merrill JO, Sullivan MD, *et al.* Opioid prescriptions for chronic pain and overdose. *Annals of Internal Medicine.* 2010; **152**(2): 8–92.

662. Simel DL, Grichnik JM. Update: melanoma. In: Simel DL, Rennie D, editors. *The Rational Clinical Examination: evidence-based clinical diagnosis.* New York: McGraw-Hill; 2009 [cited 2010 Jun 17]. Available at: www.jamaevidence.com/abstract/3482625

663. Del Mar CB, Green AC. Aid to diagnosis of melanoma in primary medical care. *BMJ.* 1995; **310**(6978): 492–5.

664. Rydholm A, Berg NO. Size, site and clinical incidence of lipoma: factors in the differential diagnosis of lipoma and sarcoma. *Acta Orthop Scand.* 1983; **54**(6): 929–34.

665. Charlton R. *Learning to Consult.* Oxford: Radcliffe Publishing; 2007.

666. Neighbour R. *The Inner Consultation.* Oxford: Radcliffe Publishing; 2005.

667. Neighbour R. *The Inner Apprentice.* Oxford: Radcliffe Publishing; 2005.

668. Pendleton D, Schofield T, Tate P. *The New Consultation.* Oxford: Oxford University Press; 2003.

669. Maguire P, Pitceathly C. Key communication skills and how to acquire them. *BMJ.* 2002; **325**(7366): 697–700.

670. Moulton L. *The Naked Consultation.* Oxford: Radcliffe Publishing; 2007.

671. Rollnick S, Butler CC, Kinnersley P, Gregory J, Mash B. Motivational interviewing. *BMJ.* 2010; **340**(7758): c1900.

672. Evans BJ, Stanley RO, Mestrovic R, Rose L. Effects of communication skills training on students' diagnostic efficiency. *Med Educ.* 1991; **25**(6): 517–26.

673. Ericsson KA. Deliberate practice and the acquisition and maintenance of expert performance in medicine and related domains. *Acad Med.* 2004; **79**(10 Suppl): S70–81.

674. Ericsson K, Prietual M, Cokely E. The making of an expert. *Harvard Business Review.* 2007 Aug. Available at: http://hbr.org/2007/07/the-making-of-an-expert/ar/1

675. Glaser AN. Communicating with deaf people. Turn the computer screen round (letter). *BMJ.* 2010; **341**: c5989.

676. Welsby PD. Communicating with deaf people. Stethoscope is a hearing aid (letter). *BMJ.* 2010; **341**: c5985.

677. Wright EB, Holcombe C, Salmon P. Doctors' communication of trust, care, and respect in breast cancer: qualitative study. *BMJ.* 2004; **328**(7444): 864–7.

678. Antonovsky A. *Health, Stress, and Coping.* San Francisco: Jossey-Bass; 1979.

679. Schilte AF, Portegijs PJM, Blankenstein AH, van der Horst HE, Latour MBF, van Eijk JTM, *et al.* Randomised controlled trial of disclosure of emotionally important events in somatisation in primary. *BMJ.* 2001; **323**(7304): 86.

680. Thomas KB. General practice consultations: is there any point in being positive? *BMJ* (Clinical research ed.). 1987; **294**(6581): 1200–2.

681. Taylor SE, Kemeny ME, Reed GM, Bower JE, Gruenewald TL. Psychological resources, positive illusions, and health. *Am Psychol.* 2000; **55**(1): 99–109.

682. Seligman ME, Csikszentmihalyi M. Positive psychology: an introduction. *Am Psychol.* 2000; **55**(1): 5–14.

683. Stone J. *Functional and Dissociative Neurological Symptoms: a patient's guide.* [cited 2010 Dec 5]. Available at: www.neurosymptoms.org/

684. Salmon P, Peters S, Stanley I. Patients' perceptions of medical explanations for somatisation disorders: qualitative analysis. *BMJ.* 1999; **318**(7180): 372–6.

685. Hall JA, Roter DL, Katz NR. Meta-analysis of correlates of provider behavior in medical encounters. *Med Care.* 1988; **26**(7): 657–75.

686. Dalrymple T. *Spoilt Rotten: the toxic cult of sentimentality.* London: Gibson Square Books; 2010.

687. Winnicott IOP. Mirror-role of Mother and Family in Child Development. In: Lomas P, editor. *The Predicament of the Family: a psycho-analytical symposium.* London: Hogarth Press and the Institute of Psycho-Analysis; 1967.

688. Singh C. The role of touch in comforting the distressed patient in the general practice consultation. Poster at RCGP Annual Conference, Oct. 2010.

689. Buis C, de Boo T, Hull R. Touch and breaking bad news. *Fam Prac.* 1991; **8**(4): 303–4.

690. Kahneman D. Objective Happiness. In: Kahneman D, Diener E, Schwarz N, editors. *Well-Being: the foundations of hedonic psychology.* New York: Russell Sage Foundation; 2003.

691. Page LA, Wessely S. Medically unexplained symptoms: exacerbating factors in the doctor-patient encounter. *J R Soc Med.* 2003; **96**(5): 223–7.

692. Salmon P, Dowrick CF, Ring A, Humphris GM. Voiced but unheard agendas: qualitative analysis of the psychosocial cues that patients with unexplained symptoms present to general practitioners. *BJGP.* 2004; **54**(500): 171–6.

693. Albarran JW, Clarke BA, Crawford J. 'It was not chest pain really, I can't explain it!' An exploratory study on the nature of symptoms experienced by women during their myocardial infarction. *J Clin Nurs.* 2007; **16**(7): 1292–301.

694. Treasure T. Pain is not the only feature of heart attack. *BMJ.* 1998; **317**(7158): 602.

695. Jones MM, Somerville C, Feder G, Foster G. Patients' descriptions of angina symptoms: a qualitative study of primary care patients. *BJGP.* 2010; **60**(579): 735–41.

696. Patient UK. *Angina.* [cited 2010 Oct 10]. Available at: www.patient.co.uk/health/Angina.htm

697. Ring A, Dowrick C, Humphris G, Salmon P. Do patients with unexplained physical symptoms pressurise general practitioners for somatic treatment? a qualitative study. *BMJ.* 2004; **328**(7447): 1057.

698. Kessler D, Hamilton W. Normalisation: horrible word, useful idea. *BJGP.* 2004; **54**(500): 163–4.

699. Griffiths F, Green E, Tsouroufli M. The nature of medical evidence and its inherent uncertainty for the clinical consultation: qualitative study. *BMJ.* 2005; **330**(7490): 511.

700. Lundahl BW, Kunz C, Brownell C, Tollefson D, Burke BL. A meta-analysis of motivational interviewing: twenty-five years of empirical studies. *Research on Social Work Practice.* 2010; **20**(2): 137–60.

701. Rabinowitz I, Luzzati R, Tamir A, Reis S. Length of patient's monologue, rate of completion, and relation to other components of the clinical encounter: observational intervention study in primary care. *BMJ.* 2004; **328**(7438): 501–2.

702. Stevens R, Mountford A. On time. *BJGP.* 2010; **60**(575): 458–60.

703. Rosenberg MB. *Nonviolent Communication: a language of life.* Encinitas, CA: PuddleDancer Press; 2003.

704. Center for Nonviolent Communication. [cited 2010 Dec 8]. Available at: www.cnvc.org/

705. Wilbush J. Clinical information—signs, semeions and symptoms: discussion paper. *Journal of the Royal Society of Medicine.* 1984; **77**(9): 766–73.

706. Tate P. *The Doctor's Communication Handbook.* Oxford: Radcliffe Publishing; 2003.

707. Brookes I, editor. *The Chambers Dictionary.* Edinburgh: Chambers Harrap Publishers Ltd; 2003.

708. Bayliss R. Pain Narratives. In: Greenhalgh T, Hurwitz B, editors. *Narrative Based Medicine: dialogue and discourse in clinical practice.* London: BMJ Books; 1998.

709. Denney M. The Well AiT Clinic: question and answer session at RCGP Annual Primary Care Conference, Harrogate: 9 Oct 2010.

710. Dorward P. Personal communication. May 2010.

711. Kay S, Purves I. The Electronic Medical Record and the "Story Stuff": a narrativistic model. In: Greenhalgh T, Hurwitz B, editors. *Narrative Based Medicine: dialogue and discourse in clinical practice.* London: BMJ Books; 1998.

712. Cape J, Geyer C, Barker C, Pistrang N, Buszewicz M, Dowrick C, *et al.* Facilitating understanding of mental health problems in GP consultations: a qualitative study using taped-assisted recall. *BJGP* 2010; **60**(580): 837–45.

713. Morris PE, Fritz CO. How to improve your memory. *The Psychologist.* 2006; **19**(10): 608–11.

714. Pashler H, McDaniel M, Rohrer D, Bjork R. Learning styles: concepts and evidence. *Psychologic Science in the Public Interest.* 2008; **9**(3): 106–19.

715. Cornoldi C, De Beni R, Mammarella IC. Mental Imagery. In: Roediger III HL, editor. *Learning and Memory: a comprehensive reference.* Maryland Heights, MO: Academic Press; 2008.

716. Deming WE. *Out of the Crisis.* Cambridge, MA: MIT Press; 1982.

717. Sadler DR. Formative assessment and the design of instructional systems. *Instructional Science.* 1989; **18**: 119–44.

718. Silverman J, Kinnersley P. Doctors' non-verbal behaviour in consultations: look at the patient before you look at the computer. *BJGP.* 2010; **60**(571): 76–8.

719. Hay GI. Looking at the patient. *BJGP.* 2010; **60**: 293.

720. Fitter A. *Collins Gem Trees: how to identify the most common species.* London: HarperCollins UK; 2004.

721. Holden P, Sharrock JTR, Burn H, Birds RSFTPO. *The RSPB Guide to British Birds.* New Edition. London: Macmillan Press Ltd; 1994.

722. Schwartz A, Elstein AS. Clinical problem solving and diagnostic decision making: a selective review of the cognitive research literature. In: Knottnerus JA, Buntinx F,

editors. *The Evidence Base of Clinical Diagnosis: theory and methods of diagnostic research*. Oxford: John Wiley and Sons; 2009.

723. Elstein AS, Schwartz A. Evidence base of clinical diagnosis: clinical problem solving and diagnostic decision making: selective review of the cognitive literature. *BMJ*. 2002; **324**(7339): 729–32.

724. Verghese A, Horwitz RI. In praise of the physical examination. *BMJ*. 2009; **339** (Dec 16_3): b5448.

725. Hamilton W. Colorectal Cancer. In: Hamilton W, Peters TJ, editors. *Cancer Diagnosis in Primary Care*. London: Elsevier Health Sciences; 2007.

726. Grover SA, Barkun AN, Sackett DL. Original article: does this patient have a splenomegaly? In: Simel DL, Rennie D, editors. *The Rational Clinical Examination: evidence-based clinical diagnosis*. New York: McGraw-Hill; 2009 [cited 2010 Nov 7]. Available at: www.jamaevidence.com/content/3487283

727. *International Association for the Study of Pain*. [cited 2010 Oct 19]. Available at: www. iasp-pain.org/AM/Template.cfm?Section=Pain_Defi...isplay.cfm&ContentID= 1728 - Pain

728. *Programme Appraisal Criteria: criteria for appraising the viability, effectiveness and appropriateness of a screening programme*. UK National Screening Committee; 2011 [cited 2011 Jan 11]. Available at: www.screening.nhs.uk/criteria#fileid9287

729. Waugh N, Scotland G, McNamee P, Gillett M, Brennan A, Goyder E, *et al*. Screening for type 2 diabetes: literature review and economic modelling. *Health Technol Assess*. 2007; **11**(17): iii–iv, ix–xi, 1–125.

730. Manser R, Irving LB, Stone C, Byrnes G, Abramson MJ, Campbell D. Screening for lung cancer. *Cochrane Database of Systematic Reviews*. 2004; **1**: CD001991.

731. Jensen G, Resnik L, Haddad A. Expertise and clinical reasoning. In: Higgs J, Jones MA, Loftus S, Christensen N, editors. *Clinical Reasoning in the Health Professions*. Philadelphia: Elsevier Health Sciences; 2008.

732. Roth T. Talking therapies. *The Psychologist*. 2010; **23**(6): 488–91.

733. Simel DL. Update: primer on decision accuracy. In: *The Rational Clinical Examination: evidence-based clinical diagnosis*. New York: McGraw-Hill; 2009.

734. Burkes M. Advice to new ST1s in general practice. *BJGP*. 2010; **60**: 63.

735. Long S, Neale G, Vincent C. Practising safely in the foundation years. *BMJ*. 2009; **338**(Apr 03_1): b1046.

736. NICE. CG47 Feverish illness in children: quick reference guide. 2007 [cited 2010 Oct 18]. Available at: http://guidance.nice.org.uk/CG47/QuickRefGuide/pdf/English

737. Harnden A. Recognising serious illness in feverish young children in primary care. *BMJ*. 2007; **335**(7617): 409–10.

738. Thompson MJ, Ninis N, Perera R, Mayon-White R, Phillips C, Bailey L, *et al*. Clinical recognition of meningococcal disease in children and adolescents. *Lancet*. 2006; **367**(9508): 397–403.

739. Herman J. A paper that changed my practice: Optional illness. *BMJ*. 1997; **315**(7108): 0g.

740. Balint M. Conclusions—what can be done? In: Balint M, editor. *Treatment or Diagnosis: a study of repeat prescriptions in general practice*. London: Tavistock Publications; 1970.

741. Carel H. *Illness*. Durham, NC: Acumen; 2008.

742. Stewart M, Brown JB, McWhinney I. *The Fifth Component: enhancing the patient-doctor relationship*. In: *Patient-Centered Medicine: transforming the clinical method*. Thousand Oaks, CA: Sage Publications, Inc.; 1995.

743. Grey-Thompson T. *Sustaining Motivation*. Presentation at Royal College of General Practitioners Annual Primary Care Conference. Oct 2010.

744. Rudebeck CE. Imagination and empathy in the consultation. *BJGP*. 2002; **52**(479): 450–3.

745. Heath I. Ways of Dying. In: *Matters of Life and Death: key writings*. Oxford: Radcliffe Publishing; 2008.

746. Baskerville S. *Taken into Custody: the war against fathers, marriage, and the family*. Nashville, TN: Cumberland House Publishing; 2007.

747. Donut E. *Seven Tales of Revenge*. We Wi Szokli Publishing; 2007 [cited 2010 Nov 25]. Available at: www.lulu.com/product/file-download/seven-tales-of-revenge/596555 0?productTrackingContext=search_results/search_shelf/center/1

748. Boyd K, Mason B, Kendall M, Barclay S, Chinn D, Thomas K, *et al*. Advance care planning for cancer patients in primary care: a feasibility study. *BJGP*. 2010; **60**(581): 881–3.

749. Pinnock H, Kendall M, Murray SA, Worth A, Levack P, Porter M, *et al*. Living and dying with severe chronic obstructive pulmonary disease: multi-perspective longitudinal qualitative study. *BMJ*. 2011; 342: d142.

750. Papadakis MA, Teherani A, Banach MA, Knettler TR, Rattner SL, Stern DT, *et al*. Disciplinary action by medical boards and prior behavior in medical school. *N Engl J Med*. 2005; **353**(25): 2673–82.

751. Wenghofer E, Klass D, Abrahamowicz M, Dauphinee D, Jacques A, Smee S, *et al*. Doctor scores on national qualifying examinations predict quality of care in future practice. *Med Educ*. 2009; **43**(12): 1166–73.

752. Yates J, James D. Risk factors at medical school for subsequent professional misconduct: multicentre retrospective case-control study. *BMJ*. 2010; **340**: 1073.

753. Levinson W, Roter DL, Mullooly JP, Dull VT, Frankel RM. Physician-patient communication: the relationship with malpractice claims among primary care physicians and surgeons. *JAMA*. 1997; **277**(7): 553–9.

754. Cunningham W, Crump R, Tomlin A. The characteristics of doctors receiving medical complaints: a cross-sectional survey of doctors in New Zealand. *NZ Med J* 2003; **116**(1183): U625.

755. Craigforth. *Making it Better: complaints and feedback from patients and carers about NHS services in Scotland*. Scottish Health Council; 2009. Available at: www.scottishhealth-council.org/idoc.ashx?docid=d9f7e7ca-6b3f-4452-826a-d4987f03cdce&version=-1

756. Hawton K, Clements A, Sakarovitch C, Simkin S, Deeks JJ. Suicide in doctors: a study of risk according to gender, seniority and specialty in medical practitioners in England and Wales, 1979–1995. *Journal of Epidemiology and Community Health*. 2001; **55**(5): 296–300.

757. Hutt P, Heath I, Neighbour R. *Confronting an Ill Society: David Widgery, general practice, idealism, and the chase for change*. Oxford: Radcliffe Publishing; 2005.

758. Berger J, Mohr J. *A Fortunate Man*. New York: Pantheon Books; 1982.

759. BMA. *Doctors for Doctors Unit*. www.bma.org.uk/sc/doctors_health/.

760. *The Doctors Support Network*. [cited 2010 Jul 3]. Available at: www.dsn.org.uk/

761. *The Royal Medical Benevolent Fund*. [cited 2010 Jul 3]. Available at: www.rmbf.org/

762. *The Sick Doctors Trust*. [cited 2010 Jul 3]. Available at: www.sick-doctors-trust.co.uk/

763. *Consultation for Doctors by Doctors—MedNet*. [cited 2010 Jul 3]. Available at: www.tavistockandportman.nhs.uk/mednet

764. *National Clinical Assessment Service.* [cited 2010 Jul 3]. Available at: www.ncas.npsa. nhs.uk/

765. Remedios L, Deshpande A, Harris M. Helping international medical graduates (IMGs) to success in the nMRCGP. *Educ Prim Care.* 2010; **21**(3): 143–4.

766. GMC. *Speaking the Same Language.* GMCtodayonline. 2010 Jun 2 [cited 2010 Aug 14]. Available at: www.gmc-uk.org/publications/7143.asp

767. Jaques H. UKCAT. *BMJ Careers.* 2010 Oct 23; GP129–30.

768. Universities and Colleges Admissions Service. UCAS similarity detection service— guidance for applicants. [cited 2010 Jun 9]. Available at: www.ucas.com/students/ applying/howtoapply/personalstatement/similaritydetection

769. Patterson F, Ferguson E, Lane P, Farrell K, Martlew J, Wells A. A competency model for general practice: implications for selection, training, and development. *BJGP.* 2000; **50**(452): 188–93.

770. Cooper N, Forrest K, editors. Ch 5. Putting a curriculum into practice. In: *Essential Guide to Educational Supervision in Postgraduate Medical Education.* Oxford: John Wiley and Sons; 2009.

771. Working Party of the Royal College of General Practitioners. *The Future General Practitioner: learning and teaching.* London: British Medical Journal; 1972.

772. Hodges B. Medical education and the maintenance of incompetence. *Medical Teacher.* 2006; **28**(8): 690–6.

773. *Royal College of General Practitioners—RCGP Curriculum Site: Trainee ePortfolio.* [cited 2010 Dec 11]. Available at: www.rcgp-curriculum.org.uk/eportfolio.aspx

774. Hafferty F. Beyond curriculum reform: confronting medicine's hidden curriculum. *Academic Medicine.* 1998; **73**(4): 403–7.

775. Goleman D. *Emotional Intelligence.* New York: Bantam Books; 2006.

776. Sullivan F, Wyatt JC. How decision support tools help define clinical problems. *BMJ.* 2005; **331**(7520): 831–3.

777. Jacobson L, Hawthorne K, Wood F. The 'Mensch' factor in general practice: a role to demonstrate professionalism to students. *BJGP.* 2006; **56**(533): 976–9.

778. Rogers CR. *A Way of Being.* Boston, MA: Houghton Mifflin Company; 1995.

779. Davis DA, Mazmanian PE, Fordis M, Van Harrison R, Thorpe KE, Perrier L. Accuracy of physician self-assessment compared with observed measures of competence: a systematic review. *JAMA.* 2006; **296**(9): 1094–102.

780. Kruger J, Dunning D. Unskilled and unaware of it: how difficulties in recogniz- ing one's own incompetence lead to inflated self-assessments. *Journal of Personality.* 1999; **77**(6): 1121–34.

781. *Beyond the Ropes.* [cited 2010 May 15]. Available at: www.mtalearning.com/articles/ beyond-the-ropes.html

782. Miller A, Archer J. Impact of workplace based assessment on doctors' education and performance: a systematic review. *BMJ.* 2010; **341**(Sep 24_1): c5064.

783. Jamtvedt G, Young JM, Kristoffersen DT, O'Brien MA, Oxman AD. Audit and feed- back: effects on professional practice and health care outcomes. *Cochrane Database of Systematic Reviews.* 2006; **2**: Art no: CD000259.

784. Campbell C, Silver I, Sherbino J, Cate OT, Holmboe ES. Competency-based con- tinuing professional development. *Med Teach.* 2010; **32**(8): 657–62.

785. Karpicke JD, Roediger III HL. Repeated retrieval during learning is the key to long- term retention. *Journal of Memory and Language.* 2007; **57**(2): 151–62.

786. Rogers CR. *Freedom to Learn: a view of what education might become.* Columbus, OH: Charles E. Merrill Publishing Company; 1969.

787. Maskrey N. *Making Decisons Better, or how could I have been so stupid?* Presentation at Royal College of General Practitioners Annual Primary Care Conference, Oct 2010.

788. RCGP Guide to the Revalidation of General Practitioners, Version 4.0. Royal College of General Practitioners. 2010 [cited 2011 July 24]. Available at: www.rcgp.org.uk/pdf/PDS_Guide_to_Revalidation_for_GPs.pdf

789. *The Institute of Risk Management—About Us.* [cited 2011 Jan 30]. Available at: www.theirm.org/aboutheirm/ABwhatisrm.htm

790. *NHS Complaints: Who cares? Who can make it better? A survey of members and their experience of the NHS complaints system.* The Patients Association. [cited 2010 Jul 3]. Available at: www.patients-association.com/Research-Publications/229

791. *National Audit Office. Feeding Back? Learning from complaints handling in health and social care.* [cited 2010 Apr 20]. Available at: www.nao.org.uk/publications/0708/learning_from_complaints.aspx

792. Parliamentary and Health Service Ombudsman LAIS. *Principles of Good Complaint Handling.* 2008 Dec 1 [cited 2010 Apr 20]. Available at: www.ombudsman.org.uk/improving-public-service/ombudsmansprinciples/principles-of-good-complaint-handling-full

793. Department of Health. *The NHS Constitution: all you need to know about how the NHS Constitution affects you as a provider or commissioner of NHS care.* 2009 [cited 2010 Apr 30]. Available at: www.dh.gov.uk/en/Publicationsandstatistics/Publications/PublicationsPolicyAndGuidance/DH_099887

794. Hurwitz B. The Wounded Storyteller: narrative strands in medical negligence. In: Greenhalgh T, Hurwitz B, editors. *Narrative Based Medicine: dialogue and discourse in clinical practice.* London: BMJ Books; 1998.

795. Bowling A. *Research Methods in Health: investigating health and health services.* Maidenhead, Berkshire: Open University Press; 2009.

796. Asch SE. Opinions and social pressure. *Scientific American.* 1955; **193**(5): 31–5.

797. Walster E. Assignment of responsibility for an accident. *Journal of Personality and Social Psychology.* 1966; **3**(1): 73–9.

798. Sutherland S. *Irrationality.* London: Pinter & Martin; 2007.

799. Baumeister RF, Bratslavsky E, Finkenauer C, Vohs KD. Bad is stronger than good. *Review of General Psychology.* 2001; **5**(4): 323–70.

800. Haggerty JL. Are measures of patient satisfaction hopelessly flawed? *BMJ.* 2010; **341**(Oct 12_1): c4783.

801. Robertson N. *Improving patient safety: 'Watch me!'.* The National Confidential Enquiry into Patient Outcome and Death Prize Essay, Sep 2010.

802. Brown D. *The Meaning of Careful.* London: HCV Publishing; 2009.

803. WHO. *Patient Safety Research.* [cited 2010 Apr 18]. Available at: www.who.int/patientsafety/research/en/

804. WHO. *Review of Methods and Measures in Primary Care Research.* [cited 2010 Apr 18]. Available at: www.who.int/patientsafety/research/methods_measures/primary_care_ps_research/en/index.html

805. *Institute for Healthcare Improvement: Home.* [cited 2010 Apr 19]. Available at: www.ihi.org/ihi

806. *European Union Network For Patient Safety.* [cited 2010 Apr 19]. Available at: www. eunetpas.eu/

807. Scottish Patient Safety Programme. [cited 2010 July 24]. Available at: http:// patientsafety.etellect.co.uk/programme

808. *NHS Quality Improvement Scotland: Support for Scotland's healthcare professionals.* [cited 2010 May 13]. Available at: www.nhshealthquality.org/nhsqis/43.140.140. html

809. *National Patient Safety Agency.* National Patient Safety Agency. [cited 2010 Apr 19]. Available at: www.npsa.nhs.uk/

810. *Improving Safety in Primary Care—NHS Institute for Innovation and Improvement.* [cited 2010 May 13]. Available at: www.institute.nhs.uk/safer_care/primary_care/ improving_safety_in_primary_care.html

811. *Care Quality Commission.* Care Quality Commission. [cited 2010 Sep 2]. Available at: www.cqc.org.uk/

812. *Patient Advice and Liaison Service.* [cited 2010 Sep 2]. Available at: www.pals.nhs.uk/

813. National Patient Safety Agency. *Design for Patient Safety: guidelines for safe on-screen display of medication information Edition 1.* 2010 [cited 2010 Aug 21]. Available at: www.nrls.npsa.nhs.uk/resources/?entryid45=66713&q=0%c2%acdesign+for+patie nt+safety%c2%ac

814. National Patient Safety Agency. *Quarterly Data Summaries.* [cited 2010 Jul 3]. Available at: www.nrls.npsa.nhs.uk/resources/collections/quarterly-data-summaries/ ?entryid45=65320

815. Rubin G, George A, Chinn DJ, Richardson C. Errors in general practice: development of an error classification and pilot study of a method for detecting errors. *Quality and Safety in Health Care.* 2003; **12**(6): 443–7.

816. Barber ND, Alldred DP, Raynor DK, Dickinson R, Garfield S, Jesson B, *et al.* Care homes' use of medicines study: prevalence, causes and potential harm of medication errors in care homes for older people. *Quality and Safety in Health Care.* 2009; **18**(5): 341–6.

817. Jha AK, Prasopa-Plaizier N, Larizgoitia I, Bates DW. Patient safety research: an overview of the global evidence. *Quality and Safety in Health Care.* 2010; **19**(1): 42–7.

818. Reason J. Human error: models and management. *West J Med.* 2000; **172**(6): 393–6.

819. NHS Litigation Authority. *Apologies and Explanations.* 2009 May 1 [cited 2010 Nov 27]. Available at: www.nhsla.com/NR/rdonlyres/00F14BA6-0621-4A23-B885-FA18326FF745/0/ApologiesandExplanationsMay1st2009.pdf

820. Napley D. The ethics of the professions. *The Law Society's Gazette.* 1985 Mar 20: 818–25.

821. Ely JW, Levinson W, Elder NC, Mainous AG, Vinson DC. Perceived causes of family physicians' errors. *J Fam Pract.* 1995; **40**(4): 337–44.

822. Boshuizin HP, Schmidt HG. The development of clinical reasoning expertise. In: Higgs J, Jones MA, Loftus S, Christensen N, editors. *Clinical Reasoning in the Health Professions.* Philadelphia: Elsevier Health Sciences; 2008.

823. Shuwirth K. Can clinical reasoning be taught or can it only be learned? *Med Educ.* 2002; **36**(8): 695–6.

824. Nendaz M, Bordage G. Promoting diagnostic problem representation. *Med Educ.* 2002; **36**(8): 760–6.

825. Schwartz A, Elstein AS. Clinical reasoning in medicine. In: Higgs J, Jones MA, Loftus S, Christensen N, editors. *Clinical Reasoning in the Health Professions.* Philadelphia: Elsevier Health Sciences; 2008.

826. Dawes RM. The robust beauty of improper linear models in decision making. In: Kahneman D, Slovic P, Tversky A, editors. *Judgment under Uncertainty: heuristics and biases.* Cambridge: Cambridge University Press; 1982.

827. Norman G. Research in clinical reasoning: past history and current trends. *Med Educ.* 2005; **39**(4): 418–27.

828. Kaufman DR, Yoskowitz NA, Patel VL. Clinical reasoning and biomedical knowledge: implications for teaching. In: Higgs J, Jones MA, Loftus S, Christensen N, editors. *Clinical Reasoning in the Health Professions.* Philadelphia: Elsevier Health Sciences; 2008.

829. Goyder C, McPherson A, Glasziou P. Self diagnosis. *BMJ.* 2009; **339**(Nov 11_1): b4418.

830. Tversky A, Kahneman D. Extensional versus intuitive reasoning: the conjunction fallacy in probability judgment. *Psychological Review.* 1983; **90**(4): 293–315.

831. Gettys CF, Kelly C, Peterson CR. The best-guess hypothesis in multistage inference. In: Kahneman D, Tversky A, editors. *Judgment under Uncertainty: heuristics and biases.* Cambridge: Cambridge University Press; 1982.

832. Tversky A, Kahneman D. Evidential impact on base rates. In: Kahneman D, Slovic P, Tversky A, editors. *Judgment under Uncertainty: heuristics and biases.* Cambridge: Cambridge University Press; 1982.

833. Langer EJ. The illusion of control. In: Kahneman D, Slovic P, Tversky A, editors. *Judgment under Uncertainty: heuristics and biases.* Cambridge: Cambridge University Press; 1982.

834. Edwards W. Conservatism in human information processing. In: Kahneman D, Tversky A, editors. *Judgment under Uncertainty: heuristics and biases.* Cambridge: Cambridge University Press; 1982.

835. Fischhoff B. Hindsight [does not equal] foresight: the effect of outcome knowledge on judgment under uncertainty. *Journal ol Experimental Psychology: Human Perception and Performance.* 1975; **1**(3): 288–99.

836. Goddard AF. Planning a consultant delivered NHS. *BMJ.* 2010; **341**: 119–20.

837. Gilbert WS, Sullivan A. *The Mikado, or, The Town of Titipu.* London: Chappell; 1911.

838. Eva K, Norman G. Heuristics and biases—a biased perspective on clinical reasoning. *Med Educ.* 2005; **39**(9): 870–2.

839. Hamilton W. Introduction. In: Hamilton W, Peters TJ, editors. *Cancer Diagnosis in Primary Care.* London: Elsevier Health Sciences; 2007.

840. Weingarten MA, Guttman N, Abramovitch H, Margalit RS, Roter D, Ziv A, *et al.* An anatomy of conflicts in primary care encounters: a multi-method study. *Fam Pract.* 2010; **27**(1): 93–100.

841. Groves J. Taking care of the hateful patient. *N Engl J Med.* 1978; **298**: 317–18.

842. Money A, Hussey L, Thorley K, Turner S, Agius R. Work-related sickness absence negotiations: GPs' qualitative perspectives. *BJGP.* 2010; **60**(579): 721–8.

843. O'Brien K, Cadbury N, Rollnick S, Wood F. Sickness certification in the general practice consultation: the patients' perspective, a qualitative study. *Fam Pract.* 2008; **25**(1): 20–6.

844. *IPDAS—International Patient Decision Aids Standards.* International Patient Decision Aids Standards (IPDAS) Collaboration. Available at: www.ipdas.ohri.ca/index.html
845. Reilly BM, Evans AT. Translating clinical research into clinical practice: impact of using prediction rules to make decisions. *Ann Intern Med.* 2006; **144**(3): 201–9.
846. *Isabel.* [cited 2010 Nov 18]. Available at: www.isabelhealthcare.com/home/default
847. *National Prescribing Centre.* [cited 2010 Nov 18]; Available at: www.npci.org.uk
848. *Healthtalkonline.* [cited 2010 May 16]; www.healthtalkonline.org/.
849. Kennedy A, Reeves D, Bower P, Lee V, Middleton E, Richardson G, *et al.* The effectiveness and cost effectiveness of a national lay-led self care support programme for patients with long-term conditions: a pragmatic randomised controlled trial. *J Epidemiol Community Health.* 2007; **61**(3): 254–61.
850. Herxheimer A, Crombag R, Leonardo Alves T. Direct Patient Reporting of Adverse Drug Reactions: a fifteen-country survey and literature review. *Health Action International Europe*; 2010 [cited 2010 Sep 7]. Available at: www.haiweb.org/10052010/10_May_2010_Report_Direct_Patient_Reporting_of_ADRs.pdf
851. Kellaway L. A corporate calendar is so last year. *Financial Times.* 2010 Mar 1: 16.

Index

Figures are given in italics.

What Makes Variables Random
Probability for the Applied Researcher

What Makes Variables Random

Probability for the Applied Researcher

Peter J. Veazie, PhD

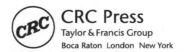

CRC Press
Taylor & Francis Group
Boca Raton London New York

CRC Press is an imprint of the
Taylor & Francis Group, an **informa** business

A CHAPMAN & HALL BOOK

CRC Press
Taylor & Francis Group
6000 Broken Sound Parkway NW, Suite 300
Boca Raton, FL 33487-2742

© 2017 by Taylor & Francis Group, LLC
CRC Press is an imprint of Taylor & Francis Group, an Informa business

No claim to original U.S. Government works

Printed on acid-free paper

International Standard Book Number-13: 978-1-4987-8108-4 (Hardback)

Library of Congress Cataloging-in-Publication Data

Names: Veazie, Peter J.
Title: What makes variables random : probability for the applied researcher /
Peter J. Veazie.
Description: Boca Raton : CRC Press, 2017. | Includes bibliographical references.
Identifiers: LCCN 2016057398 | ISBN 9781498781084 (hardback)
Subjects: LCSH: Random variables. | Variables (Mathematics) | Probabilities.
Classification: LCC QA273 .V38 2017 | DDC 519.2--dc23
LC record available at https://lccn.loc.gov/2016057398

Visit the Taylor & Francis Web site at
http://www.taylorandfrancis.com

and the CRC Press Web site at
http://www.crcpress.com

To Wendy, Matthew, and Devin

Contents

Section III Applications

Preface

A number of years ago, I noticed that the growing popularity of methods such as hierarchical modeling was accompanied by a pattern of misuse. For example, researchers were using these methods to assure appropriate standard errors, but in doing so some were confusing the statistically meaningless concept of nested data with the statistically relevant concept of a nested data generating process. This is a misunderstanding that can lead to the misapplication of the methods. As these methods became more common, so did their misuse. The underlying problematic issue arises more generally in statistical analysis when data are confused for the data generating process, and variables defined on the data are confused for random variables defined on the data generating process.

Considering the source of this confusion, I settled on what would become the title of this book: there seemed to be a lack of understanding regarding what makes variables random. Distinguishing data from the process that produced it is essential to understanding statistics as a tool for empirical analysis.

Having identified this problem, what was the solution? As many applied researchers do not have a mathematical background beyond calculus, I tried to formulate the necessary understanding of random variable in terms of a calculus-based framework. Unfortunately, this approach seemed inadequate: I was unable to use calculus alone to provide the conceptual depth required to get at what really makes variables random.

I turned to measure theory. However, I was aware that many would not be familiar with measure theory; indeed many would not have a background in real analysis. Moreover, many would likely, and rightfully, not be interested in developing such a mathematical background. I wondered whether measure theory and probability could be taught at a level sufficient to provide a conceptual tool without having to resort to the depth required for a mathematical tool. Would a measure-theoretic conceptualization in conjunction with college-level calculus be sufficient for applied researchers to better understand and better use the statistical methods with which they were already familiar? A number of years ago, I presented an 8-hour workshop focused on providing an affirmative answer to this question. Although the workshop was a successful introduction, the timeframe was insufficient to provide either the depth or scope necessary for the impact I was seeking.

Following the workshop, I expanded its notes into the book presented here. My goal was to produce a short text to augment a researcher's existing calculus-based understanding of probability. My hope is that the resulting book achieves its purpose by providing a measure-theoretic conceptualization of probability and its use in informing research design and statistical analysis.

I greatly appreciate the feedback from those who read draft sections of the text or listened to me as I incorporated its concepts into lectures on statistical methods. I am particularly indebted to Viji Kannan at the University of Rochester for her willingness to challenge the content and clarity of this text: Our discussions of measure theory and its application helped shape my thoughts about this project, its content, and its presentation.

Section I

Preliminaries

1

Introduction

For the applied researcher, mathematical probability is a tool—a means to investigate real-world phenomena. As such, many researchers learn and understand this tool in a language that facilitates direct utilization, often in terms of calculus as taught to undergraduates. Unfortunately, a strictly undergraduate-level calculus-based understanding does not always provide a sufficiently rich conceptual framework by which mathematical probability can be connected to real phenomena. Consequently, the applied researcher may engage in analysis of data without knowing what mathematical probability and statistics are representing in their investigation, thereby risking a mistaken interpretation. For example, analysts often speak of "nested data" to refer to the structure in the data they presume informs the analysis; however, nested data is not a statistically meaningful concept but rather a misconception that can be avoided with a proper understanding of probability.

Mathematicians, statisticians, and a few other disciplines will have learned mathematical probability in terms of measure theory. Not only does this mathematical perspective give them great power in constructing careful proofs in probability theory, it also provides the conceptualization that facilitates an easy translation between real-world problems and mathematical probability. Unfortunately, using measure theory operationally can be overkill for empirical analysis: understanding measure theory with sufficient mathematical rigor to use it for "doing the math" is rightfully deemed a waste of time for many applied researchers. And so, the conceptual baby is thrown out with the operational bathwater. Authors on the subject tend not to integrate the two for applied researchers. Either they conceptualize and operationalize with measure theory or they conceptualize and operationalize with standard calculus. Aris Spanos' text *Probability Theory and Statistical Inference* is a rare and excellent exception.

However, in view of the numerous calculus-based texts on probability and statistics that already exist, as well as the training many researchers may already have, another such comprehensive integrative text is not needed. What is needed is a brief text that provides a basic conceptual introduction to measure theory, probability, and their implications for applied research. Consequently, it is the goal of this short text to augment the applied researcher's existing calculus-based understanding of probability: to generate a measure-theoretic conceptualization of mathematical probability such that researchers can better use their calculus-based probability framework to design studies, analyze data, and appropriately understand results.

TABLE 1.1

Hospital Data

Physician	Patient	HbA1c	Pt Age
Harriet	James	7.7	67
Harriet	Mary	6.8	62
Harriet	John	7	73
Fred	Robert	8.3	88
Fred	Patricia	9.1	66
Lisa	Linda	9.2	86
Lisa	Barbara	7.5	63
Lisa	Michael	8.3	71
Lisa	Elizabeth	6.7	77

To achieve this goal and to make this text useful for those without the in-depth mathematical background who seek a broad-level understanding, I necessarily compromise on mathematical depth and detail. For those interested in a more mathematically rigorous treatment of the topic, see the references in the "Additional Readings" section at the end of Chapter 4, among others that can be found by searching on the terms *measure theory* and *probability*.

Imagine that you are approached by the CEO of a hospital, who wants you to evaluate the performance of the doctors in the hospital. Suppose she hands you the data in Table 1.1. The data contain patient and physician identifiers and measures for patient age and glycosylated hemoglobin (HbA1c) levels (lower numbers are better in the HbA1c range reported here).

The average HbA1c across these patients for Dr. Harriet is approximately 7.2, the average across these patients for Dr. Fred is approximately 8.7, and the average for Dr. Lisa is approximately 7.9. Dr. Harriet's patients in the data have better control of their HbA1c on average than the other physicians' patients in the data, and Dr. Fred's patients are worse on average than the other physicians' patients. You already know how to calculate these basic statistics. This book will help you understand and answer more nuanced questions such as the following:

1. Would clustering by physician be appropriate?
2. What do reported standard errors of statistics mean?
3. Would a random effects, or multilevel, model be appropriate?

The answers to these questions are the same: "there is not enough information to tell." This is because the data alone do not provide sufficient information to identify or understand the meaning of statistics as used in applied research. By the end of this book, you will understand why and be able to better design your analyses and understand your results.

Thus far, I have been careful to use the phrase *mathematical probability* rather than the term *probability*. The distinction is extremely important throughout the conceptual development in this book. The term *probability* is ambiguous. It is sometimes used to represent a mathematical structure, which only implies strict mathematical results, and it is sometimes used to mean a specific real-world concept such as a source of uncertainty. Although such substantive interpretations of probability are necessary to the work of applied research, it should not be confused with the implications of the mathematics. In this text, I encourage thinking of mathematical probability as a model of a substantive phenomenon. However, once a model is properly developed to capture a phenomenon of interest, its properties follow solely from the mathematics. The importance of this distinction will become clear throughout the book. Nonetheless, to avoid cumbersome overuse of the phrase *mathematical probability*, I will use the term *probability* in the rest of this book when the context makes it clear to which sense I am appealing.

The first section of this book comprises this introduction and a chapter reviewing set theory and functions, which may be skipped by readers who are familiar with those concepts. The second section of the book focuses on the basics of measure theory and probability. The third section focuses on the implications of measure theory to applied research—the use of a calculus-level mathematical understanding of probability informed by a measure-theoretic conceptualization.

Although I use the language of mathematics to communicate the requisite ideas, the goal of this text is to achieve a conceptual understanding of basic principles that will allow you to clearly think through research problems. I have written this book for researchers and students who already have an understanding of applied statistics in terms of undergraduate calculus. I therefore assume the reader has an understanding of probability, distributions, and statistics.

Additional Readings

The book by Aris Spanos titled *Probability Theory and Statistical Inference: Econometric Modeling with Observational Data* (Cambridge University Press, 1999) provides an introduction to probability and statistics that uses measure theory as a conceptual framework but uses basic calculus for its implementation. The book introduces probability, statistics, and statistical inference at a level useful for applied research. The intended audience of Spanos' book comprises those who have had at least a one-semester course in calculus.

For references to books on substantive theories of probability, see the "Additional Readings" section at the end of Chapter 5.

2

Mathematical Preliminaries

Before describing measure theory and mathematical probability, it would be helpful to review some basics of set theory and functions. This chapter covers the definitions and notation required to understand the remainder of the book. Readers who are familiar with set theory and functions can skim or skip this chapter without loss of continuity.

Set Theory

The essentials of set theory required to understand measure theory's relevance to applied research are captured by the following definitions.

A *set* is a collection of distinct objects (concrete or abstract). To compose a set, each object in the collection is distinct, and any object is either definitely in or definitely out of the set. The distinctiveness of the objects means that a collection of words such as {Mary, Fred, Mary} is a set that can also be represented, more efficiently, as the set {Mary, Fred}. This is because the former representation contained identical copies of the word *Mary*, whereas the latter does not, yet each contains the same distinct words. Note that it is common to use "curly" brackets (i.e., braces) to enclose members of a set.

The elements of a set need not be real; they may be imaginary, conceptual, or simply asserted to exist, as in "let A be a set of objects" or even more concisely as in "let A be a set," without further specification. It is important to remember that sets may have sets as elements, or sets of sets as elements, or sets of sets of sets as elements—you get the idea. For example, consider that the following are different sets: {1, 2, 3, 4, 5}, {{1}, {2}, {3}, {4}, {5}}, and {{{1}}, {2}, {3}, {4}, {5}}. The first set is the set of integers from 1 to 5; the second is the set of sets containing integers from 1 to 5. The third differs from the second in that the first listed member is the set containing the set that contains 1.

If an object a is one of those that compose a set A, we say "a is a *member* of set A" or "a is an *element* of set A." We denote the relation of "is a member of" or "is an element of" by the symbol $\in$. The claim that an object is not a member of a set is denoted by the symbol $\notin$. Consequently, the statement "a is a member of set A" is written as $a \in A$, and the statement "a is not a member of set A" is written as $a \notin A$.

If each member of a set B is also a member of a set A, then we can say that set B is *contained* in set A or that set A *contains* set B. In this case, B is considered a *subset* of A. Moreover, if B is contained in A, and A has at least one element that is not a member of B, then B is a *proper subset* of A. If there is no such remaining element in A (i.e., B is contained in A and A is contained in B), then A and B are considered *equal sets*. The symbol $\subseteq$ is used to denote "subset of;" for example, $B \subseteq A$ means that B is a subset of A. The symbol $\subset$ is used to denote "proper subset of;" for example, $B \subset A$ means that B is a proper subset of A, which implies that all members of B are also members of A, but there is at least one member of A that is not a member of B. The symbol $\approx$ is used to denote equal sets, as in $A \approx B$, indicating that sets A and B are equal. If it is the case that a set A is contained in another set B, and that set B is also contained in set A, then sets A and B are equal (i.e., if $A \subseteq B$ and $B \subseteq A$, then $A \approx B$). This should be evident because if A is contained in B, then B contains all elements that are in set A, but if B is also contained in set A, then A contains all elements that are in set B. Consequently, there does not exist an element in one of the sets that is not also an element of the other.

Note the distinction between the concepts "member of" (or "element of") and "subset of." The former identifies a particular object that is a component of a set, whereas the latter identifies a set whose elements are also elements of another set. For example, regarding set A defined as $\{1, 2, 3, 4, 5\}$, we can properly say that the number 2 is an element of A, and the set with 2 as its single element is a subset of A (i.e., $2 \in A$ and $\{2\} \subset A$). However, for set B defined as $\{\{1\}, \{2\}, \{3\}, \{4\}, \{5\}\}$, we can properly say that the set with 2 as its single element is an element of B, the set containing the set that contains the number 2 is a subset of B, and the number 2 itself is neither an element of B nor a subset of B (i.e., $\{2\} \in B$ and $\{\{2\}\} \subset B$, but $2 \notin B$ and $2 \not\subset B$). With respect to A, the number 2 is a member and the set $\{2\}$ is a subset; however, for set B the set $\{2\}$ is a member, and therefore the set that contains the set $\{2\}$ (i.e., $\{\{2\}\}$) is a subset of B.

In set theory, there exists a particular set that contains no members at all. This set is called the *empty set*; it is commonly denoted as $\varnothing$. It is typically a matter of mathematical convention to consider the empty set to be a subset of every set; this convention is adhered to in this book.

A set with only one element is called a *unit set* or *singleton*. For example, $\{2\}$ is a singleton containing the number 2, and $\{\{Fred, Lisa\}\}$ is a singleton containing the set $\{Fred, Lisa\}$.

The set of all subsets of a given set A is called the *power set* of A, denoted as $\wp(A)$. For example, the power set of $A = \{1, 2, 3\}$ is $\wp(A) = \{\{1\}, \{2\}, \{3\}, \{1, 2\}, \{1, 3\}, \{2, 3\}, \{1, 2, 3\}, \varnothing\}$. Note that the empty set is included because, as stated above, it is considered a subset of all sets, which means it is a subset of A and therefore belongs in the power set of A.

We use curly brackets to explicitly list the members of sets. We also use them to represent a set by denoting an arbitrary member and a rule by which the members are defined; the arbitrary member and rule are separated by a colon, which can be read as the phrase "such that." For example, $\{w: w \in A\}$ denotes the set of elements w such that w is a member of set A; or another example, $\{w: w \in A$ and $w \notin B\}$ denotes the set of elements w such that w is a member of set A and not a member of set B. With this notation in hand, we can define operations on sets (new notation for these operations is introduced in the definitions).

Let A and B be sets; then their *union* (denoted by the symbol $\cup$) is the set of elements that belong to either A or B or both:

$$A \cup B = \{w: w \in A \text{ or } w \in B\} \tag{2.1}$$

For example, if set A is {Fred, Lisa, Bill, Sue}, and set B is {Bill, Sue, Henry, Linda}, then the union of A and B is {Fred, Lisa, Bill, Sue, Henry, Linda}: the set that includes all members of each of A and B. Notice that because sets do not contain redundant labeling, even though Bill and Sue are elements of both A and B, they show up only once in the set that composes the union.

Let A and B be sets; then their *intersection* (denoted by the symbol $\cap$) is the set of elements that belong to both A and B:

$$A \cap B = \{w: w \in A \text{ and } w \in B\} \tag{2.2}$$

For example, if set A is {Fred, Lisa, Bill, Sue} and set B is {Bill, Sue, Henry, Linda}, then the intersection of A and B is {Bill, Sue}, the set that includes all the members that sets A and B share. For a graphical representation of a union and intersection of sets, see Figure 2.1.

A different notation is often used to indicate unions and intersections across indexed collections of sets. For example, consider the collection of K sets $\{A_1, A_2, \ldots, A_K\}$. Rather than listing each set connected with a union or intersection symbol, such as $A_1 \cup A_2 \cup \ldots A_K$ and $A_1 \cap A_2 \cap \ldots A_K$, a simpler notion is often adopted:

$$A_1 \cup A_2 \cup \ldots A_K = \bigcup_{k=1}^{K} A_k \tag{2.3}$$

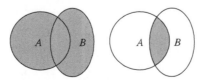

FIGURE 2.1
Union and intersection: the shaded area of the left-hand graphic depicts the union of sets A and B, whereas the shaded area of the right-hand graphic depicts the intersection of sets A and B.

and

$$A_1 \cap A_2 \cap \ldots A_K = \bigcap_{k=1}^{K} A_k \qquad (2.4)$$

For a set B, the *complement* of B (denoted by a bar placed above B) is the set of elements that are not a member of B:

$$\overline{B} = \{w : w \notin B\} \qquad (2.5)$$

Figure 2.2 presents a graphical representation of the complement of a set.

The complement of a set presupposes a *basic* or *universal* set U such that $U = B \cup \overline{B}$. Without the context of the universal set, it is difficult to identify what exactly is the complement of a set. For example, if B is defined as the set of siblings of a given family {Fred, Lisa, Bill, Sue, Henry, Linda}, what is $\overline{B}$? Is it the rest of the immediate family, all the rest of their living relatives, all people alive, all people who ever lived, all other physical objects in the world, or all physical objects plus the concepts of *liberty*, *peace*, and *blue*? Clearly, a set is understood by the content of its members; the complement of a set, which is itself a set, must similarly be understood and thereby necessitates a basic or universal set. This is clearer if the universal set, say U, is included in the definition, such as $\overline{B} = \{w : w \in U \text{ and } w \notin B\}$. For example, Figure 2.2 depicts the complement of set B as relative to the rectangle containing it, as opposed to, say, the page on which it is drawn.

Two sets A and B are considered to be *disjoint* if their intersection is the empty set, which is to say that sets A and B do not share any members:

$$A \cap B = \emptyset \qquad (2.6)$$

For example, for A defined as {Fred, Lisa, Bill, Sue} and B defined as {Henry, Linda}, the intersection of A and B is empty because neither set contains a member of the other: they are disjoint. Figure 2.3 presents a graphical representation of disjoint sets.

A collection of k sets $A_1, A_2, \ldots, A_k$ is considered to be a *disjoint collection* of sets if each distinct pair of sets in the collection are disjoint by the preceding definition. For example, consider four sets: A_1 defined as {Fred, Lisa}, A_2 defined as {Bill, Sue}, A_3 defined as {Henry}, and A_4 defined as {Linda}.

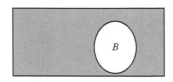

FIGURE 2.2
Complement: the shaded area represents the complement of the set B.

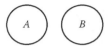

FIGURE 2.3
Disjoint sets: sets A and B do not overlap and therefore do not share any elements: they are disjoint.

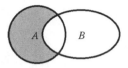

FIGURE 2.4
Relative complement: the shaded area in this graphic depicts the relative complement of the set B with respect to the set A.

None of these sets share elements with any other; they are a disjoint collection of sets.

The set of elements that are members of set A but are not members of set B is the *relative complement* of B with respect to A, sometimes called the *set difference* of the set A with respect to B (denoted by either a backslash \ or a minus −):

$$A \backslash B = A - B = A \cap \overline{B} = \{x : x \in A \text{ and } x \notin B\} \tag{2.7}$$

For example, if set A is {Fred, Lisa, Bill, Sue} and set B is {Bill, Sue, Henry, Linda}, then the relative complement of B with respect to A is {Fred, Lisa} and the relative complement of A with respect to B is {Henry, Linda}. Figure 2.4 presents a graphical representation of the relative complement.

A disjoint collection of nonempty sets $A_1, A_2, \ldots, A_k$ such that $S = \cup_{i=1}^{k} A_i$ is called a *partition* of the set S. In other words, if you chop up a set S into subsets that are mutually exclusive (i.e., each member of the set S can only be in one of the subsets) and exhaustive (i.e., each member of the set S must be in one of the subsets), then this collection of subsets is a partition of the set S. For example, if set A is {Fred, Lisa, Bill, Sue}, then the three sets A_1 = {Fred, Bill}, A_2 = {Lisa}, and A_3 = {Sue} are a disjoint collection of sets that constitute a partition of A. Figure 2.5 presents a graphical representation of a partition.

For two partitions π_0 and π_1 of a set S, π_1 is a *refinement* of π_0 if each set in π_1 is a subset of one in π_0 and at least one set in π_1 is a proper subset of one in π_0. The partition π_1 is considered to be finer than π_0, and π_0 is considered to be coarser than π_1. Essentially, a refinement of a partition π_0 is achieved by partitioning at least one of its member sets into subsets.

A sequence of sets (e.g., $A_1, A_2, \ldots, A_k$) in which each is a proper subset of the preceding one (e.g., $A_1 \supset A_2 \supset \ldots \supset A_k$) is a *nested* sequence of sets, as

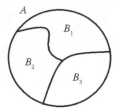

FIGURE 2.5
Partition: the sets B_1, B_2, and B_3 compose a partition of the set A (the circle).

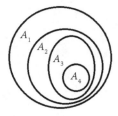

FIGURE 2.6
Nested sets: sets A_1, A_2, A_3, and A_4 compose a collection of nested sets centered on A_4 (or any subset of A_4).

shown in Figure 2.6. A sequence of such sets that can be indexed to the whole numbers, which continue infinitely, is an infinite nested sequence of sets. If the intersection of a collection of sets contains a set A, then the collection of sets is considered to be *centered* on set A. Consequently, a nested sequence of sets is centered on any subset of the last set in the sequence.

I will ostensibly define *continuous set* to mean a set such as the real line, intervals on the real line, areas of a plane, three-dimensional volumes, and higher-dimensional hyper-volumes. A characteristic of such a set is that no matter how close an inspection that you give around a point in the set, there is an infinite number of points in that region under inspection. This is a cumbersome, and pedestrian, characterization of a continuous set. Indeed, this use of the phrase *continuous set* is not true to the usual parlance of mathematics. The word *continuous* is better reserved for describing functions; however, to properly describe the notion I am presenting would require an understanding of metric spaces, limit points, and isolated points, or an understanding of sets that can support a properly defined continuous function. Given the limited reference I will make to these sets (whatever we wish to call them), it is not worth the conceptual effort to be proper. So, to restate, I will call a set that comprises a continuum of points a *continuous set*. In light of the preceding definitions, we can meaningfully speak of a nested sequence of continuous sets centered on some specified set. Figure 2.6 shows a set of nested sets centered on a set A_4.

Functions

A complete description of the mathematical concept of a function and its consequences is well beyond the scope of this book. For our purposes, we only need to have an understanding of some basics. However, before presenting a formal definition, let's consider some examples.

Example 2.1

Suppose I have two lists from an elementary school in which each student has exactly one teacher: one list contains the names of all students, the other list contains the names of all teachers. Suppose further that I identify for every student on the first list that student's teacher from the second list (see Figure 2.7). This student–teacher relationship is a function from the student list to the teacher list.

Example 2.1 is carefully constructed to highlight the main features of a function. To see what they are, consider the following contrasting examples.

Example 2.2

Suppose I have two lists from a middle school in which music is an elective that only some students take, and if a student takes music they have only one music teacher. The first list contains all the students of the school; the second list contains all the teachers. Now suppose I identify the student–music teacher relationship from the first list to the second list (see Figure 2.8). This relationship is not a function.

Unlike Example 2.1, which is a function, Example 2.2 contains students in the first list who do not have a music teacher identified in the second list.

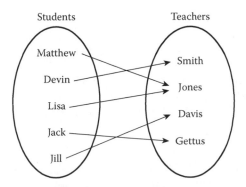

FIGURE 2.7
Function: the arrows represent a function that assigns each student to a teacher.

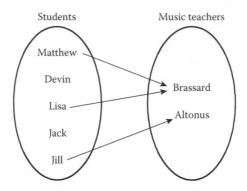

FIGURE 2.8
The arrows in this figure do not represent a function from students to teachers, because there exist some students who are not assigned a teacher. Specifically, Devin and Jack do not have a music teacher.

In order for a relationship to be a function, every member of the first list must be assigned to a member of the second list.

Example 2.3

Suppose I have two lists from elementary school: one contains the names of all students and the other contains the names of all first grade teachers. The student–teacher relationship is not a function in this case.

Example 2.3 appears subtly different from Example 2.2 in that the second list contains only a subset of teachers in the school. However, the result is essentially the same: The student–teacher relationship cannot identify a teacher for some of the students. And again, in order for a relationship to be a function, every member of the first list must be assigned to a member of the second list.

Example 2.4

Suppose I have a student list and a teacher list from a middle school in which some students have multiple teachers (see Figure 2.9). Identifying the teachers associated with each student does not constitute a function.

Example 2.4 highlights the fact that a function must assign only one element in the second list to each element in the first list (i.e., in this case a function must assign only one teacher to each student).

Example 2.5

Suppose I have a student list and an employee list from a given school. Identifying the principal associated with each student constitutes a function, even though each student is related to one and the same member of the employee list (see Figure 2.10).

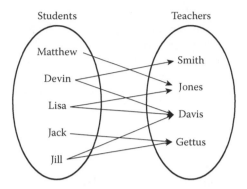

FIGURE 2.9
The arrows in this figure do not represent a function because some students (Devin, Lisa, and Jill) are assigned to more than one teacher.

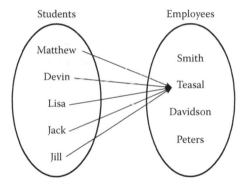

FIGURE 2.10
This figure represents a function because each student is identified with an employee—note that it does not matter that it is the same employee.

Whereas Example 2.4 did not exemplify a function because a function cannot identify each element of the first set (i.e., each student) to multiple elements of the second set (i.e., multiple teachers), Example 2.5 does exemplify a function because a function can identify multiple members of the first list (students) with the same member of the second list (employees).

A definition of a function sufficient to understand this text is as follows: Let X and Y be two sets, and let f be a relationship between the two sets that identifies one and only one member of Y with each member of X. Then f is a *function* from X to Y, written in this text as $f: X \rightarrow Y$. The set X is called the *domain* or *preimage* of function f, and the set Y is called the *codomain*. The member y of the range Y associated by function f with an arbitrary member x of the domain X is identified as $y = f(x)$. The set comprised of $f(x)$ for all x in X is called the *range* or *image* of the function f. Note the difference between the codomain and the range or image; this difference is shown in Figure 2.10. The set of employees is the codomain in this figure, whereas the set {Teasal} is the range or image.

It is important to note that the domain and codomain or range of a function are both sets, and that a set can itself contain sets. So Example 2.4 could be modified as in Example 2.6 below to achieve an appropriate function.

Example 2.6

Suppose we specify a set of students S = {Fred, Mary, Lisa, Greg} and a set of sets of teachers T = {{Mr. Smith}, {Ms. Johnson}, {Ms. Andersen}, {Mr. Smith, Ms. Johnson}, {Mr. Smith, Ms. Andersen}, {Ms. Johnson, Ms. Andersen}, {Mr. Smith, Ms. Johnson, Ms. Andersen}}. Now we can specify a function that identifies the set of teachers associated with each student. Perhaps Fred has both Smith and Johnson as teachers; our function works because the range T includes an element that is the set with both Smith and Johnson. Perhaps Mary has Mr. Smith, Ms. Johnson, and Ms. Andersen as teachers; again our function can work because the set comprising the three teachers is a member of T.

If the range of a function is equal to a set Z, then the function is said to map its domain *onto* Z (Figure 2.7 represents such a function), in which case the codomain and range are the same. If the range of a function is a proper subset of Z, then the function is said to map its domain *into* Z (Figure 2.10 represents such a function), in which case the codomain is larger than the range. For a function $f: X \rightarrow Y$, if $f(x) = f(w)$ implies $x = w$ and thereby each point in the range is associated with only one point in the domain, then f is a *one-to-one* function. If f is a one-to-one function, then there exists a function, say g, such that $g: Y \rightarrow X$ and $x = g(f(x))$ for all x in X. This function g is called an *inverse function* and is often labeled as f^{-1}, so that we would write $y = f(x)$ and $x = f^{-1}(y)$. Figure 2.11 presents an example of a one-to-one function.

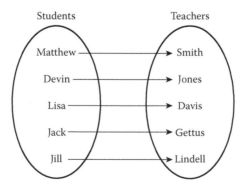

FIGURE 2.11
This figure represents a one-to-one function. This is a function from students onto teachers and each element in the domain (Students) is mapped to only one element in the range (Teachers).

Additional Readings

Stoll's book *Set Theory and Logic* (Dover edition, 1979) is an inexpensive yet fairly comprehensive and well-written introduction to set theory.

Other books that introduce set theory as well as functions include those on mathematical analysis. Bear's book *An Introduction to Mathematical Analysis* (Academic Press, 1997) is a truly simple and easy to understand introduction. Sprecher's book *Elements of Real Analysis* (Dover edition, 1987) is a more comprehensive book that includes the topics of sets and functions. Kolmogorov and Fomin's book *Introductory Real Analysis* (Dover edition, 1975) is another more comprehensive book that includes the topics of sets and functions.

Section II

Measure and Probability

3

Measure Theory

Suppose we have a set $S = \{$Fred, Lisa, Sue$\}$ and we wish to assign numbers to various members of S. If we were only interested in the individual elements of S, we might assign a function from S to some set of numbers, perhaps representing the individual weight of three individuals referred to by the names *Fred*, *Lisa*, and *Sue*. However, suppose we also wanted to assign numbers to subsets of S; perhaps we are interested in the combined weight of Fred and Lisa. In this case, we are out of luck: a function assigns an element in its range to each element of its domain and cannot make an assignment to something that is not in its domain, including subsets of the domain elements themselves. Consequently, to achieve this goal we need to specify a domain for our number assignment that contains as an element any subset of S to which we wish to assign a number. If we denote the set of subsets of S to which we wish to assign numbers as $\mathcal{A} = \{\{$Fred$\}$, $\{$Lisa$\}$, $\{$Sue$\}$, $\{$Fred, Lisa$\}$, $\{$Fred, Sue$\}$, $\{$Lisa, Sue$\}\}$, then the pair $(S, \mathcal{A})$ is a way to denote a domain $\mathcal{A}$ for number assignment reflecting information in a set S we wish to represent: specifically, we wish to define a function on the subsets $\mathcal{A}$ of the set S. Regarding $\mathcal{A}$, defined as above in terms of Fred, Lisa, and Sue, we can assign a number to each individual as we did before, but also to each pair of individuals, since $\mathcal{A}$ contains the sets $\{$Fred, Lisa$\}$, $\{$Fred, Sue$\}$, and $\{$Lisa, Sue$\}$. However, in this example we could not assign a number to the whole group because the set $\{$Fred, Lisa, Sue$\}$ is not in $\mathcal{A}$ as we have defined it above. If we wish to assign a number to the whole group, we need to include the set $\{$Fred, Lisa, Sue$\}$ in $\mathcal{A}$ as well: $\mathcal{A} = \{\{$Fred$\}$, $\{$Lisa$\}$, $\{$Sue$\}$, $\{$Fred, Lisa$\}$, $\{$Fred, Sue$\}$, $\{$Lisa, Sue$\}$, $\{$Fred, Lisa, Sue$\}\}$.

Measurable Spaces

Formally, to properly operate as we will require, the set $\mathcal{A}$ in the preceding paragraph must be more structured than indicated by the preceding example. This is done by defining what is called an *algebra* as follows.

An *algebra* $\mathcal{A}$ defined on a set S is a set of subsets of S such that the following three conditions hold:

1. $S \in \mathcal{A}$
2. If $A \in \mathcal{A}$, then $\overline{A} \in \mathcal{A}$
3. If $A \in \mathcal{A}$ and $B \in \mathcal{A}$, then $A \cup B \in \mathcal{A}$

Here, $\overline{A}$ is defined with S as its universal set; in other words $\overline{A}$ is actually the relative complement of A with respect to S (i.e., $\overline{A} = S - A$). The three conditions imply that $\mathcal{A}$ is an algebra of S if $\mathcal{A}$ includes S itself, and it is closed under complementation and union. Note that this implies $\emptyset \in \mathcal{A}$ because $S \in \mathcal{A}$, and therefore $\overline{S} \in \mathcal{A}$, but $\overline{S} = \emptyset$. Also, by this definition an algebra is closed under intersection and relative differences as well. This is the case because both intersection and relative differences can be expressed as equal to sets defined in terms of union and complementation alone: $A \cap B \approx \overline{(\overline{A} \cup \overline{B})}$ and $A - B \approx \overline{(\overline{A} \cup B)}$. You can show these equivalencies to yourself by the careful use of Venn diagrams.

Unfortunately, an algebra is not a sufficiently general structure to meet all of our needs; to meet our needs, we must modify this definition a bit to get what is called a *sigma-algebra* (also commonly denoted as a σ-algebra), defined as follows. The set $\mathcal{A}$ is a *sigma-algebra* of S if

1. $S \in \mathcal{A}$
2. If $A \in \mathcal{A}$, then $\overline{A} \in \mathcal{A}$
3. If $\{A_n: n \in \mathbb{N}\}$ is a sequence of sets in $\mathcal{A}$, then $\bigcup_n A_n \in \mathcal{A}$

This is to say that $\mathcal{A}$ is a sigma-algebra of S if it includes S, and it is closed under complementation and countable unions. The notion of a countable union in Part (c) above is simply that the union of a sequence of sets in $\mathcal{A}$ is also in $\mathcal{A}$. The detailed reasoning behind our move from unions to countable unions, and thereby from algebras to sigma-algebras, is beyond the scope of this book. Nonetheless, it turns out that sigma-algebras are sufficient for our use to represent finite, countable, and continuous sets.

For a set S and a corresponding sigma-algebra $\mathcal{A}$, the pair $(S, \mathcal{A})$ is called a *measurable space*. This pair of sets indicates that a collection of subsets of the set S has been identified to which we can assign numbers. Given the structure of a sigma-algebra, if we include a subset A of S in our sigma-algebra $\mathcal{A}$, then not only is A measurable by virtue of being an element of $\mathcal{A}$ and thereby part of a domain on which we can define a function, but consequently $\overline{A}$ is also measurable. If we also include a subset B in $\mathcal{A}$, then not only are B and $\overline{B}$ measurable but so is $A \cup B$, $A \cap B$, $A - B$, and $B - A$. Note that the smallest measurable space of a set S is $(S, \{S, \emptyset\})$; it is easy to verify that all conditions for a sigma-algebra are met by the set $\{S, \emptyset\}$.

For a set $\mathcal{C}$, representing any collection of subsets of S, let $\sigma(\mathcal{C})$ denote the intersection of all sigma-algebras that contain $\mathcal{C}$. The following two results hold for $\sigma(\mathcal{C})$: (1) $\sigma(\mathcal{C})$ is a sigma-algebra, and (2) $\sigma(\mathcal{C})$ is the smallest sigma-algebra containing $\mathcal{C}$. The set $\sigma(\mathcal{C})$ is the minimal sigma-algebra generated by $\mathcal{C}$. The details of these consequences are not of concern in this book; what *is* important is that they imply we can construct a measurable space for a set S by identifying a set $\mathcal{C}$ of subsets that we wish to measure and defining an associated sigma-algebra as $\mathcal{A} = \sigma(\mathcal{C})$. It is often easy to proceed by recursively taking all the complements, unions, intersections, and relative differences of the collection $\mathcal{C}$, and consequent sets, to get $\sigma(\mathcal{C})$. It becomes even easier to use $\sigma(\mathcal{C})$ if we identify $\mathcal{C}$ with some partition of interest. This is a natural case for applied researchers because we often think in terms of qualities that partition sets of objects. For example, consider the quality of *age* (in whole units of years) associated with people in some population: this quality can be used to partition the population into sets of people having the same age—those 1 year old, 2 years old, 3 years old, and so on. The sigma-algebra generated by this partition allows numbers to be assigned to any age subgroups of the population, since it includes the union of any age subsets.

Note that I don't need the full partition to generate the sigma-algebra; I can leave out one of the sets. In other words, if a partition comprises K sets, I can, but don't need to, generate the sub-sigma-algebra using only $K - 1$ of the sets.

Measures and Measure Spaces

In the preceding section, we defined measurable spaces as mathematical structures that allow us to assign numbers to subsets of a given set, but we have yet to define a useful assignment of such numbers. This section provides an important type of assignment, one that will underlie probability theory as well as a general calculus of integration. For a measurable space $(S, \mathcal{A})$, a function μ is called a *measure* if it has domain $\mathcal{A}$ and range contained in the extended real line such that

1. $\mu(A) \geq 0$, for all $A \in \mathcal{A}$
2. $\mu(\varnothing) = 0$
3. For any disjoint collection of sets $\{A_n : n \in \mathbb{N}\}$ in $\mathcal{A}$

$$\mu\left(\bigcup_n A_n\right) = \sum_n \mu(A_n)$$

By this definition, it is clear that a measure assigns each set in a sigma-algebra to a number in the nonnegative real line. It must assign the empty set to 0 (and may assign other sets to 0 as well), and it must assign the union of disjoint sets to the same number as the sum of what it assigns to each of the individual sets.

If $(S, \mathcal{A})$ is a measurable space and μ is a measure with domain $\mathcal{A}$, then $(S, \mathcal{A}, \mu)$ is called a *measure space*. Note that there are many ways, true to the definition of a measure, to map a given $\mathcal{A}$ to the nonnegative real line; therefore, many measure spaces can be associated with a single measurable space.

A measure space $(S, \mathcal{A}, \mu)$ has three useful properties that we are concerned with at the moment. For sets A and B and the sequence of sets $\{A_j : j \in \mathbb{N}\}$, all of which are members of $\mathcal{A}$,

1. If $A \subseteq B$, then $\mu(A) \leq \mu(B)$
2. $\mu(A \cup B) + \mu(A \cap B) = \mu(A) + \mu(B)$
3. $\mu\left(\bigcup_n A_n\right) \leq \sum_n \mu(A_n)$

Property *a* is evident if we define a set C to be the relative difference of set B with respect to set A (i.e., $C \approx B - A$). Consequently, set B is the union of the disjoint sets A and C (i.e., $B \approx A \cup C$), and the measure of B is equal to the sum of the measures of A and C [i.e., $\mu(B) = \mu(A) + \mu(C)$] from which the property is directly observed due to the fact that μ is a nonnegative function. Note that equality holds in property *a* if C is the empty set or any set with measure equal to 0.

Property *b* is evident if we note that the union of A and B can be expressed as the union of three disjoint sets—specifically, two relative differences and an intersection:

$$(A \cup B) \approx (A - B) \cup (B - A) \cup (A \cap B) \tag{3.1}$$

Being disjoint sets, the measure of the union of A and B is therefore the sum of the measure of each component:

$$\mu(A \cup B) = \mu(A - B) + \mu(B - A) + \mu(A \cap B) \tag{3.2}$$

Consequently, by adding $\mu(A \cap B)$ to both sides of Equation 3.2, the right-hand side can be expressed as follows:

$$\underbrace{\mu(A - B) + \mu(A \cap B)}_{\text{Part 1}} + \underbrace{\mu(B - A) + \mu(A \cap B)}_{\text{Part 2}} \tag{3.3}$$

However, Part 1 of Equation 3.3 is the measure of two disjoint sets that compose the set A and is therefore $\mu(A)$, and Part 2 is the measure of two disjoint sets that compose set B and is therefore $\mu(B)$. Property *b* immediately follows.

Property *c* is evident from extending property *b* over a sequence of sets and dropping the terms representing the intersections, thereby generating the inequality.

Example 3.1

Let S be the set of N people in a given room: $S = \{s_1, s_2, \dots, s_N\}$. Let C denote the set of subsets containing each individual: $C = \{\{s_1\}, \{s_2\}, \dots, \{s_N\}\}$. Then we can define a sigma-algebra on S as the sigma-algebra generated by C, which turns out to be the power set of S: $A = \sigma(C) = \wp(S)$.

Is (S, A) in Example 3.1 a measurable space? Because $\sigma(C)$ is by definition a sigma-algebra on S, then the answer is "yes" by construction—OK, that was too easy. It is more interesting to consider how we can see that (S, A) is a measurable space. Because A is the power set of S, it contains all subsets of S. The power set must therefore contain all complements, because the complement of a subset of S is also a subset of S (i.e., all the elements of S that are not in the targeted subset). The power set also contains all intersections of subsets of S because a set of elements of S that are members of any number of other subsets are still members of S and therefore compose a subset of S. Moreover, because S itself is a subset of S, and the complement of S is $\emptyset$, then both S and $\emptyset$ are also members of the power set. It is evident that all conditions for (S, A) to be a measurable space are met.

Consider a function that counts the elements of a set, for example, $\mu(\{s_i\}) = 1$ for all $i \in \{1, \dots, N\}$. Is μ a measure on (S, A) in Example 3.1? Because a set is either empty or contains a positive number of elements, then $\mu(A) \geq 0$, for all $A \in A$. Moreover, the number of elements in the empty set is 0, so $\mu(\emptyset) = 0$. Suppose A is a nonempty subset of S that is a member of A; such a subset contains a group of individuals in the classroom and is therefore the union of some sets in C, which are disjoint. The measure of A is the sum of the measures of the corresponding sets in C, which is $\mu(\cup_n A_n) = \sum_n \mu(A_n)$. The function μ is therefore a measure on (S, A).

Example 3.2

Let S be the set of N people in a given room: $S = \{s_1, s_2, \dots, s_N\}$. Let C contain the subset of women: $C = \{\{\text{women}\}\}$, where I use $\{\text{women}\}$ as shorthand for the subset of women in S. Then $A = \sigma(C) = \{S, \emptyset, \{\text{women}\}, \{\text{men}\}\}$ is a sigma-algebra on S. The pair (S, A) is a measurable space. Specify a measure μ on (S, A) such that $\mu(\{\text{women}\}) = |\{\text{women}\}| / |S|$ and $\mu(\{\text{men}\}) = |\{\text{men}\}| / |S|$, for which the parallel lines $|\cdot|$ denote the number of members of a set. Therefore $\mu(A)$ is the proportional size of A with respect to S. Because μ is a measure, then considering the union of the disjoint sets of women and men, $\mu(S) = 1$; and because $\mu(S \cup \emptyset) = \mu(S) + \mu(\emptyset)$ but the union of S and $\emptyset$ is S, then $\mu(S) = \mu(S) + \mu(\emptyset)$, which implies $\mu(\emptyset) = 0$, as we expect.

Note that in Example 3.2 we did not specify a measure that was able to assign numbers to individuals in the room, or any subsets other than those in A. Consequently, in this case the measure space (S, A, μ) is fairly limited in representing information about S; specifically, our analysis is restricted to $A \approx \{S, \emptyset, \{\text{women}\}, \{\text{men}\}\}$.

Measurable Functions

If f denotes a one-to-one function, it is common to denote its inverse (the function that maps the range of f back to its domain) as f^{-1}: we do *not* use this notational convention here! Instead, we define f^{-1} as $f^{-1}(B) = \{a: f(a) \in B\}$. In other words, f^{-1} identifies the subset of the domain for f that f maps to a specified subset of its range. Consequently, f^{-1} takes subsets of the range for f as its argument and returns subsets of the domain of f. This inverse *set function* f^{-1}, therefore, does not require the function f to be one-to-one. Suppose for example that f maps its whole domain to a single constant; f^{-1} would then map that constant back to the set that constitutes the full domain of f.

Let $(S, \mathcal{A})$ and $(T, \mathcal{F})$ be two measurable spaces. If f is a function from S to T such that $f^{-1}(B) \in \mathcal{A}$ for all $B \in \mathcal{F}$, then f is called a *measurable function* because we can define a measure on $(T, \mathcal{F})$ in terms of a measure on $(S, \mathcal{A})$, as shown below. Note that the domain of f^{-1} includes the sigma-algebra $\mathcal{F}$ associated with T, the range of f. The key to the definition of a measurable function is that for all sets in $\mathcal{F}$ (the sigma-algebra we specified as associated with the range of f) there is a corresponding set in $\mathcal{A}$ (the sigma-algebra we specified as associated with the domain of f) to which f^{-1} maps. Note, however, that it is not required that every set of S included in $\mathcal{A}$ be mapped by f^{-1} from a set in $\mathcal{F}$; only the reverse is required.

We can define a measure on $(T, \mathcal{F})$ in terms of a measure on $(S, \mathcal{A})$ as follows. Let $(S, \mathcal{A}, \mu)$ be a measure space, $(T, \mathcal{F})$ be another measurable space, and f be a measurable function from S to T. Then, we can define a function, say μ^*, on the sigma-algebra $\mathcal{F}$ as $\mu^*(B) = \mu(f^{-1}(B))$, yielding $(T, \mathcal{F}, \mu^*)$ as another measure space. The measure μ^* assigns to each set $B \in \mathcal{F}$ the number that μ assigns to the corresponding set $A = f^{-1}(B)$ in $\mathcal{A}$. So, if for each set B in $\mathcal{F}$, the inverse set function $f^{-1}(B)$ corresponds to a set A in $\mathcal{A}$, then there is the following flow between the two measure spaces:

$$(S \quad \mathcal{A} \quad \mu)$$
$$\downarrow \quad \uparrow \quad \downarrow$$
$$(T \quad \mathcal{F} \quad \mu^*)$$

indicating how the measure space $(T, \mathcal{F}, \mu^*)$ is generated from $(S, \mathcal{A}, \mu)$. The leftmost arrow represents f, the middle arrow represents the corresponding inverse set function f^{-1} as applied to events in $\mathcal{F}$, and the rightmost arrow represents the resulting specification of μ^* as an extension of μ [i.e., for each $B \in \mathcal{F}$, $\mu^*(B) = \mu(f^{-1}(B))$].

Integration

Measure theory provides a definition and understanding of integration that is more general than what is provided in typical undergraduate introductory courses. For the purpose of this book, however, we need not expound on the details; understanding basic concepts will suffice.

First, let's develop a simple understanding from the basic introductory courses. The integral of some function f with respect to its domain X is taken to be the sum (denoted by the symbol $\int$) across the domain X of the function evaluated at each element x in the domain multiplied by some small length at x (denoted as dx). Essentially, an integral is a sum of products, commonly denoted as:

$$\int f(x) \cdot dx \qquad (3.4)$$

This basic "sum of products" notion holds in the more general measure-theoretic definitions of integration as well, in which we change "length" to "measure." Before we provide that definition, however, it would be helpful to start with the basic concepts of measure spaces and measurable functions and work up from there.

Suppose we have a measure space $(S, \mathcal{A}, \mu)$ with f a nonnegative real-valued function of S measurable $\mathcal{A}$; moreover, suppose $\mathcal{A}$ is the power set of S. The function f assigns numbers to its domain S, and μ assigns numbers to its domain, each element of $\mathcal{A}$, including the singletons that comprise individual elements of S. Suppose that for each $s \in S$ and corresponding $\{s\} \in \mathcal{A}$, I took the product $f(s) \cdot \mu(\{s\})$ and then summed across all s, what would I have? I'd have a sum of products, which indeed, by the definition provided below, would be the integral of f with respect to μ. Albeit a bit more complicated, the measure-theoretic definition of integral will entail summing products of a measurable function with a corresponding measure. The greater complexity comes from the fact that $\mathcal{A}$ need not be the power set of S (or a continuous-space analog such as the Borel sigma-algebra).

From a measure-theoretic perspective, one useful definition of an integral for a nonnegative measurable function f relative to the measure of a measure space $(S, \mathcal{A}, \mu)$ is

$$\int f \cdot d\mu = \sup_{\pi \in \Pi} \sum_{A \in \pi} \left[\left(\inf_{w \in A} f(w) \right) \cdot \mu(A) \right] \qquad (3.5)$$

where Π denotes the set of all partitions of the set S in the sigma-algebra $\mathcal{A}$, inf (the infimum) denotes the greatest lower bound, and sup (the supremum) denotes the least upper bound. For finite sets, the inf and sup correspond to the minimum and maximum, respectively.

The conventional notation $\int f \cdot d\mu$, which has a familiar look to those versed in undergraduate calculus, can be a bit confusing, since the definition of $d\mu$ as a differential is a bit unclear when applied to an arbitrary measure space. Looking at the preceding definition, which contains the sum of the product of function values and measure values across partitions without reference to differentials, it might be better to denote the integral simply as $\int f \cdot \mu$. Later in the text, I will periodically use the second notation; however, for now I will use the more common first notation. Both denote the same thing.

To simplify the following discussion, it will be helpful to denote the summation as:

$$G(\pi) = \sum_{A \in \pi} \left[\left(\inf_{w \in A} f(w) \right) \cdot \mu(A) \right] \tag{3.6}$$

and therefore

$$\int f \cdot d\mu = \sup_{\pi \in \Pi} G(\pi) \tag{3.7}$$

Note, however, that there are other definitions of integrals, many of which lead to essentially the same results; others do not. For example, one could switch the sup and the inf to obtain another definition, which for smooth continuous functions would provide the same answer as the above definition when integrated with respect to a Borel sigma-algebra. For our purpose, we will use the above definition.

To see how integration works by our definition, let's break it down into steps. First, consider any particular partition π of the set S, the elements of which are contained in our sigma-algebra $\mathcal{A}$ (and is thereby subject to the measure μ). Being a partition, π comprises sets that are mutually exclusive and together make up the set S. Second, for each set A in the partition π, find the element of A that has the smallest value of the function f. Third, multiply this least value of f in A by the measure μ of the set A. Fourth, sum this product across all sets in the partition π. Fifth, repeat the second through fourth steps for all other partitions of S in the sigma-algebra $\mathcal{A}$. The integral of f with respect to μ is the largest of these sums.

Example 3.3

Consider S to be the pattern of dots on the six faces of a die, which I will denote as [1], [2], [3], ... , [6], in which [x] means the face with x number of dots. Let $\mathcal{A}$ be {S, ∅, {[1], [2], [3]}, {[4], [5], [6]}}. Let f assign the number of dots represented by each element of S (i.e., $f([x]) = x$), and let μ assign the total number of dots represented by each set in $\mathcal{A}$ (i.e., $\mu(\{[x], [y], [z]\}) = x + y + z$). First, note that there is only one partition of S represented in $\mathcal{A}$, specifically {{[1], [2], [3]}, {[4], [5], [6]}}; consequently identifying the integral of f with respect to μ does not require searching over a whole set of partitions in this example. Now, because $f([x]) = x$, the smallest f associated with {[1], [2], [3]} is $f([1]) = 1$, and the smallest f associated with {[4], [5], [6]} is $f([4]) = 4$.

Moreover, $\mu(\{[1], [2], [3]\}) = 1 + 2 + 3 = 6$ and $\mu(\{[4], [5], [6]\}) = 4 + 5 + 6 = 15$. Therefore, the integral of f with respect to μ is:

$$\int f \cdot d\mu = \sup_{\pi \in \Pi} \sum_{A \in \pi} \left[\left(\inf_{w \in A} f(w) \right) \cdot \mu(A) \right]$$

$$= f([1]) \cdot \mu(\{[1], [2], [3]\}) + f([4]) \cdot \mu(\{[4], [5], [6]\}) \qquad (3.8)$$

$$= 1 \cdot 6 + 4 \cdot 15$$

$$= 66$$

Example 3.4

Suppose in the preceding example $\mathcal{A}$ is instead defined as the power set of S, and f and μ are defined as above. There are now many partitions of S in $\mathcal{A}$. It turns out, however, that the most granular partition has the largest sum and is thereby used to calculate the integral, which in this case is

$$\int f \cdot d\mu = \sup_{\pi \in \Pi} \sum_{A \in \pi} \left[\left(\inf_{w \in A} f(w) \right) \cdot \mu(A) \right]$$

$$= \sum_{x \in \{1, ..., 6\}} f([x]) \cdot \mu(\{[x]\}) \qquad (3.9)$$

$$= \sum_{x \in \{1, ..., 6\}} x^2$$

$$= 91$$

Integrals are primarily driven by the finest measurable partitions [i.e., the finest partitions produce the largest sums $G(\pi)$]. This is the case because for two partitions π_0 and π_1, if π_1 is a refinement of π_0, then $G(\pi_1) \geq G(\pi_0)$. This can be shown by considering an arbitrary set A in π_0 and the corresponding sets A_i in π_1 that make up A. Because the sum of the measures of the π_1 sets is equal to the measure of the π_0 set under consideration, one can determine that the $(\inf_{w \in A} f(w)) \cdot \mu(A)$ term associated with $G(\pi_0)$ cannot be larger than $\sum_{A_i \in A} [(\inf_{w \in A_i} f(w)) \cdot \mu(A_i)]$ associated with $G(\pi_1)$. This is due to the fact that $(\inf_{w \in A} f(w)) \cdot \mu(A) = \sum_{A_i \in A} [(\inf_{w \in A} f(w)) \cdot \mu(A_i)]$, where the inf term is constant across the summation that is the smallest value: the sum of this smallest constant cannot be any larger than a sum that may include larger values but necessarily does not include smaller values.

Unfortunately, if π_1 and π_2 are different refinements of π_0, then even though $G(\pi_1) \geq G(\pi_0)$ and $G(\pi_2) \geq G(\pi_0)$, we do not know *a priori* whether $G(\pi_1) \geq G(\pi_2)$ or $G(\pi_2) \geq G(\pi_1)$. Similarly, we cannot judge *a priori* between two different refinements of two different partitions. In other words, we have yet to isolate a single partition π^* such that $\int f \cdot d\mu = G(\pi^*)$. However, it turns out that if we have a partition in $\mathcal{A}$ that is a refinement of all other partitions in $\mathcal{A}$, this partition is just such a π^*. This is evident because as a refinement of every partition in $\mathcal{A}$, $G(\pi^*) \geq G(\pi)$ for all π in $\mathcal{A}$, and there exists no further refinement of π^* in $\mathcal{A}$ to achieve an even greater G value.

For the measure space $(S, \mathcal{A}, \mu)$ where S is a countable set and $\mathcal{A}$ is the power set of S, the partition made up of the singletons comprising each member of S is a partition π^* such that $\int f \cdot d\mu = G(\pi^*)$. If conversely S is a continuous set (e.g., some interval on the real line), then the Borel sigma-algebra contains the necessary analog to π^* to allow integration of continuous variables (see more advanced texts in measure theory for details on Borel sets and their application).

As an aside, note that by this definition, integration automatically represents summation across discrete sets: consequently, one technically does not need to use separate notation for discrete and continuous variables—although in most cases people do so anyway, using the summation sign (Σ) for discrete sets.

At the beginning of this section, I framed the definition of an integral in terms of a nonnegative function. We can easily extend the preceding results to functions on the whole real line by partitioning the domain of the function into a set that is mapped to the nonnegative real line and another set that is mapped to the negative real line. Next, evaluate the integral of each part separately, except use the absolute value of the function for the region mapping to the negative real line. Then subtract the integral of the negative part from the integral of the positive part to achieve the full integral of the function.

The goal of this section is not to exhaust the reader's patience with excess detail; the typical undergraduate-level understanding of integration will suffice in operationalizing probability theory for most applied purposes (although the current definition is helpful when operationalizing Monte Carlo techniques for numeric integration). Rather, the purpose of this section is to set the stage for understanding a particular type of function in terms of measure theory: the density function.

Suppose we have a measure space $(S, \mathcal{A}, \mu)$ and a nonnegative measurable function f on S; the following integral defines another measure v on $(S, \mathcal{A})$:

$$v(A) = \int_A f \cdot d\mu, \quad \text{for all } A \in \mathcal{A} \tag{3.10}$$

In this case, the function f is a *density* function, and more specifically f is the density for the measure v with respect to μ.

Although density functions are not restricted to continuous measure spaces because our definition of integral encompasses finite, countable, and continuous variables, they are particularly important when characterizing continuous spaces, that is to say when we are concerned with continuous variables. When considering probability theory, we may start with the measure v and identify a density for that measure as a nonnegative function f that makes the preceding relation true, or we may start with a density f and identify the corresponding measure v.

Additional Readings

Because measures and probability are so intimately related, additional readings for this section are essentially the same as those cited in the section "Additional Readings" at the end of Chapter 4, "Probability." See that section for additional readings appropriate to this chapter.

4

Probability

If $(\Omega, \mathcal{A}, P)$ is a measure space as defined in the previous chapter and the measure P assigns 1 to the set Ω (i.e., $P(\Omega) = 1$), then P is called a *probability measure* or sometimes just a *probability*, and the triple $(\Omega, \mathcal{A}, P)$ is then called a *probability space*. Because $P(\Omega) = 1$, P assigns a number no greater than 1 to any set in the sigma-algebra $\mathcal{A}$, and the sum of probabilities assigned by P to the sets of a partition must sum to 1 across the partition, which is just what we expect from a probability. Note that for any measure space $(\Omega, \mathcal{A}, \mu)$ with $\mu(\Omega)$ finite and nonzero, a new measure can be defined by dividing μ's assignment for any set by the number that μ assigns to Ω. That is, $P(A) = \mu(A)/\mu(\Omega)$ for all sets A in the sigma-algebra $\mathcal{A}$ is a probability measure on $(\Omega, \mathcal{A})$.

Example 4.1

Let Ω be the set of possible outcomes of the flip of a coin specified as $\Omega = \{\text{heads, tails}\}$. Define $C = \{\{\text{heads}\}\}$, and therefore $\mathcal{A} = \sigma(C) = \{\Omega, \varnothing, \{\text{heads}\}, \{\text{tails}\}\}$. We can define an infinite number of probability measures on the measurable space $(\Omega, \mathcal{A})$; some are shown in Table 4.1.

Note that $(\Omega, \mathcal{A}, P)$ is a probability space by virtue of its mathematical properties alone. What $(\Omega, \mathcal{A}, P)$ is taken to mean is an entirely separate, and nonmathematical, question. The meaning of $(\Omega, \mathcal{A}, P)$ comes from our interpretation of it as a model of something in which we are interested. Researchers commonly use probability spaces to model uncertainty associated with data generating processes and to model subjective beliefs. Other interpretations exist as well. See the section "Additional Readings" at the end of Chapter 5 for references to books that discuss various interpretations of probability.

A *data generating process* is the mechanism by which observational units are obtained and measurements are made. The data generating process is typically taken to be objective. Uncertainty from a data generating process is created if the process has the potential of producing different observational units or measurements. For example, one data generating process is an equal probability random sample from a fixed population. The outcome of the process is a particular member of the population; because the process is a random sampling mechanism, it can potentially produce any one of the members. Hence, we are uncertain, *a priori*, about the result of the data

TABLE 4.1

Probabilities for Coin Flip Outcome Events

Probabilities	Ω	∅	$\mathcal{A}$ {heads}	{tails}
P_1	1	0	0.50	0.50
P_2	1	0	0.75	0.25
P_3	1	0	0.02	0.98

generating process. We use probability spaces to model this process and uncertainty.

Another common use of probability spaces is to model *subjective uncertainty*: what a person believes. For example, we may model how confident a person is that a given outcome will occur, or we may model a person's certainty in a particular value of an underlying parameter (e.g., the average height among US citizens).

Example 4.2

Suppose we wish to model the probability of outcomes associated with a flip of a coin as in Example 4.1. If the coin is fair, P_1 would represent a model of the data generating process. Of course, P_1 can also represent a model of a person who believes there is a 50% chance of heads, or who is indifferent between whether heads or tails will occur. The remaining probabilities shown in Table 4.1 could also be used for either a data generating process, if the process was not fair, or subjective uncertainty, if people believe the process was not fair.

For a probability space (Ω, $\mathcal{A}$, P) modeling a data generating process, the set Ω is often called the *outcome set* and represents the set of possible outcomes from the data generating process. The set $\mathcal{A}$ is commonly called the *event set* and represents the events to which we wish to assign probabilities. Note that events are sets of outcomes, whereas outcomes are particular possibilities: If I role a numbered six-sided die, I might get the event of an even number, which is a number in the set {2, 4, 6}, or perhaps I will get an event of less than 5, which is a number in the set {1, 2, 3, 4}, or maybe the event of a 2, which is a number in the set {2}. However, the actual outcome is a specific number from 1 to 6. The measure P is the probability measure representing the uncertainty about the occurrence of events.

You need to define P as a model of something useful for your purpose! This may be a model to represent a source of uncertainty, or it may be a model to represent a normalized frequency (no uncertainty implied, as in a population model), or yet some other interpretation.

Example 4.3

If I were a javelin thrower, then Ω might be the possible outcomes of a throw—a set of distances. If I wanted to model the probability of throwing at least 100 feet, then one of the subsets in $\mathcal{A}$ must represent the event of throwing a distance of 100 feet or more.

In many types of research, it is common to use the following specifications:

Ω is some population of interest (e.g., a population of people or hospitals).

$\mathcal{A}$ is the power set of Ω, allowing for probabilities to be assigned to any subset.

P is based on the sampling probabilities of the individuals w in the population, $w \in \Omega$. In other words, there is a sampling probability for each w in Ω reflecting the data generating process, and the $P(A)$ for all $A \in \mathcal{A}$ is derived additively across unions of the singletons $\{w\}$ for all $\{w\}$ in A.

Such a specification for $(\Omega, \mathcal{A}, P)$ is typical for representing an objective data generating process. Users of such models are often called *frequentists* because they are assumed to be interpreting P as long-run frequencies associated with the data generating process. There are other useful objective interpretations for P, the propensity interpretation of probabilities being one example, but the frequentist label has stuck. Because it seems to me that modeling the data generating process as an objective mechanism remains the most common use for specifying a probability space in applied research, this book will take the frequentist perspective for most examples. However, the general principles apply to any interpretation of probability because the mathematics do not change by virtue of the interpretation.

Conditional Probabilities and Independence

Consider a probability space $(\Omega, \mathcal{A}, P)$. If sets A and B are elements of the sigma-algebra $\mathcal{A}$ and are thereby available for number assignment by probability measure P, then, as required by our definition of a measure space, their intersection is also measurable by P. So we have a probability associated with an event of both A and B occurring, that is, $P(A \cap B)$. If the set B is such that $P(B) \neq 0$, then we can define the following ratio, which is itself a probability measure on $(\Omega, \mathcal{A})$. Let $P_B(A)$ denote this ratio:

$$P_B(A) = \frac{P(A \cap B)}{P(B)} \tag{4.1}$$

for all $A \in \mathcal{A}$ and any set $B \in \mathcal{A}$ with $P(B) \neq 0$.

Challenge 4.1

Describe a probability space for 10 people who are randomly assigned to
a treatment group or a control group with equal probability.

The triple $(\Omega, \mathcal{A}, P_B)$ is a probability space, and P_B as defined in Equation
4.1 is the *conditional probability* given B, also denoted as $P(A\,|\,B)$. Note that
conditional probabilities are only defined relative to certain subsets of Ω,
specifically sets that are members of $\mathcal{A}$ and that have a nonzero probability.
Consequently, if $\mathcal{A}$ is defined in a coarse manner (i.e. defined in terms of only
a few subsets of all the possible subsets of Ω), then only a few conditional
probabilities can be considered.

Example 4.4

For $(\Omega, \mathcal{A}, P)$ specified such that Ω is the set of individuals in a given
room and $\mathcal{A} = \{\Omega, \varnothing, \{\text{women}\}, \{\text{men}\}\}$, then the conditional probability
$P_{\{women\}}(A)$ is equal to either 1 or 0 depending on the A in $\mathcal{A}$. Nothing
more interesting can be discerned. If instead we define $\mathcal{A} = \sigma(\{\{\text{women}\},$
$\{\text{left handed}\}\})$, then $P_{\{women\}}(A)$ would assign a probability of being left-
handed among women and a probability of right-handed among women,
which would sum to 1 (assuming for simplicity there are only left- and
right-handed people).

So far, by defining a conditional probability, we have not changed the measurable space but only changed the probability measure itself. We can, however, define a new probability space with a new measurable space as well.
This can be achieved by defining a *trace* of the sigma-algebra $\mathcal{A}$ on the set B
$\in \mathcal{A}$ as the set $\mathcal{A}_B = \{B \cap A : A \in \mathcal{A}\}$. This is the set comprising the intersections
between B and all sets in $\mathcal{A}$. It can be shown that $\mathcal{A}_B$ is itself a sigma-algebra
and $\mathcal{A}_B \subseteq \mathcal{A}$. The triple $(B, \mathcal{A}_B, p)$, with $p(C) = P_B(A)$, for all $C \in \mathcal{A}_B$ such that
$C = A \cap B$, is a probability space identical to $(\Omega, \mathcal{A}, P_B)$ on all sets with $P_B(A) \neq 0$.
In other words, a conditional probability can be represented by considering
the conditioning event B as an outcome set and applying an appropriately normalized probability to the trace of $\mathcal{A}$ on B. In this case, the resulting probability
p is not a conditional probability defined on $(\Omega, \mathcal{A})$ but rather a probability on
the measurable space $(B, \mathcal{A}_B)$, yet it contains essentially the same information
regarding $\mathcal{A}_B$ as the conditional probability $P_B(A)$.

For probability spaces $(\Omega, \mathcal{A}, P)$ and $(\Omega, \mathcal{A}, P_B)$, events A and B are *independent* elements of $\mathcal{A}$ if $P(A) = P_B(A)$. This relationship for independent
events A and B requires that B have nonzero probability; it follows
however from the more general definition of independence, which is
$P(A \cap B) = P(A) \cdot P(B)$. Both imply, for B having nonzero probability, that
the probability of an event A is equal to the probability of the intersection
of A and B relative to the probability of B. In terms of a Venn diagram as

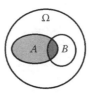

FIGURE 4.1

Independent events: events represented as the sets A and B are independent if the proportion of Ω occupied by the area of A (the combined light and dark shaded areas) is the same as the proportion of B occupied by the intersection of A and B (the dark shaded area); if not, A and B are dependent.

shown in Figure 4.1, this means the proportion of the overall area occupied by set A is the same as the proportion of set B that set A overlaps. That is, the proportion of Ω that set A covers is the same as the proportion of B that set A covers.

Product Spaces

Focusing on the data generating process as an example, we consider $(\Omega, \mathcal{A}, P)$ as a model of the uncertainty for the process that selects an outcome from Ω and thereby generates events in $\mathcal{A}$. Outcomes of the process, however, may be complex. For example, it might be that an experiment selects both a subject and an intervention to apply to that subject. The pair (subject, intervention) may vary in terms of which subject gets selected and which intervention gets applied. Another example is a data generating process that selects N subjects (i.e., gets a sample size of N). These and other complex outcomes can be factored into simpler components.

Example 4.5

Suppose we randomly select a subject from a population and give that person a randomly selected intervention from a set of possible interventions. The outcome would be a subject and intervention pair. Each component of the (subject, intervention) outcome may be represented by its own outcome space. Perhaps Φ is the set of possible subjects (e.g., the population from which a subject is to be drawn) and Θ is the set of possible interventions. It is reasonable to assume we can define corresponding measurable spaces $(\Phi, \mathcal{F})$ and $(\Theta, \mathcal{Q})$. From these individual measurable spaces, we should be able to construct a more complex measurable space $(\Omega, \mathcal{A})$. Indeed we can.

TABLE 4.2

Simple Cartesian Product

		Θ		
		θ_1	θ_2	θ_3
Φ	ϕ_1	(ϕ_1, θ_1)	(ϕ_1, θ_2)	(ϕ_1, θ_3)
	ϕ_2	(ϕ_2, θ_1)	(ϕ_2, θ_3)	(ϕ_2, θ_3)

Let $(\Phi, \mathcal{F})$ and $(\Theta, \mathcal{Q})$ be any two measurable spaces. The *Cartesian product*, or simply the *product*, of the outcome sets Φ and Θ is denoted as $\Phi \times \Theta$ and is defined as the set of all outcome pairs (w, x) such that $w \in \Phi$ and $x \in \Theta$: that is, $(w, x) \in \Phi \times \Theta$. If both Φ and Θ are finite, one could simply create a table for which the rows represent the members of Φ and the columns represent the members of Θ; the cells of the table represent the corresponding pairs (w, x). In this case, the table fills out the members of the product $\Phi \times \Theta$. Suppose $\Phi = \{\phi_1, \phi_2\}$ and $\Theta = \{\theta_1, \theta_2, \theta_3\}$, then $\Phi \times \Theta$ would contain as elements the six pairs of (ϕ_i, θ_j) shown in Table 4.2.

Because a sigma-algebra is a set (specifically, a set of sets), we can take the products of sigma-algebras as well. The product of sigma-algebras creates the set of all pairs comprising each set in one sigma-algebra with the sets in the other. The product of the two sigma-algebras $\mathcal{F}$ and $\mathcal{Q}$ can be used to generate a sigma-algebra on $\Phi \times \Theta$; the resulting sigma-algebra is denoted as $\mathcal{F} \otimes \mathcal{Q}$, such that $\mathcal{F} \otimes \mathcal{Q} = \sigma(\mathcal{F} \times \mathcal{Q})$. In other words, take all the defined events in $\mathcal{F}$, cross them with all the defined events in $\mathcal{Q}$, and take all complements and unions, according to the definition of a sigma-algebra, to produce a new sigma-algebra based on the product of the original two. Then $(\Phi \times \Theta, \mathcal{F} \otimes \mathcal{Q})$ is a measurable space corresponding to $(\Omega, \mathcal{A})$ in which $\Omega = \Phi \times \Theta$ and $\mathcal{A} = \mathcal{F} \otimes \mathcal{Q}$.

For the probability space $(\Phi \times \Theta, \mathcal{F} \otimes \mathcal{Q}, P)$, the probabilities defined as $P_\Phi(F) = P(F \times \Theta)$ for all $F \in \mathcal{F}$ and $P_\Theta(Q) = P(\Phi \times Q)$ for all $Q \in \mathcal{Q}$ are called the *marginal probabilities*. The probability $P_\Phi(F)$ is therefore the probability of an outcome in Φ that is in the set F and *any* element of Θ, whereas $P_\Theta(Q)$ is the probability of an outcome with any element of Φ and an element of Θ that is in the set Q. The marginal probabilities are associated with the probability spaces $(\Phi, \mathcal{F}, P_\Phi)$ and $(\Theta, \mathcal{Q}, P_\Theta)$, sometimes called *coordinate spaces*, which correspond to incomplete observation of the data generating process that produces $(w, x) \in \Phi \times \Theta$. However, in the former case we only observe outcome w, and in the latter case we only observe outcome x. The coordinate spaces are independent if $P(F \times Q) = P_\Phi(F) \cdot P_\Theta(Q)$ for all $F \in \mathcal{F}$ and $Q \in \mathcal{Q}$.

Note that the notation used here for marginal probabilities is the same as that used in the preceding discussion of conditional probabilities. This is purely for typographical convenience when writing the probability space associated with a conditional distribution; it is cleaner to write $(\Omega, \mathcal{A}, P_B)$ than say $(\Omega, \mathcal{A}, P(\cdot \mid B))$ for a conditional probability space. The context will make clear which probability is meant, and when both are used together the more common $P(A \mid B)$ notation will be used for conditional probabilities, as in the following paragraph.

A probability of an event in one coordinate given an event in another coordinate can also be defined on $(\Phi \times \Theta, \mathcal{F} \otimes \mathcal{Q}, P)$ using the definition of conditional probability above. $P_{\Phi \times Q}(F \times \Theta)$, also denoted as $P(F \times \Theta \mid \Phi \times Q)$, is the probability of an event F in the sigma-algebra $\mathcal{F}$, and the event of "any outcome" in the sigma-algebra $\mathcal{Q}$ given an event Q in the sigma-algebra $\mathcal{Q}$, and the event of "any outcome" in the sigma-algebra $\mathcal{F}$. If we were representing $\mathcal{F} \times \mathcal{Q}$ as a table, with the events in $\mathcal{F}$ as rows and the events in $\mathcal{Q}$ as columns, then $P_{\Phi \times Q}(F \times \Theta)$ would represent the probability of a row representing the event F given a column representing the event Q. It should be clear that because we are conditioning on a particular event in $\mathcal{Q}$, we can denote this probability as $P_{\Phi \times Q}(F)$ without confusion. The coordinate spaces are dependent if the conditional probability is not equal to the marginal probability across events.

Product spaces are more general than the two-dimensional ones discussed above. Any number of outcome sets can be components of a product space: for example, N individual outcome sets can compose an overall product set $\Phi_1 \times \Phi_2 \times \ldots \times \Phi_N$. If each is finite, then the product space can be thought of as an N-dimensional array in which each cell is a particular possible outcome such as $(\phi_1, \phi_2, \ldots, \phi_N)$.

Dependent Observations

Now we get to a question important to applied researchers that measure theory can help us sort out: when are observations dependent? Before answering, however, we need to better understand what it is that we are taking to be dependent or independent. When modeling a data generating process, the use of the term *observation* is unfortunate, as it leads one to think about a particular realization of the process: the actual result. However, our probability space is a model of the possible results from a data generating process, not an actual realization. Unfortunately, *observation* is the term in common use, so I will use it here. However, by *observation* what I really mean is "potential result of engaging a given data generating process"—that is, a specific process of observation. If we say Observations 1 and 2 are dependent, we mean that the probability associated with the potential events of data generating process 2 is dependent on the events from data generating process 1 (or vice versa). Dependence is then defined as in the preceding product space section.

When sampling a single observation from each of N populations, we might model each individual sampling process i by a measurable space $(\Omega_i, \mathcal{A}_i)$ in which Ω_i is the population and $\mathcal{A}_i$ is the power set of Ω_i. In other words, we do not necessarily consider the samples as coming from the same population. We can combine the whole group of measurable spaces as a single measurable space $(\Omega_1 \times \ldots \times \Omega_N, \mathcal{A}_1 \otimes \ldots \otimes \mathcal{A}_N)$. However, if we do sample from the same population N times, then $(\Omega_i, \mathcal{A}_i)$ is the same for each observation; that is, each observation is from the same space $(\Omega, \mathcal{A})$. In this case, we can denote $\Omega_1 \times \ldots \times \Omega_N$ as Ω^N, and $\mathcal{A}_1 \otimes \ldots \otimes \mathcal{A}_N$ as $\mathcal{A}^N$, yielding $(\Omega^N, \mathcal{A}^N)$ as the notation for a measurable space representing the data generating process that produced a sample of size N taken from the same population. Using probability P to model the uncertainty in the data generating process, we arrive at the probability space underlying a sample of size N as $(\Omega^N, \mathcal{A}^N, P)$. Because the outcome set is the product Ω^N, it has elements $(w_1, w_2, \ldots, w_N)$, and therefore P is a measure of sets of these elements and not individual w's.

Dependence between two observations i and j is then determined by considering the structure of the probability associated with the two-dimensional subspace and corresponding *bicoordinate marginal probability*, $(\Omega_i \times \Omega_j, \mathcal{A}_i \otimes \mathcal{A}_j, P_{i,j})$. As described in the preceding section, we ask whether events in these two coordinates are dependent. For frequentist modeling, this depends on knowing the data generating process: if you do not know the data generating process, you cannot know whether observations are dependent.

Example 4.6: Sampling with Replacement

Consider two observations sampled from the same population, in the same manner, using the same sampling probabilities. Our probability space representing the two-observation outcome and data generating process is $(\Omega^2, \mathcal{A}^2, P) = (\Omega_1 \times \Omega_2, \mathcal{A}_1 \otimes \mathcal{A}_2, P)$. Our question regards how P assigns probabilities to events in $\mathcal{A}_2$ given a realization of an event in $\mathcal{A}_1$. Let us consider $\mathcal{A}^2$ to be based on power sets, so any possible outcome can have a probability associated with it and any event is the sum of the probabilities of its constituent outcomes. Then this question can be thought of as whether the probabilities of the data generating process selecting individuals from the population change, given the event that a particular individual was selected on the other engagement of the data generating process. Because this design is one of sampling with replacement using the same sampling probabilities each time, the result obtained on one occasion does not affect the sampling probabilities underlying another observation. Observations are independent. Consider equal probability sampling (i.e., each member of the outcome set has the same probability of being selected): if after one member is selected it is placed back into the outcome set and again given the same equal probability of being selected, then the probability of obtaining any member of the outcome set for the second selection has not changed.

Example 4.7: Sampling without Replacement

Suppose, instead, that once someone is taken out of the population, the sampling probability associated with that person goes to 0 and the sampling probabilities associated with the remaining individuals are adjusted so the probability of someone other than the previously sampled person equals 1. The fact that the sampling probabilities change with each sampled individual means the observations are dependent. Consider an outcome set {Fred, Lisa, Mary} and corresponding sigma-algebra $\sigma(\{\{Fred\}, \{Lisa\}, \{Mary\}\})$; the measure describing equal probability sampling for the first selection is defined such that $P(\{Fred\}) = 1/3$, $P(\{Lisa\}) = 1/3$, $P(\{Mary\}) = 1/3$. If the first selection results in Mary as the outcome and she is not placed back into the pool of possible outcomes for the second selection, then the probability for the second selection implies $P(\{Fred\}) = 1/2$, $P(\{Lisa\}) = 1/2$, $P(\{Mary\}) = 0$. If instead the first result is Fred, then the probability for the second selection is $P(\{Fred\}) = 0$, $P(\{Lisa\}) = 1/2$, $P(\{Mary\}) = 1/2$, which is different—the distribution of the second observation depends on the result of the first and therefore the observations are dependent.

Example 4.8: Nested Sampling with Replacement

Suppose we take independent samples of physicians, and then take independent samples of those physicians' patients. We have just asserted that the physicians are independently sampled with replacement, and the patients within physicians are independently sampled with replacement; does this mean the observations are independent? Let's see. What is the outcome set? The data generating process produces a physician–patient pair: Considering two observations i and j, the outcome set is the same for each $\Omega = \text{PHYS} \times \text{PTS}$ (where PHYS is the population of physicians and PTS is the population of patients). To make this clear, suppose that our population of physicians comprises only two physicians and our population of patients comprises only four patients; moreover, let us assume each physician has two patients and the patients don't see other physicians. The sampling probabilities are as follows:

$$
\begin{array}{c c c c c}
 & Pt1 & Pt2 & Pt3 & Pt4 \\
Ph1 & \left(\begin{array}{cccc} p11 & p12 & 0 & 0 \end{array} \right. \\
Ph2 & \left. \begin{array}{cccc} 0 & 0 & p23 & p24 \end{array} \right)
\end{array}
$$

where the rows are physicians and the columns are patients. The probabilities across the whole table sum to 1. However, if the data generating process has generated $(ph1, pt2)$ for one outcome in a physician cluster, then the probabilities among the other outcomes in the cluster conditional on having observed $(ph1, pt2)$ are as follows:

$$
\begin{array}{c c c c c}
 & Pt1 & Pt2 & Pt3 & Pt4 \\
Ph1 & \left(\begin{array}{cccc} p11^* & p12^* & 0 & 0 \end{array} \right. \\
Ph2 & \left. \begin{array}{cccc} 0 & 0 & 0 & 0 \end{array} \right)
\end{array}
$$

where, again, the probabilities sum to 1. Given that we are sampling within a particular physician, outcomes resulting in other physicians have a probability of 0. If, instead, we observe ($ph2$, $pt4$), then the probabilities of another observation within that physician cluster become

$$
\begin{array}{c}
\begin{array}{cccc} Pt1 & Pt2 & Pt3 & Pt4 \end{array} \\
\begin{array}{c} Ph1 \\ Ph2 \end{array}
\left(\begin{array}{cccc}
0 & 0 & 0 & 0 \\
0 & 0 & p23^* & p24^*
\end{array}\right)
\end{array}
$$

However, the probabilities for observations not sampled within this instance of physician p1 remain the same at

$$
\begin{array}{c}
\begin{array}{cccc} Pt1 & Pt2 & Pt3 & Pt4 \end{array} \\
\begin{array}{c} Ph1 \\ Ph2 \end{array}
\left(\begin{array}{cccc}
p11 & p12 & 0 & 0 \\
0 & 0 & p23 & p24
\end{array}\right)
\end{array}
$$

because we return the previously selected physician to the population for sampling. From this, it is evident that observations within a sampled physician are dependent but observations across sampled physicians are independent, even though both the physicians and the patients within physicians are sampled independently. Why? These probabilities are based on a data generating process, the knowledge of which we must consider in identifying dependent observations. In this case, we must know which observations are nested within the same sampled physician; knowing this allows us to identify the dependent observation. Unfortunately, inspecting the data does not tell us this—we may well have obtained the same data by a random sample with replacement of four patients from PTS and just have happened to get two patients who have physician $Ph1$ and two patients who have physician $Ph2$. In this case, patients happen to share the same physician but are not nested within physician; observations are independent, yet the data would be the same.

I cannot stress enough, when using a probability space to model a data generating process, dependence is a function of that process and not a function of the data! Mistaking this point can lead to gross errors such as the misapplication of hierarchical models that account for "dependence" to "nested" data that are not from a nested data generating process. When using a probability space to model a data generating process, as is the frequentist tradition, it is meaningless to speak of nested data; it only makes sense to speak of nested data generating processes.

Challenge 4.2

Explain why the data generating process of the preceding example does not mean that all observations underlying your data are necessarily dependent for realizations having the same physician.

Challenge 4.3

Analyze stratified sampling with replacement in terms of dependence.

The preceding examples are illuminating and common, but also straightforward. Things get more complicated when we consider observational or administrative data in which we did not actually take a sample. As stated above, whether observations are dependent, when considering a frequentist interpretation of probability, is a function of the data generating process and identifying which observations are dependent requires knowledge of that process. This can be a problem. Consider the following examples.

Example 4.9: One Day at the Clinic

Suppose you are given a data set of patient records for all the patients who showed up at an urgent care clinic on a particular day. The clinic is attended by two physicians, of whom one does the early shift and the other does the late shift. Are observations dependent? Well, what is the data generating process? First, I would submit that we don't actually know. However, perhaps we can come up with a reasonable model of one. Let's allow for randomness in the world, an ontological commitment the assessment of which is outside the scope of this book. Otherwise the set of people who show up have a probability of 1 of being selected. We might assume that nature independently selects a set of people–time pairs and then sends those people off to the clinic at their selected times. In this case, the outcome set for each observation is PEOPLE × TIME and the probabilities of an observation from this set do not depend on any result of another observation. The observations are independent, and we would not statistically cluster by physician. Again, this is a case of data resulting from independent observations that share the same characteristic (physician).

Example 4.10: Another Day at the Clinic

Suppose instead that nature selects observations in sequence: first, one person–time pair is selected to go to the clinic, then another person is selected along with a duration of time to follow the first observation. In other words, probabilities associated with times for an observation change depending on the times selected for the other observations. Again, PEOPLE × TIME is the outcome space for each observation, but now the probabilities on the time component change conditional on the results of other observations. The observations are dependent.

"Wait a minute! We were simply given the data on all the patients that showed up on a given day, and now you are telling me that whether I treat observations as dependent changes with nature's data generating process that the data cannot fully inform?" Exactly! "But which model is correct?" An excellent question, and one that does not have a clear answer if you do not know the structure of the process that generated the data. Results may support different inferences depending on which data generating process you model.

Random Variables

Up to this point, I have not mentioned random variables, nor should you assume that I have been covertly discussing them: I have not. The preceding was about the process of observation, not random variables. However, given our understanding of probability spaces, we can now understand what a random variable is, what makes it random, and from where come its probability and distributional properties.

Let $(\mathbb{R}, \mathcal{B})$ be a measurable space such that $\mathbb{R}$ represents the real line and $\mathcal{B}$ is an appropriate sigma-algebra (commonly taken to be a special sigma-algebra called a Borel sigma-algebra, but we need not concern ourselves with this detail here). If we have $(\Omega, \mathcal{A}, P)$, a probability space, and a function X from Ω to $\mathbb{R}$ such that $X^{-1}(B) \in \mathcal{A}$ for all $B \in \mathcal{B}$, then, as stated in Chapter 3, X is a function that is measurable with respect to $\mathcal{A}$ (more concisely written as "X is measurable $\mathcal{A}$," and more precisely written as "X is measurable $\mathcal{A}/\mathcal{B}$"). Note that I did not say "X is measurable P:" that would be too restrictive. So long as $(\Omega, \mathcal{A})$ is a measurable space, then X as defined above is measurable $\mathcal{A}$, regardless of there being any measure on $\mathcal{A}$ actually specified. The function X, as described here, is called a *random variable*. The triple $(\mathbb{R}, \mathcal{B}, P_X)$, with $P_X(B) = P(X^{-1}(B))$, is a probability space representing the random variable X defined on Ω having a distribution determined by P. Note in this case the subscript X on P_X denotes the random variable that the probability is modeling, not a conditional or marginal probability as has been used previously.

The key to understanding the meaning of a random variable is to understand that its distribution is directly derived from the probabilities in the model $(\Omega, \mathcal{A}, P)$—it is not necessarily the normalized frequency of a variable across the outcome space (e.g., the population being sampled), nor is it necessarily the normalized frequency of the data.

Challenge 4.4

Suppose the expected value of a random variable does not correspond to the algebraic mean of the variable in the populations: Is the sample mean an unbiased estimator of the expectation of the random variable?

We are now in a position to understand the connection between random variables and underlying probability spaces. Let's do this by example.

Example 4.11

Suppose I wish to randomly sample a person from the US population and measure his or her weight. Further, suppose I have a sampling frame for the whole population and decide to engage an equal probability data generating process. I can model this in the following way. Let Ω represent the set of individuals in the United States. I take Ω as my outcome set because my sampling frame gives me access to everyone in the United States and hence all members are potential outcomes from my data generating process. Let $\mathcal{A}$ be the power set of Ω as my sigma-algebra, thereby letting me assign probabilities to any set of outcomes. Now, to reflect the equal probability sampling data generating process, I assign $P(\{w_n\}) = 1/N$ for all singletons $\{w_n\}$ in $\mathcal{A}$ representing each of the N persons in the population. From this I get the probability of each set in $\mathcal{A}$ by additivity, because each set in $\mathcal{A}$ is just a combination of individuals and the probability of the set is the sum of the individual probabilities. For example, a set A with 2,000 people in it would have a probability of $2000/N$.

Let X be a measurement of weight on each person in the population—note that here we are speaking of a measurement and not a measure. Being a measurement, it provides an assignment of a number on the real line: therefore, $X: \Omega \rightarrow \mathbb{R}$. If $(\mathbb{R}, \mathcal{B})$ is a measurable space such that for all B in the sigma-algebra $\mathcal{B}$ the inverse $X^{-1}(B)$ is a set that is in the sigma algebra $\mathcal{A}$, then X is a random variable measurable $\mathcal{A}$, and $(\mathbb{R}, \mathcal{B}, P_X)$ is a probability space with $P_X(B) = P(X^{-1}(B))$. The probability associated with the random variable is the probability that the data generating process will produce any of the members of the outcomes set that has the measurement (or set of measurements) on the random variable in which we are interested—outcomes with values for X that fall in set B.

What is the probability that the data generating process will generate a person who weighs between (and including) 100 and 110 lbs? First, we find the set of people whose weights are in that range [i.e., we identify the set A in $\mathcal{A}$ by $A = X^{-1}(\{100 \text{ to } 110\})$] and then get the probability associated with that set from the original space $(\Omega, \mathcal{A}, P)$. In other words, $P_X(\{100 \text{ to } 110\}) = P(X^{-1}(\{100 \text{ to } 110\}))$. Suppose there are n people in the subset of the population that weigh from 100 to 110 lbs; then $P_X(\{100 \text{ to } 110\}) = n/N$.

The key point here is that the probability measure of a random variable is a direct reflection of an underlying probability space. If the underlying probability space is used to model a different data generating process on the same population, we could get a different probability measure for X.

Challenge 4.5

For probability space $(\Omega, \wp(\Omega), P)$, where $\wp(\Omega)$ denotes the power set of Ω, $\Omega = \{\omega_1, \dots, \omega_i, \dots, \omega_{10}\}$, $P(\omega_i) = (i/55)$ and X is a random variable such that $X(\omega_i) = (11 - i)^2$.

1. What is $F(X)$ evaluated at each point in the range of X?
2. What is the probability that $20 < X < 80$?
3. What is the expected value of X?

Challenge 4.6

Show that an equal probability sample has a distribution for random variables that corresponds to the population frequency histogram of the measured variable.

Challenge 4.7

Describe a probability space for the process generating the following data, such that observations within clinics are dependent but observations across clinics are not dependent.

Clinic	Patient	HbA1c Level
1	1	8.2
1	2	7.5
2	3	6
2	4	6.6

Challenge 4.8

Describe a probability space for the process that generated the data for Challenge 4.7 such that all observations are independent.

Challenge 4.9

Describe a probability space for a process in which the observations are dependent but a random variable X is not dependent (here you will have to describe the random variable as well as the underlying probability space).

Cumulative Distribution Functions

Suppose we have a random variable X measurable $\mathcal{A}/\mathcal{B}$ that allows us to define a measure space on the real line:

$$(\Omega, \mathcal{A}, P) \xrightarrow{X} (\mathbb{R}, \mathcal{B}, P_X) \tag{4.2}$$

If X has a meaningful ordering (i.e., X is at least an ordinal-level variable) and $\mathcal{B}$ includes the sequence of intervals on the real line defined as $G = \{(-\infty, x]\}$ for all x, then the function $F_X(x) = P_X(\{(-\infty, x]\})$ is called the *cumulative distribution function* (cdf) or sometimes simply the *distribution function*. Note that this argument applies to related probability measures as well—in particular, conditional probabilities can have cumulative distribution functions. The important distinction between F_X and P_X is that the former is a function of the range of X, whereas the latter is a function of the sets in $\mathcal{B}$. As a practical matter, it is much easier to work with a function of values on the real line (e.g., F_X) than to work with a set function (e.g., P_X).

Challenge 4.10

Show that the cdf contains all the information regarding P_X and is therefore a concise means of representing the distribution of such a random variable.

Probability Density Functions

Probability measures for random variables can have corresponding density functions. Given a probability space $(\mathbb{R}, \mathcal{B}, P_X)$ for the random variable X, if there is another measure space $(\mathbb{R}, \mathcal{B}, \lambda)$ and nonnegative function f of $\mathbb{R}$, such that $P_X(B) = \int_B f \cdot d\lambda$ for all sets B in $\mathcal{B}$, then f is the probability density function for P_X with respect to λ (often called the *probability density* or just the *density* if the context makes this clear). For continuous random variables the measure λ is typically taken to be the Lebesgue measure—a detail that is unimportant for the scope of this text. Once again we have a means of arriving at probabilities in terms of functions of the range of X, in this case the density function.

If P_X has density f, then since $F_X(x) = P_X(\{(-\infty, x]\})$ and since the Lebesgue measure of an interval on the real line is simply its length that we denote as $|dx|$ for the differential dx, for continuous random variables we can write the cdf as $F_X(x) = \int_{(-\infty, x]} f(t) \cdot |dt|$. Alternatively, with a slightly different definition of integral (called the *Riemann integral*) than what we are using here, the common representation found in many textbooks would represent the integral as $F_X(x) = \int_{-\infty}^{x} f(t) \cdot dt$.

As with the cdf, the probability density is a function of X and not a function of sets in the corresponding sigma-algebra, which makes our modeling of distributions easier. Working with mathematical functions of values on the real line rather than working with functions of sets in sigma-algebras allows us to draw on the mathematical skills taught in the typical undergraduate setting.

Challenge 4.11

Show that for a discrete random variable the function $f(x) = P_X(\{x\})$ is a density for P_X with respect to λ defined as a count measure (i.e., $\lambda(A)$ is equal to the number of elements in the set A). In this case, the density $f(x)$ is called a *probability mass function*, and it is often not distinguished from $P_X(\{x\})$; however, the density $f(x)$ and probability measure $P_X(\{x\})$ are different. Explain how.

Expected Values

In terms of undergraduate calculus and the Riemann–Stieltjes integral, an expected value of a continuous random variable X (which is a general statement as a function of random variables is a random variable) is expressed as an integral with respect to its distribution function F:

$$E(X) = \int_{-\infty}^{\infty} x \cdot dF(x) \tag{4.3}$$

And because in this context the differential dF is the density times the infinitesimal differential dx,

$$dF = F(X + dx) - F(x) = \frac{F(x+dx) - F(x)}{dx} \cdot dx = f(x) \cdot dx \tag{4.4}$$

the expected value is also commonly expressed as the Riemann integral

$$E(X) = \int_{-\infty}^{\infty} x \cdot f(x) \cdot dx \tag{4.5}$$

In this text, it will be convenient, however, to consider expected values in terms of the underlying probability space and the measure-theoretic definition of integral provided in Chapter 3. Consider a random variable X defined on $(\Omega, \mathcal{A}, P)$. Because X is a measurable function of Ω, we can integrate it with respect to the measure P as shown in the section "Integration" in Chapter 3. If $\mathcal{A}$ is the power set of Ω, which thereby contains the set of singletons as the most granular partition Ω in $\mathcal{A}$, then in accordance with the definition of integral in Chapter 3 we would express the expected value of X as follows:

$$E(X) = \int_{w \in \Omega} X(w) \cdot P(\{w\}) \tag{4.6}$$

Expressing expected values of random variables in terms of integrals with respect to the underlying probability space, as in Equation 4.6, will become very helpful for understanding the implications of the complex data generating processes presented in Chapter 6.

Random Vectors

What do I have if I take more than one measurement on my study subjects? This is just an extension of the definition of random variables. Given a probability space $(\Omega, \mathcal{A}, P)$, a vector-valued function from an outcome space Ω to $\mathbb{R}^m$, where m is the number of components of the vector and thereby defines the number of dimensions of the real-valued space $\mathbb{R}^m$, is a random vector if there is a sigma-algebra on $\mathbb{R}^m$ (e.g., a generated sigma-algebra from the product of components $\mathcal{B}$) for which each included set can be identified with a set in $\mathcal{A}$ by an inverse set function.

Each component of a random vector is a random variable. Suppose we define a vector-valued function of Ω as follows:

$$X(w) = \begin{pmatrix} Height(w) \\ Weight(w) \\ SystolicBp(w) \end{pmatrix} \qquad (4.7)$$

For each w in Ω, X assigns three values, one each for the person's height, weight, and systolic blood pressure. Individually, *Height*, *Weight*, and *SystolicBp* are functions of Ω, measurable $\mathcal{A}$, and are each therefore random variables with ranges in the real line (perhaps some subset thereof). The vector-valued function X is therefore a random vector with a range in a space defined by three dimensions, each dimension being the real line (or some subset thereof).

The definition of a random vector is parallel to the definition of a random variable, except we can now allow for dependence across random variables in the random vector. By considering the marginal or conditional probabilities across the distribution of random variables in the random vector, we can consider the probability distributions for each component of the vector (i.e., each random variable) and relationships between the components of the random vector (e.g., correlations, regression equations, multivariate distribution models).

If we extend this logic further to define the full product space associated with a sample size of N, then for each observation we have a random vector of, say, m random variables, and we get an $N \times m$ random matrix comprising $N \cdot m$ random variables. Rows are random vectors representing possible measurements of characteristics of observations, whereas columns are random vectors representing possible measurements of a particular characteristic across observations.

This is a good place to pause and further consider what our data represent if our underlying probability space is modeling a data generating process. First, consider what the data are not: Imagine our data in an observation (rows) by variable (columns) format; the columns of our data table are *not* random variables, and the data themselves are *not* random variables. It is each individual "blank" cell of our table that is representing a random variable, with some distribution of possible values that could fill it (see Figure 4.2).

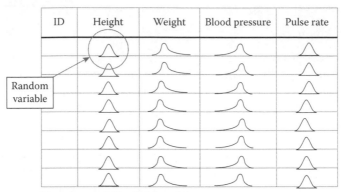

ID	Height	Weight	Blood pressure	Pulse rate

40 random variables in this matrix.

FIGURE 4.2
Random variables of a data generating process are represented by the distribution of possible values that can fill a cell in a table, not the actual data value that ends up in the cell.

Consequently, the blank table represents a random matrix, and the datum in each cell is just a particular realization of the random variable from the data generating process that underlies each cell.

This makes the concept of dependence clearer. It makes little sense to say the data are dependent: how is it that one data point, say "7," is dependent on another data point, say "33"? However, it does make sense to say that two random variables in our random matrix are dependent if the distribution of possible values that could fill one cell is different across the possible values that could fill the other cell.

Moreover, our differentiating data from the distribution of possible data provides some clarity about descriptive sample statistics and inference statistics: Descriptive sample statistics are mathematical descriptions of the data (the numbers you actually have), although data can also be modeled with a probability space (see the "Data Models" section in Chapter 5). Inference statistics are usually estimates of parameters associated with the distribution of random variables defined on probability spaces that model data generating processes.

An important consequence of understanding that each blank cell in the table represents a random variable is to note that once you run the data generating process, you only ever get one realization, one datum, for any given random variable (i.e., you only ever put one number in a cell). If you collect blood pressure measurements on a random sample of 100 people, you have one realization for each of the 100 different random variables. However, if you only have one data point for each random variable, how can you presume to have enough information to inform your understanding of each random variable's distribution? The key to accruing information is to have multiple random variables that have the same distributional characteristics.

For example, if our sample of 100 people represents realizations of 100 random variables each from an implementation of the same type of data generating process on the same population, then we have realizations from 100 random variables that each has the same distribution for blood pressure. In this case, each datum informs the same distribution, even though each is a realization from a different random variable. It is important to note the distinction between having only one realization per random variable and having multiple random variables (and thereby multiple realizations) that have the same distributional characteristic of interest.

This notion, as I've stated it, may at first seem foreign, but it is implicit in the classic manner in which the sample mean is shown in introductory statistics classes to be an unbiased estimator of a random variable's expected value. Suppose we have a data set comprising measurements on some characteristic X for n individuals (i.e., the sample size is n). The sample mean statistic, $\overline{X}$, is defined as follows:

$$\overline{X} = \frac{1}{n} \cdot \sum_{i=1}^{n} X_i \tag{4.8}$$

The expected value of the sample mean is

$$E(\overline{X}) = E\left(\frac{1}{n} \cdot \sum_{i=1}^{n} X_i\right) = \frac{1}{n} \cdot \sum_{i=1}^{n} E(X_i) \tag{4.9}$$

The very fact that the expected value of the sample mean is expressed as a function of the sum of the expected values for each X_i (see the rightmost term of Equation 4.9) implies that each of the n X_i's is taken to be a distinct random variable with its own expected value. Moreover, if each of the n random variables has the same expected value, say μ, then

$$E(\overline{X}) = \frac{1}{n} \cdot \sum_{i=1}^{n} E(X_i) = \frac{1}{n} \cdot \sum_{i=1}^{n} \mu = \frac{1}{n} \cdot (n \cdot \mu) = \mu \tag{4.10}$$

Consequently, the expected value of the sample mean, as a function of n random variables having the same expected value, is the expected value of those individual random variables. Therefore, the sample mean is considered an unbiased estimator of the expected value of X_i for all i. This conclusion, regarding the unbiased nature of the sample mean, assumes the very ideas presented above; specifically, each X_i is a distinct random variable, and these random variables share a common distributional characteristic—in this case, they each have the same expected value.

To press this point further, if we have an $n \times m$ random matrix (e.g., the potential outcomes of m measures on n observations), comprising by necessity $n \cdot m$ random variables, without further knowledge we cannot combine the resulting data to inform questions regarding underlying distributions.

Why? Because without further knowledge, we simply have a single realization from each of $n \cdot m$ completely different distributions, that is, distributions not presumed to share any characteristic of interest. We need to presume, by virtue of design or reasonable assumption, that some random variables share common characteristics in their distributions to warrant combining their corresponding data.

Dependence within Observations

Suppose we have a random vector with m elements defined on $(\Omega, \mathcal{A}, P)$, then we simply have m random variables, which are measurements on the elements of our outcome set Ω.

Example 4.12

Let Ω denote the set of individuals in a population, then the measurements of height and weight associated with each individual compose a two-component random vector of (Height(w), Weight(w)) that comprises the random variables Height(w) and Weight(w), assuming of course that they are measurable with respect to $\mathcal{A}$.

To understand whether such random variables are independent or dependent requires us to tie them back to the independence and dependence of events in $\mathcal{A}$, the sigma-algebra associated with the underlying probability space. This should not be surprising because the probabilities associated with random variables derive from the underlying probability space; as such, everything we do with our random variables must tie back to the original probability space. We take this step by noting that each random variable X generates a partition π_X on the outcome space, which can be used to generate a sigma-algebra $\sigma(\pi_X)$ that is contained in $\mathcal{A}$, assuming $\mathcal{A}$ is rich enough to support the partition. The sigma-algebra $\sigma(\pi_X)$ is termed a *sub-sigma-algebra* of $\mathcal{A}$.

Example 4.13

Let $(\Omega, \mathcal{A}, P)$ represent a data generating process that samples from a population Ω of people. Let an indicator of being female be a random variable Female associated with a given population. Female assigns two possible values: 1 if the individual is female and 0 if the individual is male. The sets Female$^{-1}(\{1\})$ and Female$^{-1}(\{0\})$ in $\mathcal{A}$ are subsets of Ω that compose a partition of Ω (everyone in Ω is a member of either in Female$^{-1}(\{1\})$ or Female$^{-1}(\{0\})$ but not in both). The sub-sigma-algebra of $\mathcal{A}$ generated by the Female partition is $\sigma(\text{Female}^{-1}(\{1\})) = \{\Omega, \varnothing, \{\text{female}\}, \{\text{male}\}\}$.

Challenge 4.12

Explain why the sigma-algebra generated from the full partition is the same as the sigma-algebra generated from all sets in the partition but one (any one).

Random variables defined on $(\Omega, \mathcal{A}, P)$ are independent if their corresponding sub-sigma-algebras are independent. In other words, the events associated with one sigma-algebra are each independent of the events in the other; the independence of events was described above. What this means is that random variables X and Y are independent if for all events $A \in \sigma(\pi_X)$ with positive measure and all events $B \in \sigma(\pi_Y)$, $P(B\,|\,A) = P(B)$, or generally defined as $P(A \cap B) = P(A) \cdot P(B)$. Another way to think of this is that the trace of $\sigma(\pi_Y)$ on A should produce the same relative "sizes" (in a Venn diagram sense) across the events in $\sigma(\pi_Y)$ for all $A \in \sigma(\pi_X)$. No matter which event A that I consider, the relative probabilities of events B remain the same.

Example 4.14

Suppose we wish to know whether a variable that indicates men versus women is independent of a variable that indicates being right-handed versus left-handed (assuming no one is ambidextrous). The top row of Figure 4.3 indicates the case in which the partition on the population generated by the sex variable and the partition generated by the handedness variable produce independent events. Note that the proportion of the circle that is right-handed is 0.5, and the proportion of right-handed

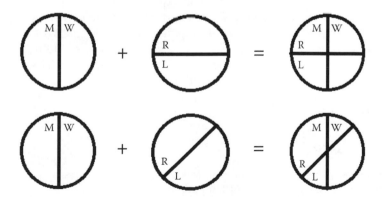

FIGURE 4.3
Independent and dependent variables: the top row depicts independent variables; the proportion of the area of the circle captured by values of one variable remains the same regardless of the value of the second variable (e.g., R takes up half of the area of both M and W). The bottom row depicts dependent variables; the proportion of the area captured by values of one variable depends on the value of the other variable (e.g., R takes up a larger portion of M than it takes up of W).

given women is also 0.5, as is the proportion of right-handed given men. The bottom row of Figure 4.3, however, shows a case in which the events are not independent. The same overall proportions hold for Sex and Handedness; however, now the proportion of right-handed given women is less than 0.5, whereas the proportion of right-handed given men is greater than 0.5. The conditional probabilities do not equal the marginal probabilities—Sex and Handedness are dependent.

Note that, assuming $\mathcal{A}$ is rich enough to support as random variables all the measurements we want, the fact that some pairs of random variables are independent and others are not independent shows that just because events in $\mathcal{A}$ are not generally independent does not mean that certain sub-sigma-algebras (ways of chopping up Ω) are not independent of other sub-sigma-algebras (other ways of chopping up Ω).

Dependence across Observations

Above I established that for frequentists the data generating process dictates whether observations are dependent. Does our determination of observational dependence translate over to random variables defined across observations? First I'll let the cat out of the bag and then I'll explain: Random variables for independent observations are necessarily independent across observations. However, random variables for dependent observations *may or may not be dependent* across observations. The consequence of this latter point is that knowing observations are independent immediately tells us that the corresponding random variables are independent across those observations, whereas knowing that observations are dependent does not tell us whether our random variables are dependent, only that they may be. Therefore, just because we use a clustered sampling design, which, as we have seen, gives us dependent observations, does not mean that the random variables of interest are dependent across observations.

Example 4.15

Suppose a data generating process was a cluster sampling design in which physicians are sampled and then patients are sampled within physician. The (physician, patient) observations are dependent within physician as discussed above. However, suppose that the distribution of patient ages is the same for each physician in the physician population being sampled. This being the case, the conditional probability for patient age (a random variable) does not change given the result of the patient age on another dependent patient observation. By contrast, suppose the distribution of HbA1c differs across physicians; consequently, across dependent observations, the resulting HbA1c for one observation informs the distribution of HbA1c for the other, and the corresponding random variables are thereby dependent.

Example 4.16

Suppose we have two physicians labeled Ph1 and Ph2 and six patients labeled pt1, pt2, pt3, pt4, pt5, and pt6; further suppose that patients pt1, pt2, and pt3 see only physician Ph1, whereas patients pt4, pt5, and pt6 see only physician Ph2. Our set of outcomes for a single sampling instance can be specified as Ω = {(Ph1, pt1), (Ph1, pt2), (Ph1, pt3), (Ph2, pt4), (Ph2, pt5), (Ph2, pt6)}. Let A be the power set of Ω, and P be a probability measure representing the sampling probabilities for a clustered sampling strategy (physicians are sampled first, then patients within physicians—each with replacement). Our measure space for a sample size of N is (Ω^N, A^N, P). Note that we could just as well specify our outcome set as all physician–patient pairs and designate P to assign a zero probability to any pair that doesn't match the above combinations, but there is no advantage to this here.

From previous examples we know the observations within physicians are dependent, so let's consider an arbitrary bicoordinate subspace representing two dependent observations, say Observations 1 and 2. Our measure space of interest here is then $(\Omega_1 \times \Omega_2, A_1 \otimes A_2, p)$. Our concern is whether random variables measured on this space are independent or dependent.

Note that an arbitrary element w of the outcome space contains two physician–patient pairs, one for Observation 1 and the other for Observation 2: $w = ((Ph_i, pt_j)_1, (Ph_k, ph_l)_2)$ with i and $k \in \{1, 2\}$, j and $l \in \{1, 2, 3, 4, 5, 6\}$. Let's define two functions on the outcomes set $\Omega_1 \times \Omega_2$. One indicates whether the patient on Observation 1 weighs less than 150 lbs; the other indicates whether the patient on Observation 2 weighs less than 150 lbs:

$$X_1(w) = \mathbf{1}_{wt((pt_j)_1) \ < \ 150lbs}(w) \tag{4.11}$$

$$X_2(w) = \mathbf{1}_{wt((pt_l)_2) \ < \ 150lbs}(w) \tag{4.12}$$

Suppose the functions in Equations 4.11 and 4.12 map to the measure space $(\mathbb{R}^2, B^2)$, with $B^2 = B_1 \otimes B_2$, such that they are measurable $A_1 \otimes A_2$. They are, therefore, random variables and we can consider their probabilities p_X as determined by p. $(\mathbb{R}^2, B^2, p_X)$ is a probability space representing the distribution of the random variables associated with the underlying data generating process.

If X_1 and X_2 are independent, then $p_X(B_2 | B_1) = p_X(B_2)$ for all $B_1 \in B_1$ with positive measure and $B_2 \in B_2$. As noted in the preceding section, the independence of random variables derives from the independence of their associated sub-sigma-algebras of events in the underlying probability space. What is the event associated with $X_1 = 1$? Suppose each patient has weight less than 150 lbs as indicated in Table 4.3, in which 1 = less than 150 lbs and 0 = greater than or equal to 150 lbs.

TABLE 4.3

Values for Indicator X of Weight Less Than 150 lbs

	Ph1			Ph2		
	Pt1	Pt2	Pt3	Pt4	Pt5	Pt6
$1_{wt<150}$	1	0	0	1	1	0

TABLE 4.4

Pairs of Observations for which $X_1 = 1$ in the Case of Different Distributions across Physicians

			Observation 1					
			Phys 1			Phys 2		
			1	2	3	4	5	6
Observation 2	Phys 1	1	1					
		2	0			╳		
		3	0					
	Phys 2	4				1	1	
		5	╳			1	1	
		6				0	0	

Patients 1, 4, and 5 have low weight, whereas Patients 2, 3, and 6 have high weight. Notice that the distributions of weight in the patient populations across physician are *not* the same. In this case, what happens if we condition on the case of $X_1 = 1$, that is, Observation 1 produces a patient with low weight. The cells containing numbers in Table 4.4 indicate all of the outcomes in $\Omega_1 \times \Omega_2$ for which this condition is true. There are nine possible outcomes for which X_1 is 1—remember that each outcome contains two physician–patient pairs and we are conditioning on the first pair.

There are five out of nine possible outcomes having a patient in the second observation with low weight, that is, five possible outcomes with $X_2 = 1$. Now let's consider when we condition on $X_1 = 0$. The columns containing numbers in Table 4.5 represent the outcomes meeting this condition. Again, there are nine possible outcomes that meet the condition, but only four out of nine have the patient in the second observation with low weight. For the two preceding tables, we see that the probability of X_2 depends on X_1; therefore, X_1 and X_2 are dependent.

Instead, suppose each patient has weight less than 150 lbs as indicated in Table 4.6. Patients 1 and 4 have low weight, whereas Patients 2, 3, 5, and 6 have high weight. Note that the distributions of weight in the patient populations across physician are the same. In this case, what happens if we condition on the case of $X_1 = 1$, that is, Observation 1 produces a patient with low weight? The cells with numbers in Table 4.7

TABLE 4.5

Pairs of Observations for which $X_1 = 0$ in the Case of Different Distributions across Physicians

			Observation 1					
			Phys 1			Phys 2		
			1	2	3	4	5	6
Observation 2	Phys 1	1		1	1			
		2		0	0			
		3		0	0			
	Phys 2	4						1
		5						1
		6						0

TABLE 4.6

Values for Indicator X of Weight Less Than 150 lbs

	Ph1			Ph2		
	Pt1	Pt2	Pt3	Pt4	Pt5	Pt6
$1_{wt<150}$	1	0	0	1	0	0

TABLE 4.7

Pairs of Observations for which $X_1 = 1$ in the Case of Same Distributions across Physicians

			Observation 1					
			Phys 1			Phys 2		
			1	2	3	4	5	6
Observation 2	Phys 1	1	1					
		2	0					
		3	0					
	Phys 2	4				1		
		5				0		
		6				0		

indicate all of the outcomes in $\Omega_1 \times \Omega_2$ for which this condition is true. There are six possible outcomes for which X_1 is 1—remember that each outcome contains two physician–patient pairs.

One-third of the possible outcomes have the patient in the second observation with low weight, that is, with $X_2 = 1$. Now consider conditioning on $X_1 = 0$. Table 4.8 represents the twelve outcomes meeting this

TABLE 4.8

Pairs of Observations for which $X_1 = 0$ in the Case of Same Distributions across Physicians

			Observation 1					
			Phys 1			Phys 2		
			1	2	3	4	5	6
Observation 2	Phys 1	1		1	1			
		2		0	0			
		3		0	0			
	Phys 2	4					1	1
		5					0	0
		6					0	0

condition. Again, one-third of the possible outcomes have the patient in the second observation with low weight. Under both conditions of X_1, the probability of X_2 remains the same: X_1 and X_2 are independent.

In both scenarios in Example 4.16, the underlying probability space was the same, representing the dependent observations of a cluster sampling design; however, the random variables in the first scenario were dependent, whereas the random variables in the second scenario were independent. For this kind of study design, independence occurs within cluster when the distribution of the variables is the same in each cluster.

Another View of Dependence

Remember the definition of a partition and note that sigma-algebras contain partitions. The simplest example of this claim is that for any set A in a sigma-algebra $\mathcal{A}$ on outcome set S, $\mathcal{A}$ also includes $\overline{A}$, the complement of that set by definition; the pair A and $\overline{A}$ is a partition of the outcome set S.

Moreover, if a partition Π is contained in the sigma-algebra $\mathcal{A}$, then the sigma-algebra generated by the partition $\sigma(\Pi)$ is contained in $\mathcal{A}$. Again, this should be clear because $\mathcal{A}$ must include all the complements and countable unions of its sets and therefore for any collection of sets in $\mathcal{A}$, $\mathcal{A}$ must include all the sets in the corresponding sigma-algebra generated from that collection. Because a partition of Ω in $\mathcal{A}$ is a collection of sets, the sets in the sigma-algebra generated by the partition are also in $\mathcal{A}$.

For a probability space $(\Omega, \mathcal{A}, P)$ with a partition Π of Ω contained in $\mathcal{A}$, the space $(\Omega, \sigma(\Pi), p)$ is a probability space with $p = P$ for all $A \in \sigma(\Pi)$. In other words, we don't change the numerical assignment of probability; we merely cull from $\mathcal{A}$ a sub-sigma-algebra generated by a particular partition. In mathematical terms, we say that p is the *restriction* of P to the measurable space $(\Omega, \sigma(\Pi))$. It should not be surprising that we can do this, because a partition of Ω is a collection of disjoint sets that cover Ω and the sum of P across the sets that make up Ω is 1.

Suppose we wish to consider the dependence status of two random variables associated with observations i and j from $(\Omega^N, \mathcal{A}^N, P)$, which is to say we consider random variables defined on $(\Omega_i \times \Omega_j, \mathcal{A}_i \otimes \mathcal{A}_j, p)$. The dependence status of random variables across observations depends on whether the observations are dependent. Remember that observations are dependent if

$$\exists A_i \in \mathcal{A}_i \; \exists \, A_j \in \mathcal{A}_j(p(A_j|A_i) \neq p(A_j)) \tag{4.13}$$

This is to say that the distribution of events on observation j is not the same as the distribution conditional on some event A_i. For simplicity of notation, take A_i and A_j to be a pair of events for which the preceding inequality holds. Then, it must be the case that $p(A_j \,|\, A_i) \neq p(A_j \,|\, \overline{A}_i)$; therefore, the sets of the partition $(A_i, \overline{A}_i)$ are contained in $\mathcal{A}_i$ across which the conditional distributions of events in $\mathcal{A}_j$ differ.

More generally, suppose we have a partition $\Pi = (\pi_1, \pi_2, \ldots)$ contained in $\mathcal{A}_i$ such that the following two conditions hold:

1. $p(A_j \,|\, \pi_k) \neq p(A_j \,|\, \pi_m)$ for all distinct pairs π_k and π_m in Π.
2. $p(A_j \,|\, B) = p(A_j \,|\, \pi)$ for all $B \in \mathcal{A}_{i\pi}$ and for all $\pi \in \Pi$, where $\mathcal{A}_{i\pi}$ is the trace of $\mathcal{A}_i$ on π.

Although Condition 1 is overly strict, as we only need two sets of the partition for which the probabilities are not equal, this specification is useful in identifying the minimal partition that drives dependence. Condition 1 states that observations i and j are dependent by virtue of events in the partition Π contained in $\mathcal{A}_i$; if there were sets in the partition for which Condition 1 did not hold, we would simply replace them with their union to get another partition for which the condition did hold. Condition 2 states that events are independent within each set of the partition. If Condition 2 does not hold for any set π of the partition Π, then we subdivide that π further to achieve a finer-grained partition until Condition 2 is met (assuming the algebra is sufficiently rich). One way to think of this is that the nature of dependence across observations is characterized completely by the partition Π of Ω_i that is contained in $\mathcal{A}_i$.

Let Z be a random variable that assigns to each element of the outcome set a number identifying the set of the partition Π to which it belongs. Moreover, assume there are at least two sets in the partition with nonzero probabilities. Because Π characterizes the dependence structure, we should expect that Z, which numerically indexes Π, does so as well. This is indeed the case.

Let X_i and X_j be random variables: are they dependent? The joint probability of these two random variables is

$$p(X_i, X_j) = \sum_{Z_i} p(X_i, X_j | z_i) \cdot p(z_i) \tag{4.14}$$

which by Condition 2 above, which states that X_i and X_j are independent conditional on each z_i, is

$$p(X_i, X_j) = \sum_{Z_i} p(X_i | z_i) \cdot p(X_j | z_i) \cdot p(z_i) \tag{4.15}$$

By definition, if X_i and X_j are independent, then Equation 4.15 must reduce to

$$p(X_i, X_j) = p(X_i) \cdot p(X_j) \tag{4.16}$$

otherwise the random variables are dependent.

If the distribution of either one of the random variables does not change across Z_i, then X_i and X_j are independent. For example, suppose the distribution of X_j does not vary across the partition characterizing the dependence between the observations [i.e., $p(X_j | z_i) = p(X_j)$], but the distribution of X_i does vary [i.e., $p(X_i | z_i) \neq p(X_i)$]. Then

$$p(X_i, X_j) = p(X_j) \cdot \sum_{Z_i} p(X_i | z_i) \cdot p(z_i) = p(X_j) \cdot p(X_i) \tag{4.17}$$

Moreover, X_i and X_j are independent. If neither of the random variables X_i and X_j is independent of z_i, then the two random variables are dependent and the equation

$$p(X_i, X_j) = \sum_{Z_i} p(X_i | z_i) \cdot p(X_j | z_i) \cdot p(z_i) \tag{4.18}$$

gives us insight into the reason for dependence: random variables are dependent when their distributions vary across the partition indexed by the random variable Z that characterizes the dependence between observations.

Note, however, that for a random variable to be dependent on the indicators of a partition, it is not required that the distribution of the random variable be different across all components of the partition. It is only required that there exists at least one component of the partition for which the distribution of the random variable is different. This will be important when analyzing the dependent structure of study designs such as the cluster-randomized clinical trial in which clusters are sampled, the whole cluster is assigned to a treatment or control condition, and individuals within the cluster are sampled for measurement (or all individuals sampled within a cluster are assigned a treatment as designated by the assigned cluster-level treatment designation).

A few paragraphs above I mentioned in the condition, "Moreover, assume there are at least two sets in the partition with nonzero probabilities." What if instead there is a particular z for which $p(z) = 1$? Well, then the preceding equation becomes

$$p(X_i, X_j) = p(X_i|z) \cdot p(X_j|z) \tag{4.19}$$

Equation 4.19 doesn't look exactly like our criterion for independence: are X_i and X_j independent? They are if $p(X_i|z) = p(X_i)$ and $p(X_j|z) = p(X_j)$, which is indeed the case. This is easy to show, so I will leave it as a challenge.

Challenge 4.13

Show for the preceding case that indeed $p(X_i|z) = p(X_i)$ and $p(X_j|z) = p(X_j)$ if there is a particular z with $p(z) = 1$. Hint: this is easily shown intuitively by Venn diagrams on the underlying probability space.

Example 4.17

For a cluster sample in which patients are nested within physicians, our partition is determined by physician, and z_i is a variable that identifies the physician for observation i. The data generating process, by virtue of being a cluster sampling process, is such that z_i also indicates the physician of observation j. Consequently, if the distribution of the qualities measured by the X's varies across physician, then the random variables are dependent. Note that the random variables X_i and X_j need not measure the same qualities on the two observations. Preceding examples used weights on each patient; however, it could just as well be observation i's weight and observation j's patient satisfaction. If both vary by physician, then they are dependent.

The key point of this section is that random variables are not dependent if the observations are not dependent, and random variables *may* be dependent if the observations are dependent. If there is a partition on the outcome set across which the conditional distributions of random variables differ, then the random variables are dependent. A corollary to this last point is that the intraclass (or intracluster) correlation does not determine whether observations are dependent, only whether random variables are dependent given the *a priori* determination that the observations are dependent. If we know that the data generating process is such that the observations are independent, the corresponding random variables are independent regardless of the intraclass correlation, and the intraclass correlation should not be taken as evidence for dependence.

Densities Conditioned on Continuous Variables

It is common to speak of conditional probabilities, densities, and moments as if they were conditioned on a single point in a continuous space. For example, treating weight as a continuous variable, we might say the probability density of systolic blood pressure given weight equal to 210 pounds has a particular distribution, perhaps a normal distribution. However, our measure-theoretic understanding of random variables suggests that such statements are wrong. The easiest way to see this is by considering the following two equations regarding the joint distribution of two random variables Y and X, where B denotes a measurable set in the range of Y and x is a single point:

$$P(B|\{x\}) = \int_{y \in B} f(y|x)dy \qquad (4.20)$$

and

$$P(B|\{x\}) = \frac{P(B, \{x\})}{P(\{x\})} \qquad (4.21)$$

Equation 4.20 simply establishes f as what we would like to consider the usual conditional probability density of Y, given that X is equal to some value x that can produce the probability on the left-hand side of the equation. However, Equation 4.21 shows that this conditional probability is in fact not defined because the probability measure of a point in a continuous space is usually considered to either be zero or not defined (depending on the measure of the corresponding density). Consequently, the probability in the denominator of the right-hand side of the second equation, $P(\{x\})$, is zero or not defined and consequently neither is the conditional probability on the left-hand side. Therefore, even though the function f on the right-hand side of the first equation is nonnegative, integrates to 1, and calculates to a number, it cannot be the desired conditional probability density, because, as stated, the conditional probability it purports to support does not actually exist. Therefore, the first equation above is not actually a meaningful equation.

To add to the confusion, which I will clear up below, the joint probability density $f(y, x)$ and marginal densities $f(y)$ and $f(x)$ are well defined, as is the equation $f(y, x) = f(y|x) \cdot f(x)$. The conditional function is the ratio of two probability densities, $f(y|x) = \frac{f(y, x)}{f(x)}$, and is itself a density for some measure on Y, X, or both, just not the probability measure we might presume for the conditional probability of interest. However, clearly our disputed function $f(y|x)$ serves a purpose. So, what is it? Well, though $f(y|x)$ is not the presumed conditional probability density function, it is a function of Y and X that relates a marginal density to a joint density.

This is all well and good when we are using $f(y|x)$ to connect a marginal distribution to a joint distribution, but we use such conditional "probability densities" in applied research for more than specifying joint distributions (specifically, researchers are often interested in the parameters of conditional distributions). For example, they are presumed to underlie regression functions such as

$$E(Y|X=x) = \int y \cdot f(y|x)dy \qquad (4.22)$$

However, the fact that $f(y|x)$ is not a probability density should lead us to suspect that the function $E(Y|X=x)$ is not actually a conditional expectation—indeed, as argued above, it is not! What we should be speaking of is $E(Y|X \in \Delta_x)$, where Δ_x denotes a measurable set of points containing x with positive measure.

To understand the role of $f(y|x)$ in quantities of interest, consider the conditional probability $P(A|\Delta_x)$, where A is a measurable set associated with Y, and again Δ_x denotes a measurable set of points containing x for which $P(\Delta_x)$ is not zero:

$$P(A|\Delta_x) = \frac{P(A, \Delta_x)}{P(\Delta_x)} \qquad (4.23)$$

This is a well-defined equation with the left-hand side a proper conditional probability statement. The numerator on the right-hand side can be expressed as

$$P(A, \Delta_x) = \int_A \int_{\Delta_x} f(y, x)dxdy \qquad (4.24)$$

where $f(y, x)$ is the joint probability density that is the product of our disputed $f(y|x)$ and the marginal density $f(x)$:

$$P(A, \Delta_x) = \int_A \int_{\Delta_x} f(y|x) \cdot f(x)dxdy \qquad (4.25)$$

By bringing the constant $P(\Delta_x)$ under the integral, we can thereby express $P(A|\Delta_x)$ as

$$P(A|\Delta_x) = \int_A \int_{\Delta_x} f(y|x) \cdot \underbrace{\left(\frac{f(x)}{P(\Delta_x)}\right)}_{\text{Part 1}} dxdy \qquad (4.26)$$

$$\underbrace{\phantom{P(A|\Delta_x) = \int_A \int_{\Delta_x} f(y|x) \cdot \left(\frac{f(x)}{P(\Delta_x)}\right) dxdy}}_{\text{Part 2}}$$

where Part 1 of the right-hand side is a legitimate conditional density of X given $X \in \Delta_x$, and Part 2 is therefore the expected value of $f(y|x)$, with respect to the distribution of X given $X \in \Delta_x$ for any value of Y. Consequently,

$$P(A|\Delta_x) = \int_A E_X(f(y|x)|X \in \Delta_x)dy \qquad (4.27)$$

which, by our definition for probability densities, implies that $E_X(f(y|x)|$ $X \in \Delta_x)$ is the conditional probability density that corresponds to the conditional probability measure $P(A|\Delta_x)$. So, the conditional probability $P(A|\Delta_x)$ has a legitimate probability density, which we can label $f(y|\Delta_x)$, that is the conditional expectation of $f(y|x)$ taken with respect to the conditional distribution of X given $X \in \Delta_x$.

Now, if we consider $f(y|\Delta_x)$ with respect to a nested sequence of convex sets centered on the singleton $\{x\}$ starting from Δ_x equal to some set, say $\Delta_x{}^*$, such that the sequence converges to the singleton $\{x\}$, then $f(y|\Delta_x)$ with respect to this sequence will approach $f(y|x)$; technically, we would take the limit of this sequence, assuming the limit exists. Consequently, we can use $f(y|x)$ to approximate $f(y|\Delta_x)$ if Δ_x is a really small set with positive measure containing x, and our common use of $f(y|x)$ as if it were the probability density of interest, though technically wrong, is vindicated as an approximation in this case. Note that in empirical work Δ_x is naturally taken to be a set of X values within the unit of measurement around the measured value x—which may not be small enough for a good approximation.

Note the technical consequence of this section's discussion regarding our definitions of regression functions. Specifically, regression functions that are defined as functions of continuous random variables are in fact not actually conditional expectations; instead, they are limits of conditional expectations with respect to sequences of sets that converge to the singular set containing the point being conditioned on, which is not measurable. Nonetheless, it is often convenient to write expressions such as $E(Y|X \in \Delta_x)$ as $E(Y|X)$: I will use this convention where it is not confusing.

Statistics

Statistics is a term used to label a field of study and an activity, but formally a statistic is a type of measurable function. For example, suppose we have a data generating process underlying N observations that we model as $(\Omega^N,$ $\mathcal{A}^N, P)$. The outcome set in this example is the product of N sets: $\Omega^N = \Omega_1 \times \Omega_2 \times \ldots \times \Omega_i \times \ldots \times \Omega_N$, in which $\Omega_n = \Omega$ for all $n \in \{1, 2, \ldots, N\}$. An individual element of Ω^N is a group of N elements, one from each component set of Ω^N: that is, $(w_1, w_2, \ldots, w_N) \in \Omega^N$. Suppose we measure a characteristic X on each of the N individuals that comprise an outcome $(w_1, w_2, \ldots, w_N)$; X then underlies N random variables:

$$(\Omega^N, \mathcal{A}^N, P) \xrightarrow{X_1, \ldots, X_N} (\mathbb{R}^N, \mathcal{B}^N, P_X)$$

We therefore have N random variables X_1 to X_N.

Because $(\mathbb{R}^N, \mathcal{B}^N, P_X)$ is a probability space, we can define a random variable with respect to it by a measurable function from $\mathbb{R}^N$ to $\mathbb{R}$, the real line. The average of the N random variables is a common example:

$$\hat{\mu} = \frac{1}{N} \sum_{i=1}^{N} X_i \qquad (4.28)$$

In this case, $(\mathbb{R}^N, \mathcal{B}^N, P_X) \xrightarrow{\hat{\mu}} (\mathbb{R}, \mathcal{B}, P_\mu)$ and $\hat{\mu}$, by virtue of P_μ, has a probability density f_μ and distribution F_μ. The function, $\hat{\mu}$, of the random variables X_1 to X_N is called a *statistic*; its probability P_μ, and consequently its distribution, reflects P from the original probability space via its connection through P_X. If the original probability space is solely modeling a data generating process, then the distribution of $\hat{\mu}$ is called its *sampling distribution*. This distribution reflects the values of $\hat{\mu}$ that are possible due to the different sets of N observations obtainable by the data generating process. The standard deviation of the distribution for $\hat{\mu}$ is its standard error. See the "Interpreting Standard Errors" section of Chapter 6 for a discussion of the relationship between standard deviations and standard errors in probability spaces that do not solely model data generating processes.

It is interesting to note that, although statistics are often defined as the sum of functions of random variables, such as the sample mean of the preceding example, it is not necessary that each individual component of the sum be a random variable. This is evident in the maximum likelihood estimator. Suppose we define two random variables, Y and X, for each of N observations. This results in $2 \cdot N$ random variables (i.e., an (X, Y) pair for each observation). For $ll(Y_i, X_i; \theta)$ denoting the log-likelihood component associated with observation i, the maximum likelihood estimator is defined as follows:

$$\hat{\theta} = \underset{\Theta}{\operatorname{argmax}} \sum_{i=1}^{N} ll(Y_i, X_i; \theta) \qquad (4.29)$$

Assuming appropriate conditions are met that guarantee a maximum for all possible outcomes and θ values, then $\hat{\theta}$ is a random variable: $(\mathbb{R}^{2N}, \mathcal{B}^{2N}, P_{YX}) \xrightarrow{\hat{\theta}} (\mathbb{R}, \mathcal{B}, P_\theta)$. However, in this case, each log-likelihood component of the sum shown above is not a random variable that maps to the real line because θ is unspecified (although $ll(Y_i, X_i; \theta)$ is a random function of θ). Nonetheless, $\hat{\theta}$ is a random variable with properties that make it useful for using the data-specific values of $\hat{\theta}$ (i.e., an estimate) to inform hypothesis tests and estimation goals (e.g., under certain conditions being consistent for the θ value that parameterizes the distribution underlying the log-likelihood).

Some reflection should reveal the distinction between the role of the likelihood function in determining the maximum likelihood statistic and the role of the likelihood in classic Bayesian analysis. As a statistic, its role is purely instrumental: as it turns out, by proof, this function has properties we desire of an estimator that make it useful, but there are often other estimators that we could just as well use. Indeed, once I know the estimator has the properties I want (e.g., being consistent and asymptotically efficient), I do not really care about the inherent meaning of the underlying function, except as required for proper specification. In a classic Bayesian analysis, however, the likelihood function is not a statistic, but rather is part of the specification of a joint probability distribution that dictates the meaning of the posterior distribution being sought. In the Bayesian analysis the likelihood provides meaning to the posterior.

What's Wrong with the Power Set?

In the preceding sections, I usually jumped straight to specifying my sigma-algebra as the power set of a finite outcome set of interest. Is this always wise? For most of our purposes as applied researchers, I argue it is useful, but first let's see why it can be a problem. Some contend that the power set can be too large to assign probabilities and therefore should not be specified when the outcome set is anything but small. This contention presupposes that you are assigning the probabilities to the events of this sigma-algebra; if true, I agree. Typically when you endeavor to make assignments to the base-level probability space (as opposed to a random variable generated space), you are doing certain types of experiments or discerning a measure of subjective uncertainty.

Example 4.18: Particle Beam Deflection

Suppose two young physicists, Matthew and Devin, hypothesize that under certain conditions a beam of particles shot toward a wall will be deflected to the left of the vertical centerline. Also suppose the wall shows where the beam hits. The outcome space for this experiment can be specified by the cells of a fine grid on the surface of the wall (say each cell is 0.000000001 inches square).

Matthew decides to take the event set to be the power set of the outcome set, and he therefore has a super-large set of events. If Matthew wishes to directly assign frequentist probabilities to the event space as operationalized via multiple independent runs of the experiment, he would need to rerun the experiment an extremely large number of times to get a good estimate of the probabilities associated with each event. Once done, he can test his hypothesis.

Devin, by contrast, realizes that her hypothesis is simply left of center versus right of center, so she specifies her event space to be $\sigma(\{\text{left of center}\}) = \{\{\text{The Whole wall}\}, \varnothing, \{\text{left of center}\}, \{\text{right of center}\}\}$. Devin needs only to track the proportion of points that are left of center to fill out her probability measure.

Devin will be home for dinner tonight; Matthew won't even make his retirement party.

When using experiments to directly assign the probability measure of an event space, the power set can indeed be too large for practical use, and careful consideration of what you are really interested in becomes a very important practical matter.

If instead we are interested in features of random variables, rather than directly identifying the probabilities of the underlying probability space, then we can simply use the data. The underlying probability space generates the random variables, the distribution of which is reflected in samples from the data generating process. So long as we use the same data generating process we suppose we are modeling, then information in the data (realizations of random variables) is sufficient to estimate and test other quantities of interest.

Example 4.19

Continuing the preceding example, Matthew may keep his specification of the event space but then measure a random variable that indicates left of center and use an estimator of the proportion of points with the value of the random variable associated with left of center. Now Matthew can go home for dinner as well.

Do We Need to Know P to Get P_X?

It may seem from the preceding sections of this book that we must actually calculate the probabilities P_X of random variables X from the underlying probability P, thereby requiring us to know P in order to determine the distribution of X. This is not so. Although the distribution of X comes from P, it is still the distribution of X and we can discern it from a sample (using data generating processes that produce a series of random variables having the same distribution) without knowing or assigning P. Or we can hypothesize a distribution for X and use data from random variables having the same distribution to test the hypothesis. In other words, nothing said so far precludes our usual approaches to modeling random variables from the data comprising realizations of random variables from a data generating process. However, our model specification and interpretation of results strongly depend on the preceding discussion.

It's Just Mathematics—The Interpretation Is Up To You

One should never lose sight of the fact that the mathematical probability theory underlying our analyses is just mathematics; it provides little insight without an interpretation in terms of what we seek to understand.

Also, because it is just mathematics, how one makes the interpretation is not perfectly constrained by fixed rules.

Whereas it is common to model our base-level probability space in terms of capturing the units on which we are going to make measurements (height, weight, etc.), we could just as well start at a different level.

Example 4.20

Rather than letting $(\Omega, \mathcal{A}, P)$ model the population of interest as a set of individuals, I could just as well consider the outcome space to be {woman, man} and the equal probability sample of the population will produce one or the other outcome, with properly associated probabilities. Of course, the disadvantage of this is that we may find it difficult to understand the probabilities, as they are not derived from the simple assignment of $1/N$; nonetheless, one would not be sent to jail for taking this approach. Of course, the only sensible random variable would be an indicator variable (say, woman = 1 and man = 0), whereas using the previous model I can consider any possible measurement on humans—a considerably richer model.

Although modeling the data generating process often means specifying the objects of measurement as the outcome set, modeling subjective beliefs can take the more abstract approach.

Example 4.21

If I wished to model your confidence in the average height of people in the United States, I would specify my outcome set as the positive real line and determine a probability measure that reflects your confidence that the average height is in the various intervals in some appropriate sigma-algebra. Perhaps I use $(\mathbb{R}^+, \{\mathbb{R}^+, \varnothing, \{0 \text{ to } 6 \text{ ft}\}, \{\text{greater than } 6 \text{ ft}\}\}, P)$ as my probability space and P assigns your confidence judgments that the average height is less than 6 ft and greater than 6 ft.

Example 4.22

Suppose I am a frequentist wishing to investigate failure times in randomly selected individuals. If I consider that each person has a fixed failure time, then I might simply model the data generating process on the population of people as done above and consider failure time as a random variable. On the other hand, if I consider that nature assigns failure times for each individual by some random process, and as such each individual may have any possible failure time, then I might model my outcome set as the product $(\Omega \times \mathbb{R}^+)$. In other words, the data generating process combines my process of randomly selecting a person and nature's random assignment of failure time. The corresponding random variable is the observed failure time. The subtlety here is that the outcome is (w, t), for which many possible t's could have shown up even with the same w. The random variable is $X((w, t)) = t$.

The next section of the book provides examples of various uses and interpretations for probability models—some common, some not.

Additional Readings

Billingsley's book, titled *Probability and Measure* (Wiley Interscience, 1995), is an excellent text on probability theory presented in terms of measure theory. Resnick's book, titled *A Probability Path* (Birkhauser, 1999), is another such book.

For those interested in the topic from the disciplinary perspective of econometrics, Dhrymes' book *Topics in Advanced Econometrics: Probability Foundations* is worth reading. However, across both statistics and econometrics, my personal favorite is Davidson's book *Stochastic Limit Theory: Advanced Texts in Econometrics*—in my opinion, one of the best works on the subject.

Moving from probability to statistics, Schervish's book *Theory of Statistics* (Springer, 1995) provides an introduction to statistics in a measure-theoretic framework. It presupposes an understanding of measure theory and probability; however, it provides introductions to the topics in appendices.

Section III

Applications

5

Basic Models

The preceding chapters presented a conceptual introduction to measure-theoretic mathematical probability. This chapter will introduce uses of probability spaces as models for common research designs. We will start with the conceptually simple (i.e., modeling measurement error) and progress to a study design that may defy the usefulness of probability spaces as a modeling paradigm (i.e., modeling natural data generating processes for observational data).

Experiments with Measurement Error Only

Perhaps the simplest scientific use of a probability space is to model the variability associated with measurement in the context of a fully controlled experiment of a deterministic process. Consider an experiment in which all conditions are fully controlled except for chance error in the measurement instrument itself. In other words, for each run of the experiment, the physical outcome is the same, but the measurements may vary by chance. If we run the experiment N times, we record N measurements that may differ due solely to measurement error. How do we use this set of data to draw inferences regarding the underlying process?

We can model the measurement process for the experimental setup as a probability space: let Ω denote an outcome set comprising possible states that the measurement instrument can take, let $\mathcal{A}$ be an appropriately rich sigma-algebra, and let P denote a probability measure that models the objective uncertainty associated with the state of a given measurement outcome being in the sets of $\mathcal{A}$. Then $(\Omega, \mathcal{A}, P)$ is a probability space representing the uncertainty of the measurement process of the experiment. Suppose we define a function, labeling it Y, from each state of the measurement instrument to numbers on the real line. Now, if $\mathcal{B}$ is a sufficiently rich sigma-algebra on $\mathbb{R}$ such that the range of the function $Y^{-1}(B)$ for all $B \in \mathcal{B}$ is contained in $\mathcal{A}$, then $(\mathbb{R}, \mathcal{B})$ is a measurable space and Y is measurable $\mathcal{A}$: Y is therefore a random variable representing variation in the measurement process. If we let $p(B) = P(Y^{-1}(B))$ define a measure on $(\mathbb{R}, \mathcal{B})$, then $(\mathbb{R}, \mathcal{B}, p)$ is a probability space associated with the random variable Y. Characteristics of p provide information useful for making inferences about the experiment accounting for measurement error.

For N independent runs of the experiment, there is one realization from each of N random variables from the probability space. If the experimental runs are identical, it is reasonable to presume that each of these random variables has the same distribution, and we can use statistics (a function of the N random variables, which consequently is itself a random variable) to estimate properties of p and thereby provide information for making inferences. For example, the histogram of the data reflects p from the N realizations from the probability space. If we are interested in the expected value of Y taken with respect to p as a summary of the experimental outcome, then the sample mean and confidence interval provide a reasonable estimate of this quantity, as shown in any introductory statistics text. If our interest is not in the estimate itself, but instead we are interested in testing a particular hypothesis, then we can proceed with statistical hypothesis testing. For example, suppose we have a theory that implies a state corresponding to a perfect measurement of less than 10. If we are correct in assuming that the measurement instrument provides unbiased results, then the mean of the distribution for Y with respect to p will also be less than 10. We record the measurements for N independent runs of the experiment and calculate a sample mean of 9. This result conforms to our prediction, but can we rule out the alternative explanation that the true value is 10 or greater and we got a sample mean of 9 by virtue of measurement error alone? Here we have a classic setup for a statistical test to rule out an alternative explanation for the data.

Experiments with Fixed Units and Random Assignment

Another use of probability spaces is to model uncertainty associated with random assignment of research subjects to experimental conditions. In this setup the probability space is not used either to model uncertainty regarding which research subjects are used (they are considered fixed) or to model measurement error, which is considered to be zero. Instead, the probability measure is defined to represent the uncertainty that a subject is assigned to each possible experimental condition. In this case, for each subject, we may define an outcome space of $\Omega = \{C_1, C_2, \ldots, C_K\}$, in which each element is a particular experimental condition with a corresponding sigma-algebra $\mathcal{A}$ as the power set of Ω. For an experiment with N subjects, $(\Omega^N, \mathcal{A}^N)$ is a measurable space representing the possible configuration of experimental conditions assigned across the group of subjects. For P, a probability measure representing the probability of assignment to conditions for the N subjects, $(\Omega^N, \mathcal{A}^N, P)$ is the probability space that models assignment.

Unfortunately, using $(\Omega^N, \mathcal{A}^N, P)$ as our model is restrictive in its representational benefits. The outcome space Ω^N contains information regarding experimental conditions but does not have individual-specific information. In other words, we can define random variables that indicate what condition was assigned, but it is not apparent how outcomes are available for each individual in each condition. Consider only one subject (i.e., $N = 1$) with one treatment (T) and a control (C) assignment possible: the probability space is $(\{T, C\}, \mathcal{A}, P)$. A random variable is an $\mathcal{A}$-measurable function of $\{T, C\}$. It is not clear how we obtain the person-specific measures based on T or C alone: Suppose T is a particular medication and we are interested in a subject's blood pressure. Our random variable assigns a number to the condition of taking the medication and a number to the condition of not taking the medication. However, do such conditions have a blood pressure? No. Neither medications nor the condition of taking medications is the kind of things that can have a blood pressure. Of course, we can simply declare the function and, making its assignment correspond to a particular subject's measurements, multiple subjects would then require multiple functions; however, this makes the model somewhat opaque. So, for didactic purposes, an alternative would be to consider our outcome space to comprise the set of all qualities of the subject (say subject s) under condition T and the set of all qualities under the condition C: $\Omega = \{\{X_s\}_T, \{X_s\}_C\}$. As before, there are only two elements to this outcome set: one element is the set of characteristics associated with subject s under condition T, and the other is the set under condition C. Meaningful random variables are now more evident: some obvious ones include measurements on the real line of the X qualities as well as treatment assignment.

Sticking to our one-subject experiment with only two treatment conditions, suppose we model the experiment with $(\Omega, \mathcal{A}, P)$ for $\Omega = \{\omega_1, \omega_2\}$ with ω_k being either the simple indicator of treatment and control or the sets of qualities under treatment and control conditions. For an appropriately defined random variable Y, the parameters of the distribution of Y are readily calculated. For example, the expected value of Y is $Y(\omega_1) \cdot P(\{\omega_1\}) + Y(\omega_2) \cdot P(\{\omega_2\})$. For those qualities that do not change, $Y(\omega_1) = Y(\omega_2)$, and the expectation is simply the value; for those qualities that differ across treatment groups, the randomization-weighted average becomes the expectation.

For example, let $\Omega = \{\{\text{male, blood pressure, } T\}, \{\text{male, blood pressure, } C\}\}$, in which case the outcome space is the sex and blood pressure state of the individual under treatment condition T and control condition C. Define $\mathcal{A}$ to be the power set of Ω, and P is 0.5 for each element of the most granular partition of Ω in $\mathcal{A}$ (i.e., equal probabilities of being assigned to treatment or control). Now let us define three random variables: Y = 1 if male, 0 otherwise; X = blood pressure measurement (suppose it is 130 under the treatment condition and 150 under the control condition); and Z = 1 if treatment condition, 0 otherwise. The expected value of Y is $1 \times 0.5 + 1 \times 0.5 = 1$, and the variance of Y is $(1 - 1)^2 \times 0.5 + (1 - 1)^2 \times 0.5 = 0$. The expected value of X is $130 \times 0.5 + 150 \times 0.5 = 140$, and the variance of X is $(130 - 140)^2 \times 0.5 + (150 - 140)^2 \times 0.5 = 100$. The expected value of Z is $1 \times 0.5 + 0 \times 0.5 = 0.5$, and the variance of Z is $(1 - 0.5)^2 \times 0.5 + (0 - 0.5)^2 \times 0.5 = 0.25$. The treatment effect on sex is $E(Y \mid Z = 1) - E(Y \mid Z = 0)$, which is 0 (i.e., sex does not change), whereas the treatment effect on blood pressure is $E(X \mid Z = 1) - E(X \mid Z = 0)$, which is -20.

Of course, knowledge of the variable values associated with each outcome in the outcome space is typically unknown except for the few outcomes that are measured. Consequently, multiple experiments with random variables having the same distribution (or shared parameters of interest) are typically used so that statistics are available to estimate desired quantities.

Observational Studies with Random Samples

A common study design among applied researchers is to collect a sample from a population and measure their characteristics. For example, perhaps we wish to know the distribution of blood pressure among the adult population in the United States. We might propose to measure the blood pressure of all adults in the population, but that would likely be impractical. So, instead we might propose to collect a sample of adults from the population and measure their blood pressures. However, now the set of blood pressures we obtain will likely vary depending on the sample we happen to get, and the sample we happen to get will likely vary due to how we go about obtaining the sample. Consequently, there may be variation in the observed numbers (e.g., sample averages and variances) due to the mechanism of sampling, that is, due to the data generating process. How can we account for this variation? One strategy is to base our analysis on a probability space that models the data generating process producing this variation.

To proceed with this example, suppose we have a sampling frame of all people in the United States (e.g., a list of unique identifiers and viable contact information). Suppose we plan to randomly select a sample of individuals from the frame such that each person has an equal chance of being selected. For simplicity in this example, let us further suppose we plan to sample with replacement (i.e., after selecting a name, we put the name back so it could possibly be selected again). Moreover, again for simplicity, suppose that we can compel the measurement of all those whom we select and that measurements are precise. We can model this process by letting the outcome set be the population of the United States and the associated event set be the power set of the outcome set; we define the probability measure based on the sampling probability associated with each unit set in the event set (i.e., each individual in the population):

Ω is the population of people in the United States.

$\mathcal{A}$ is the power set of Ω, allowing for probabilities to be assigned to any subset.

P is based on the sampling probabilities of the individuals w in the population, $w \in \Omega$, that is, $P(\{w\}) = 1/N$ for all unit sets $\{w\}$ in $\mathcal{A}$, and N denotes the number of people in the population.

By these definitions, $(\Omega, \mathcal{A}, P)$ provides a model of the data generating process that will allow us to account for variation in sampling. If we define $Y(w)$ to be a real-valued function on Ω to reflect a measure of systolic blood pressure, then for Y measurable $\mathcal{A}$, we have $(\mathbb{R}, \mathcal{B}, p)$, with $p(B) = P(Y^{-1}(B))$ for all $B \in \mathcal{B}$, as a probability space that defines the distribution of the random variable representing blood pressure measurements, and we can use our usual statistical methods to estimate parameters of this distribution or test hypotheses.

If instead we generate the data by taking a random sample of states (with replacement, for simplicity) and then we take a random sample of individuals from within each state (again, with replacement), we would have a simple cluster (or nested) sampling design. The outcome set of this data generating process may be defined as the product set of states S and US population Ω (i.e., $S \times \Omega$), the event set is again the power set of the outcome set, and P represents the cluster data generating process. For example, P is such that $P(\{s, w\}) = P_S(\{s\}) \cdot P_{s \times \Omega}(\{w\} \mid \{s\})$, which is the probability of obtaining a state s in the first step of the data generating process multiplied by the conditional probability of obtaining individual w given one has obtained state s in the first step of the data generating process. The random variable Y then reflects the distribution of blood pressure associated with P, which in this case is the distribution associated with a cluster sampling design.

Consider a third strategy. Suppose we engage the strategy of the first example, but in this case we cannot compel participation in our study: each individual may or may not agree to participate. In this case, our outcome set may be modeled as $\Omega \times$ {agree to participate, not agree to participate}, our event space is again the power set associated with this outcome set, and our probability is defined as $P(\{w, a\}) = P_\Omega(\{w\}) \cdot P_{w \times A}(\{a\})$, the probability of selecting an individual w multiplied by the conditional probability of agreeing to participate given that the individual is selected. The random variable for blood pressure now has a distribution reflecting the combination of how we select individuals and whether those individuals are inclined to participate in our study. If those with high blood pressure are less inclined to participate, then the distribution of y will reflect this by shifting toward lower values of blood pressure, and vice versa if those with high blood pressure are more inclined to participate.

These examples highlight an important point: Statistical analyses provide estimates or tests of the parameters associated with random variables, and these random variables derive their distributions from the underlying probability space being used. Consequently, when modeling different data generating processes that are implemented on the same population, there may be different distributions for the same type of measurement (e.g., blood pressure). Using an unbiased estimator for each random variable will provide unbiased information about the parameters related to the data generating process, but it may not necessarily correspond to the underlying population. If you wish to estimate the average blood pressure in the population, but you use the third data generating strategy (i.e., the one with self-selection), then the unbiased estimator of the mean for the random variable Y may not be unbiased for the population average itself (perhaps only those with low blood pressure are willing to participate). Again, your statistics are estimating parameters of a probability space modeling a particular data generating process, which may not correspond to the population-level information that you seek. Consequently, it is necessary to design the data generating process and analytic strategy so that functions of the related parameters correspond to the population quantities of interest.

Experiments with Random Samples and Assignment

If we collect a random sample of individuals and then randomly assign each individual to one of a set of conditions, then our model of the data generating process is based on the product outcome space of both the random assignment and random sample models considered separately above. For example, suppose we collect a sample of individuals from a population Ω and assign each individual to a treatment or control condition from the set $T = \{$treatment, control$\}$. We can model this data generating process using the outcome set specified as $\Omega^* = \Omega \times T$. With an appropriately defined sigma-algebra, the probability can be written as the product of the marginal probability of selecting an individual from Ω and the conditional probability of treatment given the individual selected: $P(\{w, t\}) = P_\Omega(\{w\}) \cdot P_{w \times T}(\{t\})$. If treatment assignment is independent of individual selection, then as we know this probability reduces to the product of the two marginal probabilities: $P(\{w, t\}) = P_\Omega(\{w\}) \cdot P_T(\{t\})$.

We should keep in mind that the structure of $P(\{w, t\})$ (i.e., whether it reduces to the product of marginals or not) for each observation does not bear on our judgment of whether *observations* are independent or not. Such dependence is a question to be asked of the bicoordinate probabilities associated with the higher-order measurable space $(\Omega^{*N}, \mathcal{A}^N)$ reflecting the data generating process underlying the selection of a sample of N outcomes. As presented in preceding sections, this case is one in which observations are independent, and consequently the random variables across observations are independent as well.

Suppose, instead, that our data generating process is based on cluster sampling with random assignment of conditions. Perhaps we take a random sample of elementary schools (with replacement) from the population of elementary schools in the United States, we then take a sample of children (with replacements) from each school's population of students, and finally we randomly assign each student to an experimental condition. Our outcome set is made up of the US population of elementary schools (S), the US population of elementary schoolchildren (C), and the set of experimental conditions (T): $\Omega = S \times C \times T$. Our event set is the sigma-algebra generated by the product of the sigma-algebras defined for each component of the outcome set: $\mathcal{A} = \mathcal{A}_S \otimes \mathcal{A}_C \otimes \mathcal{A}_T$. Moreover, our probability is constructed to model the cluster sampling and random assignment so that our random variables will reflect this data generating process and our corresponding standard errors will represent variation in the estimators due to the sampling uncertainty of the data generating process: $P = P_S \cdot P_{C|S} \cdot P_{T|C,S}$, which is the product of the probability of getting a particular school with the probability of obtaining a particular child within that school and the probability of assigning a particular treatment to that child. If treatment assignment is random without regard to school or child, then P reduces to $P_S \cdot P_{C|S} \cdot P_T$.

Again, dependence between observations is identified by considering the bicoordinate probabilities associated with the higher-order measurable space $(\Omega^N, \mathcal{A}^N)$. As preceding sections have shown, for cluster samples, observations within clusters are dependent and observations across clusters are independent (when equal probability sampling is done with replacement). Random variables for observations across clusters are independent. By contrast, dependence of random variables for observations within clusters will depend on whether the distribution of the random variables is the same across all clusters: if so, the corresponding random variables are independent; if not, they are dependent for observations within a cluster—in this case, within a school.

Would the situation change if we engage a cluster randomized trial in which we obtain a sample of schools, randomly assign the school to an experimental condition, and randomly select a sample of students within each of the selected schools? All students within a given school will be subject to the same experimental treatment. In this case, the probability space representing each observation would be similar to that presented in the preceding paragraph.

Table 5.1 presents the sampling probabilities of particular school (S), experimental condition (T), and child (C) combinations. Remember, the probabilities in the table sum to 1.

TABLE 5.1

Probabilities for First Observation of Cluster Randomized Trial

School	Experimental Condition	Children							
		C_1	C_2	C_3	C_4	C_5	C_6	C_7	C_8
S_1	T_0	p_{101}	p_{102}	p_{103}	p_{104}	0	0	0	0
	T_1	p_{111}	p_{112}	p_{113}	p_{114}	0	0	0	0
S_2	T_0	0	0	0	0	p_{205}	p_{206}	p_{207}	p_{208}
	T_1	0	0	0	0	p_{215}	p_{216}	p_{217}	p_{218}

TABLE 5.2

Probabilities for Second Observation of Cluster Randomized
Trial given that First Observation is (S_1, T_0, C_3)

School	Experimental Condition	Children							
		C_1	C_2	C_3	C_4	C_5	C_6	C_7	C_8
S_1	T_0	P_{101}	P_{102}	P_{103}	P_{104}	0	0	0	0
	T_1	0	0	0	0	0	0	0	0
S_2	T_0	0	0	0	0	0	0	0	0
	T_1	0	0	0	0	0	0	0	0

TABLE 5.3

Probabilities for Second Observation of Cluster Randomized
Trial given that First Observation is (S_2, T_1, C_5)

School	Experimental Condition	Children							
		C_1	C_2	C_3	C_4	C_5	C_6	C_7	C_8
S_1	T_0	0	0	0	0	0	0	0	0
	T_1	0	0	0	0	0	0	0	0
S_2	T_0	0	0	0	0	0	0	0	0
	T_1	0	0	0	0	P_{215}	P_{216}	P_{217}	P_{218}

Given that we obtained (S_1, T_0, C_3) on one observation, the conditional
probability of another observation within the same cluster becomes as represented in Table 5.2, and again the probabilities sum to 1.

By contrast, the probabilities associated with the second observation given
the first observation obtained (S_2, T_1, C_5) are presented in Table 5.3 in which
the probabilities sum to 1.

In Tables 5.2 and 5.3, the probability distributions vary by which school and
condition was obtained in the first observation: the observations are dependent
within school and condition. Of course, since each school is assigned only one
treatment condition, this reduces to dependence within school. Similar to the
usual cluster sample design, observations within cluster are dependent, whereas observations across clusters are independent. The corresponding random
variables are dependent if their distributions vary across school and condition.

Observational Studies with Natural Data Sets

Another common source of data that requires careful consideration is what
I call a *natural data generating process* (NDGP): this is a data generating process that is not designed but is presumed to underlie data that are simply

collected as they occur. Examples include data from all patients that visited a clinic in some time period; New York's Statewide Planning and Research Cooperative System, which collects patient-level detail on patient character-istics, diagnoses and treatments, services, and charges for every hospital dis-charge, ambulatory surgery patient, and emergency department admission in New York State; and the National Cancer Institute's Surveillance, Epi-demiology, and End Results registries, which collect data on each cancer patient in participating regions of the United States.

The distinguishing feature of such data sets is that they result from meas-urements on individuals who were not selected by virtue of some designed data generating process but rather who happen to "show up" by virtue of some unknown natural process and be recorded: those individuals in a pop-ulation who happen to seek care from a given clinic at a given time; those individuals in New York who happen to be admitted to a hospital; those individuals in certain US regions who present with cancer to the medical sys-tem. What at first may seem like a trivial question is in fact a perplexing problem: how do we model an NDGP? This is a question that may not have a satisfactory answer, leaving us with a suspicious interpretation of analyses. Examples 4.9 and 4.10 in Chapter 4 presented two simple scenarios with NDGPs. Let's consider some other examples.

Suppose we are interested in modeling the natural probability that a per-son gets some specified illness in a given year and that we have access to data on each person in a population regarding whether that person got this illness. We are not asking about the proportion of people who actually got sick in that year. Instead, we presume that those who happened to get sick could well not have gotten sick, and those who did not get sick could well have. Our interest is in modeling the natural uncertainty about an indi-vidual getting this illness and estimating a corresponding probability parameter.

We could begin by specifying the population as the outcome set, the power set as the event set, and a probability modeling nature's selecting of individ-uals. For a large population, this probability space might be a reasonable approximation, but the specification is flawed in its particulars. Suppose our outcome set is the population, our probability measure represents an NDGP that assigns a probability to each person in the population of getting sick, and nature engages this NDGP a number of times to generate the peo-ple who get sick. However, what is the probability that someone will get sick each time the NDGP is engaged? By the definition of a probability space, it is one: someone must get sick each time the NDGP is engaged. Moreover, only one person gets sick each time the NDGP is engaged; therefore, we need to model a process by which a number of people may get sick. Because the number of people who get sick is uncertain, we need to augment the sick-generating NDGP with a number-of-people-generating NDGP in which nature picks the number N of people who will get sick and thereby the number of times the sick-generating NDGP is engaged. If N is 0, then the sick-generating NDGP is never engaged; if N is 1, then it is engaged once, and so on. If not this strategy, then some other clever organization of probability models that serve the same function must be developed (e.g., using the power set of the population as the outcome set would allow for nature's selecting any number of people to be sick).

An alternative is to model each person's natural uncertainty separately. In a simplified form, perhaps the outcome space for each person is defined as $S = \{$not sick, sick$\}$ with corresponding algebra $\mathcal{A} = \{S, \varnothing, \{$not sick$\}, \{$sick$\}\}$ providing us with a measurable space on which each person w has a probability p_w defined that reflects their natural susceptibility to getting sick. Consequently, for each person w in population Ω, we have a probability space $(S, \mathcal{A}, p_w)$. The product space across Ω provides the overall probability space reflecting the population: $(S^N, \mathcal{A}^N, P)$, in which P reflects the combination of the p_w's across the individuals in population Ω. Now that each person may or may not get sick, it is possible for any number of people to get sick, or no one at all.

Unfortunately, without additional constraints, this specification is not amenable to analysis. If each person has an idiosyncratic probability of getting sick, then there are N probability parameters and N observations. If, by contrast, it is reasonable to model the probability of an arbitrary person getting sick as a function of specific characteristics and a small set of fixed common parameters, we can use the information across the whole population to estimate those parameters.

As a simple example, suppose $p_w = p$ for all $w \in \Omega$ (i.e., everyone has the same probability of getting sick). Moreover, suppose this illness is such that each person's probability is independent of whether others get sick. Then $(S^N, \mathcal{A}^N, P)$ is a probability space with P equal to a product measure comprising individual probabilities p of getting sick and $(1 - p)$ of not getting sick. Because the data comprise realizations of random variables with a common p, we can estimate p from the data. For example, by maximum likelihood our estimator of p is $\hat{p} = N_s/N$, in which N_s is the number of people in the population who got the specified illness. The variance of our estimator is $\mathrm{var}(\hat{p}) = (p \cdot (1 - p))/N$. Note that the usual "large sample" asymptotic properties of maximum likelihood estimation hold in terms of population size rather than the usual consideration of sample size.

Contrast this with the goal of estimating the proportion of people who got sick in the population. We then calculate the proportion as $\pi = N_s/N$, which is the same quantity that our estimator $\hat{p}$ would produce as an estimate, except that in the case of π, we do not have an estimate of a data generating process parameter. Instead we have the actual proportion—a population parameter. Whereas the estimator $\hat{p}$ has a variance associated with possible realizations of which people could become sick in the population, π does not have such a variance associated with it. By one account we can say that the proportion of people who got sick was π; by another account we can say the probability of a person getting sick is estimated as $\hat{p}$, which will have a variance of $\text{var}(\hat{p})$. The difference between these two accounts derives from what is being modeled, not from the data.

Now let's consider we have an equal probability random sample (generated with replacement) of n people from the population. The estimator $\tilde{p} = n_s/n$, in which n_s is the number of people in the sample who were sick, provides an estimate of a parameter for the sampling data generating process, which corresponds to π and has a variance $\text{var}(\tilde{p}) = (\pi \cdot (1 - \pi))/n$. On the other hand, if we consider $\tilde{p}$ as an estimator of the probability of a person getting sick, then, unfortunately, it is likely to be biased due to the difference between the equal probability sampling and the unequal probabilities of getting sick (an interesting mirror image of classic self-selection bias, which would require similar strategies to handle).

Our assumption that $p_w = p$ for all $w \in \Omega$ does not at all seem plausible for any real illness. After all, how likely is it that each individual has the same probability of getting a particular illness? If this assumption is sufficiently in error, then $\hat{p}$ becomes meaningless as an estimator of an individual's probability of getting sick, whereas both π and $\tilde{p}$ remain meaningful in their original interpretations. To be clear, in this case $\hat{p} = N_s/N$ makes no sense but $\pi = N_s/N$ does. How can two quantities that are the same differ in being meaningful or not? They do so because they differ in meaning: $\hat{p}$ estimates a parameter of an NDGP that represents the natural probability of a person getting sick, whereas π is the proportion of people who got sick. Similarly, $\tilde{p}$ is an estimator of a sampling data generating process, which, if the data generating process is indeed as we specified, is also consistent for π and retains its meaning accordingly.

Suppose we have a vector of characteristics x for each individual in the population such that the natural probability of an arbitrary individual w getting sick can be reasonably modeled as a function g of characteristics x and corresponding parameter θ: $p_w = g(x_w, \theta)$. In other words, probabilities of getting sick vary across individuals in the population because individuals have different characteristics as measured by x. Note that by our current specification of $(S^N, \mathcal{A}^N, P)$, our only random variable is an indicator of illness. So, what is x? Well, it is not a random variable, but it is an individual-specific observed parameter that specifies the individual probabilities. Now the probability space $(S^N, \mathcal{A}^N, P)$ can be the basis for estimating the common unobserved parameter θ, which in combination with an individual's specific x would provide us with an estimate of that person's probability of getting sick. Moreover, the point and interval estimators of θ will give us information about how these natural probabilities of getting sick are related to the idiosyncratic parameters x.

In the preceding example, I assumed observations were independent. However, how might we determine whether observations ought to be modeled as dependent? Determining whether two arbitrary individuals i and j are dependent requires considering the bicoordinate subspace $(S_i \times S_j, \mathcal{A}_i \otimes \mathcal{A}_j, p)$.

We can represent the meaningful components of the Cartesian product of events as a simple two-by-two table:

$$
\begin{array}{c c c c}
 & & \multicolumn{2}{c}{j} \\
 & & s & ns \\
 & s & p_{s,s} & p_{s,ns} \\
i & & & \\
 & ns & p_{ns,s} & p_{ns,ns} \\
\end{array}
$$

Does the probability of illness for individual j given that individual i is ill differ from the probability of illness for individual j given that individual i is not ill? The answer depends on the data generating processes.

Assume that we are interested in an illness stemming from exposure to an environmental toxin. It might be reasonable to presume that, although P_i and P_j may both be high or low for individuals with similar exposures, the probability of illness for one individual is the same regardless of whether the other was selected by nature to be ill; therefore, the probabilities are independent. As an aside, consider how our judgment in this regard might change if we were modeling subjective beliefs about how likely these people were to get ill rather than the frequentist approach taken here.

What if we were interested in an infectious disease? Now we might consider that these two observations are dependent if the process by which nature assigns illness to one also impacts the other. In a fully connected society (i.e., there is a pathway of individuals that connects everyone in the population), we might consider every pair of observations as dependent, with the degree of dependence a function of how many pathways connect the individual's. However, identifying that the state of illness is dependent between all pairs of individuals is not of much help because we only have one observation per person. We need to model the dependence if it is to be useful in our analysis. Perhaps categorizing by family or neighborhood would work, or perhaps using some distance measure.

The preceding example focused on having data on the full population; however, it is more common that we have data on only some of the population, as mentioned in the introduction to this section. To illuminate issues regarding modeling an NDGP in this case, let's revisit the examples provided in Chapter 4.

Consider that you have all the study-relevant patient data for a specific day of a health care clinic. The physician who attended in the morning did a better job at treating the outcome of interest than the physician who attended in the evening. How do we determine whether the observations of the NDGP are dependent?

If nature independently samples N people with replacement from a population Ω and independently samples a time of the day, with replacement, from a set T, for each person and then sends the N people to the clinic at their designated times, then it should be clear that the observations are independent. The probability of a person–time pair of one observation does not depend on the actual person–time event occurring on any other observation. However, if nature does a sequential sampling strategy by which people are sent to the clinic in the order of the sequential sample, then the probabilities associated with events on the outcome set ($\Omega \times T$) changes with the sequence. For example, if the first observation has a time of 10 am, then the probabilities associated with events on the outcome set ($\Omega \times T$) for the second observation must assign zero to all event with T less than 10 am. The third observation is constrained by the previous, and so on. The observations are dependent. Are the outcome variables dependent? Because physician shift is fixed according to time of day (morning/evening) and the morning physician does better than the evening one on a particular outcome, the distribution of outcomes changes with each observation in the sequence indicating dependence in the outcome variables. Note, as I've mentioned at various points in this chapter, that the data could well be the same for both processes and therefore cannot differentiate the models in this case.

Population Models

The preceding models use probability spaces to represent sources of uncertainty. However, remember that mathematical probability is not substantively interpreted in itself and is therefore not restricted to modeling uncertainty. In fact, the main targets of investigation are often in terms of a probability model having a different interpretation.

As researchers, we are typically not interested in the parameters of a data generating process (except perhaps in the case of a natural data generating process); a random variable from a sampling process is seldom inherently interesting. Most likely, we are using sample information about a parameter of the data generating process to provide information about a target population. We are interested in parameters of a population model.

A *population model* is a probability space defined to represent the normalized histogram of variables and their relationships in a given population. In this case, the outcome space (Ω) is defined as the population of interest, the event space is the power set of the outcome space ($\mathcal{A} = \wp(\Omega)$), and the probability ($P$) is defined such that $P(\{w\}) = 1/N$ for all elements w in Ω, in which N denotes the total number of elements in Ω. It is important to note that the probability is not modeling a data generating process: the $1/N$ does not denote an equal probability sampling strategy. Instead, it defines a weight that allows us to represent the associated random variables according to their actual normalized frequencies and relations in the population. The probability space (Ω, $\mathcal{A}$, P) is then a population model, and the parameters of associated distributions for random variables on this probability space are called *population parameters*.

Suppose we were interested in the relationship between body mass index and systolic blood pressure in the United States. We can use a population model (Ω, $\mathcal{A}$, P) in which Ω represents the population of people in the United States, and the other components of the probability space are defined as above. Let measures of body mass index (BMI) and systolic blood pressure (BP) be random variables that are measurable with respect to $\mathcal{A}$. Then the joint distribution of BMI and BP in the population derives from P, which is defined to assure that the joint distribution reflects the normalized histogram of BMI and BP across the population. Consequently, the parameters of this joint distribution are population parameters that represent the actual distribution of BMI and BP as they exist in the population. For example, the regression $E(BP \mid BMI \in b)$ (i.e., the expected value of BP given that BMI has a value in some small interval of values denoted by b) reflects the average BP in the subpopulations having the specified BMI values.

Note that, although the random variables are likely to have standard deviations, there is no meaningful sense of a standard error associated with random variables of a population model because these models are not representing data generating processes. If you could measure the BMI and BP for all persons in the population of interest, then the parameters of their distribution in the population may be directly evaluated—there is no sampling error and consequently no standard errors (which are data generating process concepts). See Chapter 6 for further discussion of standard errors.

Data Models

Probability measures can also be used to model data, but here we must be careful not to confuse a model of data with a model of a data generating process. Whereas a model of a data generating process represents uncertainty regarding the possible outcomes the process could obtain, a model of data does not represent such uncertainty, because the outcome set represents the data in hand rather than a set of possible outcomes.

Suppose we define an outcome set as comprising the data elements in a table of data and the corresponding event set as the power set. Leaving aside the question of what definition of a probability measure would be useful, we immediately run into the question of what useful random variable could be defined. Because the elements on the outcome set are numbers, presumably the random variables would be functions of those numbers. However, by our specification, the outcome set is an undifferentiated set of numbers (no longer labeled by variable names, etc.); consequently, it is unclear what purpose such functions would serve.

It can be better to partition the data by the objects being represented. For example, it is common for rows of a data table to represent measurements

TABLE 5.4

Representation of a Data Set in Terms of Rows and Columns

	Height	Weight	Blood Pressure	Cholesterol
Row 1	66	150	120	190
Row 2	60	155	143	225
⋮	⋮	⋮	⋮	⋮
Row n	72	210	138	250

on specific objects (e.g., people or hospitals): each row is a vector of measures for a different object (e.g., blood pressure or number of beds). In this case, we can model data in an indirect fashion by defining the outcome set as the designated partition. For example, the set of rows in the data set: $\Omega = \{r_1, \ldots, r_n\}$ for n rows (e.g., see data in Table 5.4). Now we can define random variables as functions of the specific elements of the vectors (rows in the table), labeling them according to their meaning (blood pressure, age, etc.). Our probability space is then $(\Omega, \mathcal{A}, P)$, in which the set Ω is the data partition of interest, the sigma-algebra $\mathcal{A}$ is sufficiently rich for our purpose (e.g., the power set), and P reflects a useful probability measure. The random variables will then have corresponding distributions reflecting data that preserve a useful interpretation, being functions of specified measurements (e.g., again, blood pressure and age) across the partition representing the objects that were measured.

What would be a useful definition of P? Perhaps the most useful and common definition is to set $P(\{r\})$ equal to $1/n$ for all n elements r of the outcome set Ω, which, for example, may be the rows of a data table. This specification will allow our random variables to represent the normalized histogram of measures in the data across the partition. In fact, by defining our probability space this way, we are treating the set of objects (i.e., the elements of a partition) on which we have measurements (data) as its own population and are defining a corresponding population model as defined in the preceding section. This data model is the basis for the sample descriptive statistics.

Another useful definition of P is as renormalized sampling probabilities of a data generating process that produced the data. Such a data model allows for random variables that reflect an underlying population from which a nonequal probability data generating process obtained the sample. Herein lies the basis for probability-weighted statistics of a data model.

Connecting Population and Data Generating Process Models

If we do not have access to measures on all members of the population, and therefore cannot directly calculate parameters of a population model, we may resort to defining a data generating process by which we can collect a sample to inform our questions. Suppose we are interested in the parameters of a population model (Ω, $\mathcal{A}$, P) in which $P(\{w\}) = 1/N$ for all w in Ω to facilitate describing the normalized histogram of characteristics in the population. We do not have access to the full population, but we can obtain data from an equal probability sample with replacement. The measure space for each observation of the data generating process is (Ω, $\mathcal{A}$, p) in which $p(\{w\}) = 1/N$ for all w in Ω. Because p, which models a data generating process, assigns the same probabilities to each set in $\mathcal{A}$ as does P, which is instrumentally defined for a population model to be $1/N$ for all unit sets, then the distributions for all random variables of the data generating process model are the same as those for the random variables of the population model. Collecting information about the data generating process model can inform the population model.

If instead p is a model of sampling with other than equal probabilities, then we can create random variables associated with (Ω, $\mathcal{A}$, p) that inform population parameters. For example, suppose we define a measurable function X on (Ω, $\mathcal{A}$), and we are interested in its mean with respect to (Ω, $\mathcal{A}$, P), the population model—that is, we want the mean of X in the population. We have a data generating process that produces X as a random variable on (Ω, $\mathcal{A}$, p) for which p does not assign equal probabilities to each possible person in the population such that the distributions of X related to P and p are not the same. If we define a random variable as follows:

$$Z(w) = X(w) \cdot \frac{P(\{w\})}{p(\{w\})} \tag{5.1}$$

then the expected value of Z with respect to p is equal to

$$E_p(Z) = \sum_{\Omega} \left(\left(X(w) \cdot \frac{P(\{w\})}{p(\{w\})} \right) \cdot p(\{w\}) \right) \tag{5.2}$$

but the probabilities p in Equation 5.2 cancel such that the summation reduces to the simpler summation

$$\sum_{\Omega} \left(\left(X(w) \cdot \frac{P(\{w\})}{p(\{w\})} \right) \cdot p(\{w\}) \right) = \sum_{\Omega} (X(w) \cdot P(\{w\})) \tag{5.3}$$

which is equal to the expected value of X with respect to the probability P:

$$\sum_{\Omega} (X(w) \cdot P(\{w\})) = E_P(X) \tag{5.4}$$

Weighting by a function of sampling probabilities provides a random variable with a mean equal to the population mean (actually, and more generally, P can be any probability and not merely one associated with a population model). Although statistical estimation is not the focus of this book, note that when P represents a population model, or more generally when $P(\{w\})$ is a constant across all $\{w\} \in \mathcal{A}$, P drops out of most estimators, leaving $1/p(\{w\})$ as the relevant factor, called the *sampling weight*.

Connecting Data Generating Process Models and Data Models

A fundamental connection between a model of a data generating process and a model of data is represented in Figure 5.1. The top section of Figure 5.1 indicates that we specified a model of a data generating processes as $(\Omega, \mathcal{A}, p)$, which will be used to specify n different random variables X_1 to X_n (representing the same type of measurement—e.g., blood pressure for each). Because each random variable reflects the same model of a data generating process and the same type of measurement, each of the n random variables has the same distribution F. One realization for each random variable is possible; consequently, we can obtain a single data point for each random variable: datum x_1 for random variable X_1, datum x_2 for random variable X_2, and so on. Put together, this set of data generating processes, random

---

Model of the data generating process

DGP models	Random variables	Data points
$(\Omega, \mathcal{A}, p) \rightarrow$	$X_1 \sim F \rightarrow$	x_1
$(\Omega, \mathcal{A}, p) \rightarrow$	$X_2 \sim F \rightarrow$	x_2
$\vdots$	$\vdots$	$\vdots$
$(\Omega, \mathcal{A}, p) \rightarrow$	$X_n \sim F \rightarrow$	x_n

$$(\Omega^n, \mathcal{A}^n, P) \rightarrow \{X_1, \dots, X_n\} \sim F(X_1, \dots, X_n) \rightarrow \{x_1, \dots, x_n\}$$

Full DGP model	Random vector	Data set

Model of the data

Data model	Random variable

$$(\{x_1, \dots, x_n\}, \mathcal{F}, P^*) \rightarrow X^* \sim F^*_n \equiv \text{Normalized histogram}$$

Connecting DGP and data

$$\lim_{n \to \infty} F^*_n \rightarrow F$$

FIGURE 5.1
Connecting a data generating process model to a data model.

variables, distributions, and data compose the overall measure space (Ω^n, $\mathcal{A}^n$, P) with corresponding random vector $(X_1, X_2, \ldots, X_n)^{\mathrm{T}}$, having a joint distribution $F(X_1, X_2, \ldots, X_n)$, and resulting dataset $\{x_1, x_2, \ldots, x_n\}$.

We can model the resulting data with the probability space $(\{x_1, x_2, \ldots, x_n\}, \mathcal{F}, P^*)$ as in the middle section of Figure 5.1. As a data model, the outcome set represents the data, $\mathcal{F}$ is the power set of the data, and P^* is equal to $1/n$ for all sets containing individual data elements representing the objects that were measured. P^* does not represent a data generating process. It is specified, as with common population models, to allow the distribution of X^* to represent the normalized histogram across the data. In the preceding general discussion of data models, it was better to define the outcome set as a partition of the data. By contrast, in this example, each data point represents the same quality (e.g., blood pressure) and thereby the meaning of each datum is not ambiguous, and the random variable of interest on this space will simply be the identity function $X^*(x_i) = x_i$. Thus, we can just as well use the actual set of data as the outcome space for Figure 5.1 without generating ambiguity. The random variable X^* has a distribution F_n^*, which represents the normalized histogram of the x_i in the data.

At this point the only evident connection between the data generating process model and the data model is merely the fact that the latter uses the data from the former as its outcome set. However, a more important connection exists. If the data are realizations of random variables having the same distribution, then as n gets large and continues to increase (formally, we'd say as n goes to infinity), the histogram of X^* (and therefore its distribution) will get closer to the histogram of each X (and therefore its distribution). This is formally stated as the limit, as n goes to infinity, of F_n^* is equal to F (or more precisely, F_n^* becomes arbitrarily close to F). In practical terms, this fact is the basis for asymptotic properties underlying classic bootstrap estimation in which samples are taken from the data as if the data constituted the distribution from which the original sample was taken.

To restate, one connection between a data generating process model and the model of its corresponding data is that as the sample size increases, the distribution in the data begins to look like the distribution associated with the data generating process. Therefore, resampling (i.e., bootstrapping) from large data sets can mimic the process underlying the original sample and provide a means of estimating the variation in an estimator due to the data generating process. Note that we have introduced the notion of sampling from the data itself, which can be modeled as another sampling process.

An extension of this connection between models of data generating processes and models of data is found in estimation by method of moments. The idea behind the method of moments estimator is to estimate parameters of interest by equating moments of a distribution from a data generating process with moments of the distribution from the data (called the *sample moments*) and to solve these equations for the data generating process parameters of interest. For the simplest of examples, suppose the mean of a random variable X from a data generating process is μ, and the mean of the corresponding X^* from the data is $\overline{X} = \frac{1}{n}\sum_{i=1}^{n} x_i$. The method of moments estimate for μ is determined by setting μ equal to the corresponding sample moment $\overline{X}$,

$$\mu = \frac{1}{n}\sum_{i=1}^{n} x_i \qquad (5.5)$$

and solving for the parameters of interest, which is trivial in this case, because μ is the parameter of interest and Equation 5.5 already presents the solution. In more complex cases, the parameters of interest may be functions of numerous moments, and multiple equations may be needed if there are multiple parameters of interest.

Note that the x_i's are specific elements of the outcome space; they do not comprise n random variables in the data model. There is one random variable X^* (to use the notation of the preceding example) that has a distribution with expected value equal to $\overline{X} = \frac{1}{n}\sum_{i=1}^{n} x_i$. Therefore, this connection alone is not sufficient to determine all information we typically require: it cannot provide information regarding variation due to the data generating process because it does not contain random variables of the data generating process. In order to obtain standard errors, we do not solely need an estimate based on the data model alone; we need an estimator. Moreover, that estimator needs to be a function of random variables associated with the data generating process, not with the data model, which being a type of population model has no sense of standard error applicable to it. Consequently, in the method of moments, we determine the estimator by substituting into the equation the random variables from the data generating process that produced each data point. So, we substitute the random variables X_i from the data generating process into the equation for each datum x_i in the data that it underlies. This yields

$$\hat{\mu} = \frac{1}{n}\sum_{i=1}^{n} X_i \qquad (5.6)$$

Now Equation 5.6 is an estimator that is a function of random variables from the data generating process model, but the form of the function comes from the data model. The estimator, being a function of random variables modeling the data generating process and not data, has a corresponding standard error reflecting variation in possible estimates due to sampling.

A more complicated example of method of moments is found in determining an estimator for a linear regression function. Consider the regression function of $E(Y \mid X) = X' \cdot \beta$ defined for a data generating process model and the corresponding error term $\varepsilon = Y - X' \cdot \beta$, which has expectation equal to 0. For the data model, $\varepsilon^* = y - x' \cdot b$ in which x and y denote a matrix and vector of data values, respectively. We are interested in obtaining an estimator for the parameter β in the data generating process model. We can equate the data generating process moments of the covariance between X and ε, with its counterpart in the data model: $\text{Cov}(X, \varepsilon) = \text{Cov}(X^*, \varepsilon^*)$. Letting $\sigma_{x,\varepsilon}$ denote $\text{Cov}(X, \varepsilon)$ from the data generating process model and noting that the $\text{Cov}(X^*, \varepsilon^*)$ in the data model is $\frac{1}{n}x'(y - x \cdot b)$, we have

$$\frac{1}{n}x'(y - x \cdot b) = \sigma_{x,\varepsilon} \tag{5.7}$$

which, solving for b, gives

$$b = (x'x)^{-1}x'y - n(x'x)^{-1}\sigma_{x,\varepsilon} \tag{5.8}$$

and after plugging in the corresponding random matrix X and vector Y from the data generating process (DGP) that produced the data, we have

$$\hat{\beta} = (X'X)^{-1}X'Y - n(X'X)^{-1}\sigma_{x,\varepsilon} \tag{5.9}$$

Unfortunately, Equation 5.9 is a function of unknown parameters $\sigma_{x,\varepsilon}$. To obtain an actual estimator, we need additional information: for example if it is reasonable to presume that $\sigma_{x,\varepsilon}$ is a vector of 0s (i.e., X and ε are uncorrelated in the data generating process model) and therefore the second term on the right-hand side of the above equation is 0, we get the usual ordinary least squares linear regression estimator for β:

$$\hat{\beta} = (X'X)^{-1}X'Y \tag{5.10}$$

This may seem a bit complicated. A simpler approach is to initially consider the covariance of the random variables X with ε to be 0 in the data generating process model (what is called the *moment condition*), impose the same constraint on the data model, solve for the data model's analogous parameter (in this case b), and then substitute the DGP's random variables that generated the data into the equation to produce the usual ordinary least squares estimator.

Models of Distributions and Densities

In Chapter 4, I mentioned that an advantage of cumulative distribution functions and probability density functions is that, unlike probability measures, they are expressed as functions of the range of random variables rather than functions of sets in sigma-algebras. This advantage is particularly evident when we seek to model these functions. Mathematical models of real-valued variables are extremely common, relatively easy to work with, and likely to be familiar to most researchers.

Suppose we have a probability model of a data generating process $(\Omega, \mathcal{A}, p)$ on which we have defined a random variable X. The probability measure p implies X has some distribution F, but we may not know F (otherwise, we would not need to collect data). Moreover, although, as discussed in the preceding section, F^* from our data model will converge to F as n goes to infinity, it is not likely to be a simple function of the data's random variable X^*, and most certainly not in most realistic finite samples. Suppose we draw one million samples from a uniform distribution on the unit interval. Notwithstanding the distribution of the data generating process, the distribution of the data itself, F^*, is not likely to have a uniform distribution. Figure 5.2 shows a histogram of a variable (labeled u) from such a sample. Note that the bars of the histogram vary around 1, sometimes a little high, sometimes a little low—not by much, but they vary nonetheless. The distribution F^* of the data model is not uniform. If it were, it would be a constant, not plus or minus a little. Indeed, trying to capture F^* from Figure 5.2 may require a fairly complicated equation of u. Looking at the uneven sawtooth pattern, it would likely require an extremely high-order polynomial to capture this interval exactly—if it were possible at all (note that our density must work

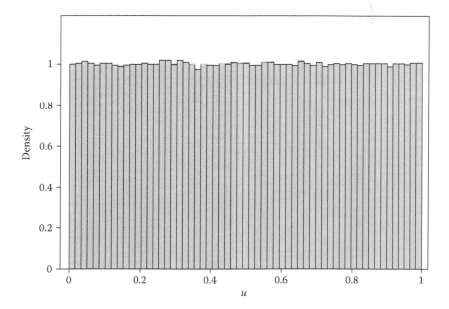

FIGURE 5.2
Histogram of one million draws from a uniform distribution on the unit interval.

point by point and not just for the arbitrary bins graphically presented in the figure). However, we may consider the variability around 1 to be sufficiently small to ignore and instead choose to model F^* as $M^*(u) = u$ (i.e., to model F^* as a uniform distribution on the unit interval). In this case, as we expect of models, our model is wrong in some respects but presumably accurate enough in some other respect that serves our purpose.

What is our purpose? Well, of course, that depends on what we are doing, but such models are commonly used to inform our understanding of F—the distribution of the random variable from the data generating process. Does this mean we presume F has a simple functional form and that since F^* converges to F, so will an appropriately specified model M^* of F^*? Although this is perhaps a common approach, it is not necessary; indeed, it would be safer to not make such a presumption.

Because a model in this case will not perfectly capture that which is being modeled, there must be criteria by which we select our model and determine whether it is sufficiently faithful in representing the features of interest. Applying a criterion to modeling F and optimizing across possible models with respect to that criterion would identify some model M reflecting features of F that we presumably seek. (I am glossing over the mathematical requirements, the technical details of which are beyond the scope of this book.) Unfortunately, as with F, we do not have M. However, if M^* is determined by the same criterion that we would apply to M, if only we could, then, as presented in Figure 5.3, we might reasonably expect M^* to converge to M as n goes to infinity. Suppose that a data generating process is represented by the probability space $(\Omega, \mathcal{A}, p)$, which implies a distribution F for our random variables of interest; using criterion c we would model F, or some relevant feature, as M_c. If we engage the data generating process n times, we obtain a data set D modeled with the probability space $(D, \mathcal{F}, P^*)$, which implies distribution F^* for its corresponding random variables. Applying criterion c, we can model F^* as M_c^*. As n goes to infinity, if F^*

$$
\begin{array}{cc}
\text{DGP} & \text{Data} \\
\text{model} & \text{model} \\
\end{array}
$$

$$(\Omega, \mathcal{A}, p) \Rightarrow (D, \mathcal{F}, P^*)$$

$$F \xleftarrow{\ n \to \infty\ } F_n^*$$

$$M_c \xleftarrow{\ n \to \infty\ } M_c^*$$

FIGURE 5.3

Depiction of the connection between a data generating process (DGP) and a data model. Data realizations from the data generating process are modeled by P^*. The distribution of random variables, F^*, defined on the data model converges to the distribution of the random variables that generated the data, F, as the sample size increases. Consequently, a model based on criterion c, M_c^*, of F^* converges to a similarly specified model M_c of F as the sample size increases.

converges to F, then M_c^* converges to M_c. Consequently, our modeling process applied to data will converge to the model we would achieve if applied to F and our model of data features inform features of the data generating process.

Unfortunately, in applied research we work with finite samples, and M_c^* is data specific. The closer we model F_n^*, the more likely it will *not* represent M_c but take on the detailed characteristics of F^* from the data instead of F from the data generating process—this is called *over-fitting* of data. One approach to this problem is to use a fit criterion such as the Akaike Information Criterion (AIC) or the Bayesian Information Criterion (BIC) (among many others). This approach, which I will not discuss further, is to apply a criterion that penalizes the complexity of the model to avoid selecting one that matches F_n^* too closely.

Another approach is to statistically test whether the data are inconsistent with a hypothesized F. However, to do so in practice is to actually test a model M of F (or parameter thereof), which leads to a conundrum. Because we assume, *a priori*, that M is in fact not F but is only an approximating model, the test that F is M is unnecessary: we already presume M is not F and given enough information we could confirm this. How then can we proceed to use data as evidence to investigate our questions about F? Some suggest nonparametric statistics, which avoid much of the modeling burden, but such a strategy can come at a great cost in terms of untestable assumptions, the need for larger data sets, and sometimes greater computational complexity. Although in some situations using a fit criterion or nonparametric statistics may be reasonable, I suggest we need not abandon all hope in testing parametric models, but we need to have a better understanding of what is achieved by doing so.

Rather than seek to identify F as it is in its intimate detail, we can seek to identify the models of F that are consistent with results from the data generating process (Ω^n, $\mathcal{A}^n$, p) and rule out models that are inconsistent with data. This strategy does not consider a model as a hypothesized F (we assume a model is not in fact F) but instead considers a model as a counterfactual approximation to F. Note here that we are considering the full data generating process and are thereby concerned with n as well as F. Essentially we are concerned with identifying the models of F that a given sample size cannot rule out, called *statistically adequate models*. We presume, of course, that a larger sample will garner greater refinement in discerning models, but for any given sample size the data may well be consistent or inconsistent with various models. Moreover, for smaller sample sizes the data will be consistent with more models (i.e., fewer models can be ruled out by statistical testing).

Figure 5.4 presents data from a data generating process with a sample size of 100. Table 5.5 presents tests for three nested regression models: a linear function of X (Block 1), a quadratic polynomial (Block 2), and a cubic polynomial (Block 3). Because these tests of a polynomial require comparison to the next highest polynomial, a fourth-order polynomial (Block 4) is

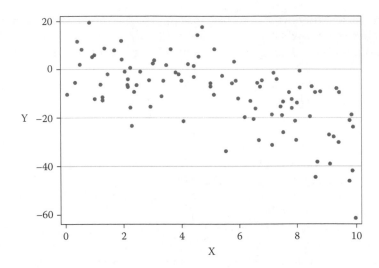

FIGURE 5.4
Scatter plot of Y versus X of 100 samples.

TABLE 5.5

Test Results for Nested Regression Models

Block	F	Block df	Residual df	Pr > F	R^2	Change in R^2
1	62.97	1	98	0.000	0.39	
2	10.75	1	97	0.002	0.45	0.06
3	0.71	1	96	0.401	0.46	0.01
4	0.03	1	95	0.875	0.46	0.00

included to facilitate testing the cubic model; also note that Block 1, being the linear model, is used to test whether the regression is merely a constant. The data provide evidence to rule out a constant mean and a model of the regression function for Y as a linear function of X, but not sufficient evidence to rule out a quadratic polynomial of X, or a cubic polynomial of X (note that I do not take insignificant findings as evidence for hypotheses being tested). In this case, we may infer that F is sufficiently different from a constant mean (the test reported for Block 1) and a linear model (the test reported for Block 2), such that a data generating process with sample size of n can discern it, but F is not sufficiently different from the higher-order polynomial models that the data generating process can discern this.

If the p-value of a specification test for M is small, then either the data are a rare case from an F that is approximately M, or the data are a common case from an F that is not approximately M. Because, by definition, it is likely that the data are a more common case than a rare case, it is reasonable to presume that F is sufficiently dissimilar to M and therefore rule out M as a statistically adequate model.

It may be that the data are consistent with a nonsingleton set of models: in the preceding example they are consistent with the higher-order polynomials. Adjudicating among such a set is typically accomplished by using criteria accounting for fit with the data and/or functional simplicity. However, because no model in this set was empirically ruled out and is thereby consistent with the data, we should be careful picking just one by nonstatistical criteria without investigating whether the substantive inferences based on these models differ from that of the model we otherwise prefer.

This logic of inference extends to testing functions of parameters associated with a statistically adequate model. Suppose we identify M as a statistically adequate model and seek to use it for testing a hypothesis regarding F. If the p-value is small, based on M, then F must be sufficiently different than the hypothesized characteristic to warrant ruling out that hypothesis. For example, suppose we have the following hypothesis regarding F:

$$\frac{\partial E_F(Y|X)}{\partial X} > 0 \tag{5.11}$$

If M is a statistically adequate model and a test of whether

$$\frac{\partial E_M(Y|X)}{\partial X} > 0 \tag{5.12}$$

garners a small p-value, then we have evidence that, although M is a statistically adequate model of F, the characteristic $\partial E_F(Y|X)/\partial X$ is sufficiently different from the hypothesis that the data from a data generating process with sample size n can discern this fact. We can then rule out the hypothesis as characterizing F even though it was based on a test of M. If the p-value is large, then the characteristic is not sufficiently different from the hypothesis that it can be discerned by the data generating process, and therefore it cannot be ruled out. The statistical test is based on the counterfactual M rather than F: we ask how likely it is that we would get data at least as extreme as what we observed if F was M, even though we presume it is not. However, we use this information to draw inferences regarding F.

It is important to note that according to this logic, data provide stronger evidence by virtue of ruling out models or characteristics of a distribution. Data provide disconfirming evidence for a model or characteristic by ruling it out, and data provide confirming evidence for a model or characteristic by not ruling it out while ruling out the alternatives. Data do not provide evidence to adjudicate among models that are all consistent with the data. Consequently, disconfirming evidence is typically stronger than confirming evidence. If many models or characteristics are ruled out, then each model, individually, is taken to be unlikely. However, if many models or characteristics are not ruled out (i.e., they are statistically adequate), then each model is only one of many candidates. Fit criteria may be used to distinguish these models, but their epistemic value does not accrue from an understanding of the underlying data generating process.

Arbitrary Models

The preceding models provide (simplified) examples of probability models in common usage. However, because mathematical probability is a calculus awaiting interpretation, we can apply it in other ways that may be useful. Suppose I wish to investigate characteristics of the United States House of Representatives. I might proceed with a population model defined with an outcome set Ω comprising the members of the House, the power set of Ω as the event set $\mathcal{A}$, and a probability P that assigns $1/N$ to each unit set (each individual member) in which N denotes the number of members of the House. In this case, $(\Omega, \mathcal{A}, P)$ would be a probability space that would allow me to characterize the normalized histogram of random variables measured on members of the House—that is, the population model of the House of Representatives.

If we define two random variables on the corresponding measurable space as X denoting a measurement of each member's support for universal health care and Y denoting the measurement of each member's years in Congress divided by the total person-years across all members of Congress (perhaps taken to be a measure of relative influence in the House). Then the expectations $E_P(X)$, $E_P(Y)$, and $E_P(X \cdot Y)$ represent the average support for universal health care across the House, the average influence across the House, and the average effective support for universal health care in the House.

Suppose, however, that I am instead interested in investigating total support for universal health care. I may then use Y (defined as a measure on $\mathcal{A}$) as my probability rather than $1/N$ and define my probability space as $(\Omega, \mathcal{A}, Y)$. Now $E_Y(X)$ becomes the total influence-weighted support for universal health care. Consider the difference:

$$E_P(X \cdot Y) = \frac{1}{N} \sum_{\Omega} X_w \cdot Y_w \tag{5.13}$$

whereas

$$E_y(X) = \sum_{\Omega} X_w \cdot Y_w \tag{5.14}$$

The expectation associated with the population model in Equation 5.13 provides the average effective support for universal health care among the members of the House, whereas the expectation in Equation 5.14 associated with $(\Omega, \mathcal{A}, Y)$ provides the effective support for universal health care.

Of course, in this case we can use $(\Omega, \mathcal{A}, P)$ to get the same result by taking the expectation of a variable $W = N \cdot X \cdot Y$, but it is less intuitive and ad hoc.

By using $(\Omega, \mathcal{A}, Y)$, it is easy to evaluate effective support directly. Suppose X has a range of $[-1, 1]$, in which -1 corresponds to full support for efforts against universal health care, 1 corresponds to full support for efforts toward universal health care, and 0 corresponds to no support either way. The effective support for efforts in favor of universal health care is the probability (again, defined in terms of Y) of X greater than 0, whereas the effective support for efforts against universal health care is the probability of X less than 0.

Suppose we define another random variable Z as a measurement of support for efforts to decrease federal power. Analysis based on our population model $(\Omega, \mathcal{A}, P)$ may result in a decreasing regression function of $E_P(X \mid Z)$, as shown in Figure 5.5a, indicating that the average support for universal health care decreases with support for decreasing federal power. However, an analysis based on $(\Omega, \mathcal{A}, Y)$ could result in an increasing regression function of $E_Y(X \mid Z)$ as shown in Figure 5.5b, in which the size of the dots reflects the relative influence of the House member. By this analysis, the effective support for universal health care is positively related to support for decreased federal power. This difference is driven by the correlation between X and Z among those who have more years of experience in the House.

Another example is the use of probability spaces to help conceptualize the explanatory power of a theory. Suppose we wish to explicitly define

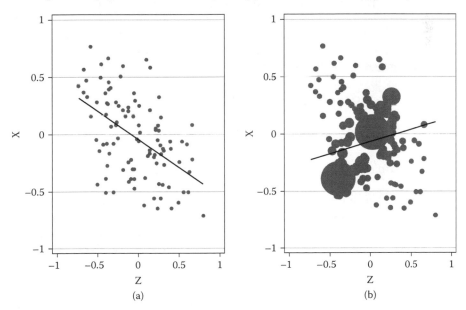

FIGURE 5.5
(a) The relationship between X and Z based on $(\Omega, \mathcal{A}, P)$; (b) the relationship between X and Z based on $(\Omega, \mathcal{A}, Y)$. The solid lines in each panel represent the regression lines.

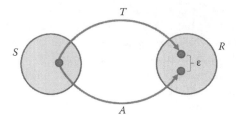

FIGURE 5.6
Two maps, T and A, from S to R in which ε represents a difference, assuming R is a metric space.

explanatory power. We could do so in different ways but each drawing on the same initial representation. Define S to be the set of real-world situations that fall within the scope of a given theory. Also define R to be another set of situations that will represent possible results that follow from each situation in S. We may then consider a map $T: S \to R$ representing the resulting situation predicted by the theory for each situation in S. We may also define a map $A: S \to R$ representing the actual resulting situation that follows from each situation in S (see Figure 5.6).

To clarify our understanding, we can define a probability space $(S, \mathcal{A}, P)$ for which $\mathcal{A}$ is the power set of S and $P(\{s\}) = 1/|S|$. We can define a second measurable space $(R, \mathcal{F})$ and two random variables T and A measurable $\mathcal{A}$. Consequently, the vector (T, A) is a random vector from $(S, \mathcal{A}, P)$ to $(R^2, \mathcal{F}^2, p)$ in which p is the corresponding probability defined in terms of P. Based on this representation, we can provide definitions for explanatory power in terms of agreement (the extent to which T and A agree on the results for situations in S) or disagreement (the extent to which T and A disagree regarding the results for situations in S).

Regarding agreement, we might define

$$\text{Power}_1 = \sum_{r \in R} p(T = r, A = r) = \sum_{r \in R} P(T^{-1}(r) \cap A^{-1}(r)) \qquad (5.15)$$

Power_1 sums the intersections of sets $T^{-1}(r)$ and $A^{-1}(r)$ in S across all r in R. Figure 5.7 shows these sets for an arbitrary r. The definition of power in Equation 5.15 provides the proportion of situations in S for which the theory agrees with actual results.

Alternatively, we can create a definition based on disagreement by defining another random variable $D = (T(s) - A(s))^2$ measurable $\mathcal{F}^2$ on $(R^2, \mathcal{F}^2, p)$ to $(\mathbb{R}, \mathcal{B}, p_D)$ in which $\mathbb{R}$ is the real line, $\mathcal{B}$ is the Borel sigma-algebra, and p_D is derived from the preceding probability spaces. We can then define

$$\text{Power}_2 = E_{p_D}(D) \qquad (5.16)$$

Power_2 represents the expected squared difference in results between what the theory predicts and what would actually happen.

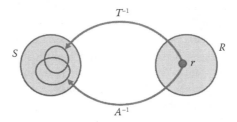

FIGURE 5.7
The overlapping subsets in S corresponding to the pre-images of T and A corresponding to a single point r in their range.

We can see that Power$_1$ is simpler to understand than Power$_2$ because it directly represents agreement, which matches the colloquial sense of explanatory power (an increase in Power$_1$ corresponds to what we would consider an increase in explanatory power). On the other hand, Power$_2$ is interpreted in the opposite direction (an increase in Power$_2$ is interpreted as a decrease in explanatory power). This analysis provides another reason, however, for favoring Power$_1$ over Power$_2$, one that does not turn on semantics (we could have sought a concept for explanatory deficit): Power$_2$ requires a more complicated random variable D that allows for differences to be calculated (which can be thought of as requiring a distance metric defined on R rather than merely allowing it to be a set). Power$_1$ does not require us to define such a distance metric.

We could have defined the indicator of whether T and A map to the same result as $D = \mathbf{1}(T(s) = A(s))$. The measurable space that D maps into could then be simplified to $(\{0, 1\}, \mathcal{P}, p_D)$, where $\mathcal{P}$ is the power set of $\{0, 1\}$: that is, $\{\{0, 1\}, \{0\}, \{1\}, \varnothing\}$. This definition of D avoids the requirement of a distance metric and makes the interpretation of Power$_2$ the same as that of Power$_1$: the proportion of situations in S for which T and A agree.

The main point here is not that such models are in common use but rather to emphasize that, from the mathematical perspective, probability spaces are uninterpreted objects that carry with them the full scope of probability results. The utility and meaning of those results depends solely on the interpretation of the probability space that the analyst provides—in other words, meaning depends on what the probability space is being used to model and is not inherent in the mathematical definition of probability itself.

Additional Readings

This chapter provided examples of how probability spaces can be used to model some specific research problems based on my perspective that probability is a mathematical structure that the researcher can use under any useful interpretation. I answered the question of what probability is by reference to its mathematical definition. What it can be used for is only limited by the imagination of the user, who need only provide a coherent interpretation and legitimate rationale for its application. There is, however, considerable literature on differing views regarding the proper answer to the question regarding what probability is. These views take a substantive meaning as definitional of the term and consider mathematics as constraining how it is applied. Consequently, if there is to be only one substantive meaning of probability, it should not be a surprise that there is considerable argument over what that definition ought to be.

Gillies' book *Philosophical Theories of Probability* (Routledge, 2000) and Mellor's *Probability: A Philosophical Introduction* (Routledge, 2005) both provide fairly easy-to-read overviews to the primary competing theories. The books *Probability is the Very Guide of Life: The Philosophical Uses of Chance*, edited by Kyburg and Thalos (Open Court, 2003), and *Philosophy of Probability: Contemporary Readings*, edited by Eagle (Routledge, 2011), provide compilations of papers discussing some key contested issues.

There are also books that consider the various definitions of probability in the context of science, such as Suppes' book, titled *Representation and Invariance of Scientific Structure* (CSLI Publications, 2002). Moreover, there are books that consider, and advocate, various definitions of probability for the purpose of accruing and using scientific evidence. Earman's book, titled *Bayes or Bust? A Critical Examination of Bayesian Confirmation Theory* (MIT Press, 1992), gives an analysis of Bayesian theory as an epistemological tool for accruing evidence. Mayo's book, titled *Error and the Growth of Experimental Knowledge* (University of Chicago Press, 1996), provides a defense of the frequentist definition of probability. Similarly, *Error and Inference: Recent Exchanges on Experimental Reasoning, Reliability, and the Objectivity and Rationality of Science* (Cambridge University Press, 2010), edited by Mayo and Spanos, provides an updated defense of the frequentist definition of probability and the consequent statistical tools used in science. This book is in the form of position chapters by Mayo and Spanos, challenges from various contributing authors, and responses by Mayo and Spanos. The book *The Nature of Scientific Evidence: Statistical, Philosophical, and Empirical Considerations* (University of Chicago Press, 2004), edited by Taper and Lele, provides a compilation of chapters that argue for specific approaches to scientific evidence—many explicitly adopting a specific definition of probability, while others are less explicit in doing so.

For an excellent book on method of moments and its generalization, see Hall's *Generalized Method of Moments* (Oxford, 2005).

6

Common Problems

In this chapter, I will address some vexing problems that motivated writing this book. The structure of this chapter is different from the preceding ones in that much of the presentation is framed by presenting problem statements and providing corresponding solutions in which I clarify the issues and the approach to resolving them.

This chapter addresses some of the most challenging conceptual errors that applied researchers face. You will likely see many of them as extensions of the topics discussed in the preceding chapter. However, here they will be elaborated upon within the context of a research problem.

Interpreting Standard Errors

By now it should be clear that in statistics, all probability-related characteristics of random variables stem from the underlying probability space; consequently, the interpretation of such characteristics comes from the interpretation of the underlying probability space. If you are using a probability space to model uncertainty of an objective process by which the data are generated, then the standard deviation of your random variables represents variations associated with the possible realizations of the random variable from that process. In other words, from a strictly frequentist theory of probability you would interpret your random variables in terms of the values you could get if the process were repeated an infinite number of times; from a propensity theory of probability, you would interpret your random variables in terms of the inherent potential of a given process to produce particular values. If you used a probability space to model your subjective uncertainty about some outcome, answer, or quantity, then you would interpret your random variables in terms of your beliefs about the potential value of the quantities being considered.

A statistic, being a function of random variables, is itself a random variable; therefore, it has a distribution associated with its underlying probability space. The standard error of a statistic is typically defined as its standard deviation (assuming it has one), our estimator of which is often used in conjunction with the original statistic to define another statistic with a known distribution, or known limiting distribution of a function of the statistic.

This definition is suitable for most purposes, but we run into some difficulty in more complicated situations, particularly when the underlying probability measure can be factored into a part that represents a data generating process and a part that does not. This will become clear as we discuss the problems presented below.

To frame this distinction, consider that the phrase "standard error" is meaningful solely in terms of capturing a consequence of a data generating process. I interpret the standard error as reflecting the variation in a statistic due to the possibility of obtaining different data sets from a data generating process. For example, suppose I sample patients associated with each of the primary care physicians of a given healthcare organization. Physicians are not sampled because all physicians are determined to be used; only patients are sampled. My probability space can be defined as $(\Omega \times S, \mathcal{A}_\Omega \otimes \mathcal{A}_S, P)$ in which Ω denotes the population of patients and S denotes the set of physicians in the organization. The probability measure for an arbitrary patient–physician pair (w, s) can be factored as $P(\{(w, s)\}) = P(\{w\} \times S \mid \Omega \times \{s\}) \cdot P(\Omega \times \{s\})$ in which the conditional probability reflects the probability of the data generating process obtaining individual w from a physician s, and the marginal probability is the probability associated with the population model of physicians. In other words, setting $P(\Omega \times \{s\}) = 1/N_S$ reflects the set of N_S physicians and allows for representing their normalized histogram of characteristics. It does not model a data generating process and is not, therefore, a sampling probability. Consequently, sample variation of any random variable is due solely to the part of the probability measure, that is, modeling the data generating process (i.e., due to $P(\{w\} \times S \mid \Omega \times \{s\})$), and not due to the part modeling the physician population (i.e., not due to $P(\Omega \times \{s\})$).

The preceding example shows that the standard deviation of an estimator may not be its standard error defined to reflect variation due to a data generating process. The standard deviation will reflect the variance derived from the overall probability measure, P, whereas the standard error should only reflect the source of variance due to the possible outcomes of generating the data, $P(\{w\} \times S \mid \Omega \times \{s\})$ in this example. The standard error should be interpreted as reflecting how much we roughly expect an estimate to deviate from the estimator's mean value *due to the variation in possible samples we could obtain from a given data generating process*. If a standard error of an unbiased estimator for mean blood pressure is 5, then we roughly expect the estimate to be wrong by approximately 5 units due to sampling. I use the phrase "roughly expect" because the standard error is based on the square root of an expected value and not the expected absolute deviation directly.

To drive this point home, the standard deviation is a mathematical property of a probability distribution, and it retains its meaning regardless of whether the probability space is modeling something of substantive interest to a researcher or modeling nothing substantive as might interest a pure mathematician. The standard error, on the other hand, is strictly a contextually interpreted concept; it has no meaning in the absence of its representation of variation due to a data generating process. The standard deviation and the standard error are the same only in the case that the underlying probability measure is solely representing variation in the data generating process, which is the most common case in applied research. Consequently, one cannot properly identify a standard error without first knowing what the probability measure of a probability space is modeling.

In summary, if you have not thought about what you are modeling with the probability space that underlies your random variables, then they are not interpreted, and it is hard to tell what makes your variables random and what the appropriate standard errors are. You may then make the mistake that some do when faced with the mistaken argument in the following problem.

Problem 6.1

Critique the following passage from Goodman SN (1999) "Toward Evidence-Based Medical Statistics. 1: The P Value Fallacy" *Ann Intern Med.* 130:995–1004.

"A classic statistical puzzle … involves two treatments, A and B, whose effects are contrasted in each of six patients. Treatment A is better in the first five patients and treatment B is superior in the sixth patient. Adopting Royall's formulation (6), let us imagine that this experiment was conducted by two investigators, each of whom, unbeknownst to the other, had a different plan for the experiment. An investigator who originally planned to study six patients would calculate a p-value of 0.11, whereas one who planned to stop as soon as treatment B was preferred (up to a maximum of six patients) would calculate a p-value of 0.03 (Appendix). We have the same patients, the same treatments, and the same outcomes but two very different p-values (which might produce different conclusions), which differ only because the experimenters have different mental pictures of what the results could be if the experiment were repeated. A confidence interval would show this same behavior."

Solution: Goodman makes the fallacy of misclassification in his presumed argument. His argument is based on a model of subjective uncertainty, whereas the two investigators presumably based their decisions on models of data generating processes. The standard errors associated with the first investigator's estimator reflect the variation in the effect measure due to the potential for a given process that samples six subjects. The standard errors associated with the second investigator's estimator reflect the variation in the effect measure due to the potential for a given process that samples subjects until treatment B is preferred. These are indeed distinct processes that in fact have different standard errors. Goodman considers the difference to be in the mental pictures of the investigators, from which I infer Goodman is thinking of a subjective measure. While Goodman contends the results "differ only because the experimenters have different mental pictures of what the results could be if the experiment were repeated," I imagine the investigators would contend that the results differ because they were using different procedures, and each procedure in fact has a different distribution of possible outcomes. If you doubt this, set up a Monte Carlo experiment in which you could simulate each of these two processes. You will find the standard errors are in fact different—regardless of your mental picture. Goodman's concern over having "the same patients, the same treatments, and the same outcomes but two very different p-values" exhibits confusion between data, which are not random variables in the context of the investigation, and the actual random variables that reflect the data generating process. Moreover, there is a lack of understanding that data cannot change the characteristics of random variables representing a data generating process.

Notational Conventions

Before addressing key issues that measure theory can help us sort out, we need notational conventions. For the purpose of the remainder of this book, it will help to simplify our notation for probability measures defined on measurable spaces having product sets for their outcomes and to have a notational language that clearly and coherently uses indexing of variables and values.

In Chapter 4, conditional probabilities on a probability space such as $(\Omega \times S, \mathcal{A}, P)$ are denoted as $P(\{w\} \times S \mid \Omega \times \{s\})$ to indicate the probability of obtaining an outcome containing w given the outcome contains s, and the marginal probability of an outcome containing w can be denoted as $P(\{w\} \times S)$. For greater concision, however, in the rest of this chapter these will be denoted as $P(\{w\} \mid \{s\})$ and $P(\{w\})$, respectively. Although technically incorrect, this notation will make it easier to more concisely represent the problems addressed.

A variable is a function that is denoted by capital letters. Sets are also denoted by capital letters. The context of their use will distinguish them. For example, a function X from some domain D to some range R is a variable representing the mapping $X: D \rightarrow R$. A vector or matrix of variables will be denoted as a bold capital letter, such as $\mathbf{X}$.

The value of a variable applied to an arbitrary element of its domain is denoted by a lowercase letter with a subscript indicating the arbitrary element. For variable X with domain D, the value of X applied to element $d \in D$ is $x_d = X(d)$. In this case, x_d is the specific value in the range of the variable X evaluated at the element d in D. The equal sign appropriately denotes the mathematical equivalence of the left- and right-hand sides of the preceding equations. Nonetheless, the left- and right-hand sides are conceptually different, just as $X(d) \equiv d^2$ leads to $4 = X(2)$ in which the left-hand side is a number and the right-hand side is a function evaluated at a number. The meaning of the squared function evaluated at 2 is not the same as the meaning of the number 4.

We often choose different letters or words to denote different variables; for example, three variables may be denoted by X, Y, and Z. Alternatively, particularly when we wish to denote many variables, we can differentiate variables by an index rather than letters. Instead of a set of three variables being denoted as $\{X, Y, Z\}$, we may denote them as $\{X_1, X_2, X_3\}$. More generally, we may specify an index set and specify individual variables by virtue of the indices rather than different uppercase letters. For example, suppose we determine an index set of $\mathbb{I} = \{1, 2, 3, 4, 5, 6, 7, 8, 9, 10\}$, the set of variables $\{X_i : i \in \mathbb{I}\}$ contains 10 separate variables. An index set need not be numerical, and if it is numerical it need not be either discrete or finite. However, for our purpose, they will usually be numerical and both discrete and finite.

To be useful in applied research, the index set is often defined as the range of a one-to-one function that maps from a conceptually understood domain. The inverse of the function thereby provides an interpretation of the index set. For example, suppose I wish to index variables associated with each member of a set Ω that comprises individuals of a particular population. Then, a one-to-one index function $\mathcal{J}^{-1}: \Omega \to \mathbb{I}$ defines $\mathbb{I}$ as an index set for Ω, and $\mathcal{J}: \mathbb{I} \to \Omega$ provides an interpretation for each element $i \in \mathbb{I}$ in terms of the meaning ascribed to Ω. As another example, suppose I define O as the set of data generating processes and $\mathbb{I}_N$ the set of numbers from 1 to N, where N is the number of elements in O. The function $\mathcal{J}^{-1}: \Omega \to \mathbb{I}_N$ defines $\mathbb{I}_N$ as the index set for N data generating processes, that is, the set of occurrences of the data generating process that will ultimately produce a data set of N results. $\mathcal{J}: \mathbb{I}_N \to \Omega$ provides an interpretation for each element $i \in \mathbb{I}_N$ as the observation number associated with a particular data generating process.

Note that for clarity I write the interpretation function as $\mathcal{J}$ and the indexing function as its inverse $\mathcal{J}^{-1}$ rather than the reverse as might be expected given their introduction above. This is because it will be easier to speak of the interpretation function and therefore I use the simpler notation to denote it. Being a one-to-one function, this is arbitrary. Suppose Ω is a set denoting three people {Fred, Ethel, Hildegard} and a corresponding index set is $\mathbb{I} = \{1, 2, 3\}$. An interpretation of $\mathbb{I}$ could be $\mathcal{J}(1) = $ Fred, $\mathcal{J}(2) = $ Ethel, and $\mathcal{J}(3) = $ Hildegard. In this case, a variable X_2 would be interpreted as the variable X associated with Ethel.

Note that $\mathcal{J}: \Omega \to \Omega$ is possible and can be useful when arbitrary, rather than explicit, indices are being discussed. However, it can be useful to index a nonnumerical set by a numerical one; for example, if Ω is nonnumerical (e.g., a set of people who compose a population of interest), then it can be useful to index it with a numerical set $\mathbb{I}$ (e.g., $\mathcal{J}^{-1}: \Omega \to \mathbb{I}$) thereby having an interpretation $\mathcal{J}: \mathbb{I} \to \Omega$, as in the example presented in the preceding paragraph.

The advantage for the applied researcher of using the same uppercase letter (or letters, or word, or even words) in denoting different variables via an index i is not merely efficiency in denoting many variables, but also in allowing the researcher to use the uppercase component to denote a specific concept and leaving it to the indices to denote the different variables. For example, suppose I wanted to define variables that captured blood pressure and stress level for 10 different people. I may use the letter B to denote the concept of blood pressure and S to denote the concept of stress. Defining a set $\mathbb{I}$ that indexes the 10 people, I can denote variables for blood pressure and stress associated with each person as B_i and S_i for $i \in \mathbb{I}$. Therefore, the symbols for each variable have conceptual information that can carry throughout an analysis. In this example, wherever we see a "B" we know it is referring to a random variable representing blood pressure, and wherever we see an "S," we know it is referring to a random variable representing stress.

Variables can also be distinguished with multiple indices, as long as the combination of indices provides a unique (one-to-one) identification: $\mathcal{J}^{-1}$: $\Omega \rightarrow \mathbb{I} \times \mathbb{T}$ with corresponding interpretation $\mathcal{J}$: $\mathbb{I} \times \mathbb{T} \rightarrow \Omega$. For example, we can use two sets $\mathbb{I} = \{1, 2, \ldots, N\}$ and $\mathbb{T} = \{1, 2, \ldots, T\}$ to identify a set of variables $\{X_{it} : i \in \mathbb{I}, t \in \mathbb{T}\}$. Suppose I wish to define variables that represent the temperature at each point of the earth's surface. I can define a set $\mathbb{O}$ that indexes longitude and a set $\mathbb{A}$ that indexes latitude. Note that in this case both index sets are continuous. With these indices, I can then define a set of variables $\{T_{oa} : o \in \mathbb{O}, a \in \mathbb{A}\}$ that represent these temperature variables. As another example, the indexing may be hierarchically structured as shown in Table 6.1. Rather than a single index i with index set $\mathbb{I}$, two indices j and k, with index sets $\mathbb{J}$ and $\mathbb{K}$, are used such that k is nested within j. Note in the table that each element of Ω is uniquely indexed by the (j, k) pair.

If, unlike in Table 6.1, the number of k elements associated with each i index varies, then we would require a set of index sets, one for each i: $\{\mathbb{K}_i : i \in \mathbb{I}\}$.

By this indexing scheme, if we were to denote a specific variable such as for $i = 2$ and $j = 3$, we would have T_{23}, which could mistakenly be interpreted as an index value 23 for a single indexed variable T_i. We require additional notation to avoid this ambiguity, such as putting a comma between the numbers; however, in this text, in which we will work only with arbitrary indices

TABLE 6.1

Single and Paired Index Sets

Ω	$\mathbb{I}$	$\mathbb{J}, \mathbb{K}$	
	i	j	k
w	1	1	1
w'	2	1	2
w''	3	1	3
w'''	4	2	1
w''''	5	2	2
w'''''	6	2	3

denoted by single letters, we can dispense with additional notation for this purpose.

For random variables defined on probability spaces, we will add one more notational nuance. Remember that when a data generating process underlies our collection of N samples, we represent it by a probability space such as $(\Omega^N, \mathcal{A}^N, P)$ that comprises the N probability spaces $(\Omega, \mathcal{A}, P_i)$ for each $i \in \mathbb{I}$ in which the interpretation of $\mathbb{I}$ is the set of processes that will each produce an outcome from Ω. Each of these component probability spaces will have random variables defined on them that we may wish to distinguish via indexing by i. But suppose that we wish to use indexing to further distinguish the variables within the observation. For example, we may be measuring blood pressure at three different fixed times on any person w that the data generating process obtains. We could denote them as $Y1_i$, $Y2_i$, and $Y3_i$ or we could use an index set $\mathbb{T} = \{1, 2, 3\}$ interpreted as the set of times and denote them as Y_{it} for $t \in \mathbb{T}$. However, it will become useful to distinguish the observation indexing (using i in this example) from the within-observation indexing (using t in this example). We do this by separating them with a comma: for example, $Y_{i,t}$. In a more general sense, suppose we use two indices (e.g., i and k) to identify observations (i.e., individual runs of a data generating process) and one index to identify repeated measures (e.g., t), our random variables would be written as $Y_{ik,t}$. The indexing to the left of the comma will typically reflect the structure of the data generating process, whereas the indexing to the right of the comma will distinguish variables within observation.

This nuanced notation provides a different meaning for Y_{it} and $Y_{i,t}$. The first can represent an observation defined by a random selection of a person and then a random selection of a time at which to measure Y for that person. Note that t is not specifying the time in this case but an index of the occurrence, or operation, of selecting a time. The second can represent a random selection of a person and the measure of Y at a predetermined time.

So far, we have identified two types of indices, one that applies to variables, which denotes distinct variables, and one that applies to values, which denotes arbitrary elements of a variable's domain. We can add nuance if needed. Consider two variables X_1 and X_2 with the same domain:

$$X_1: D \rightarrow R \tag{6.1}$$

$$X_2: D \rightarrow R \tag{6.2}$$

Using the preceding, indexing for arbitrary values of the variables in Equations 6.1 and 6.2 leads to the notation

$$x_d = X_1(d) \tag{6.3}$$

$$x_d = X_2(d) \tag{6.4}$$

which is ambiguous in the denoted values. Consequently, when using indexed variables, their corresponding values can be uniquely specified by the following notation:

$$x_{1:d} = X_1(d) \tag{6.5}$$

$$x_{2:d} = X_2(d) \tag{6.6}$$

or, for all i's in index set $\mathbb{I}$:

$$x_{i:d} = X_i(d) \tag{6.7}$$

Functions may take multiple arguments, and consequently so can variables. A variable may therefore be defined with a product set as its domain. For example, consider the function $X: D \times F \rightarrow R$. In this case, X is a variable that identifies each pair $(d, f) \in D \times F$ with an element in its range R. The corresponding value is then denoted as $x_{df} = X(d, f)$. If on the other hand, $X(d, f) = X(d, f')$ for all $f \in F$ and all $f' \in F$, then we denote $X(d, f)$ simply as $X(d)$ in contexts where this notational simplicity is clear.

We can now express notation more generally. Using all of the nuances expressed above, we would have

$$x_{ij,st:df} = X_{ij,st}(d, f) \tag{6.8}$$

which would indicate an arbitrary value and corresponding random variable with a Cartesian product having elements (d, f) in a domain and indexed by i and j to distinguish variables across observations and s and t to distinguish variables within observation. This can seem complicated, but we will usually leave off the variable index on the value (corresponding to the lowercase labels) when the context makes it clear to which variable the value applies: for example, in the preceding case, we would typically denote the value as x_{df}. It is, however, important to preserve the notational nuance for the variables (corresponding to the uppercase labels).

Variables may be functions of other variables. In this case, the arguments for the left-hand side variable must be the same as the full set of arguments on the right-hand side (except for right-hand side arguments that are integrated out). For example, consider the following equation of variables in which α and β are constants:

$$Y(d, f) = \alpha + \beta \cdot X(d) + \mathcal{E}(f) \quad \text{for all } d \in D \text{ and } f \in F \tag{6.9}$$

Although X and $\mathcal{E}$ have different domains in this example, Y has a Cartesian product for a domain (i.e., $D \times F$) that comprises the domains of the right-hand side variables. This should be intuitively clear because the variation in Y is due to the variations in both X and $\mathcal{E}$, which are due to the arbitrary elements across their respective domains. Alternatively, and more accurately, X and $\mathcal{E}$ are each function of $D \times F$, but each only varies according to one of its arguments.

Because the left-hand side domain is determined by the domains of the right-hand side variables, we can drop the left-hand side denotation of domain elements, unless needed for clarity. Equation 6.9 could simply be written as

$$Y = \alpha + \beta \cdot X(d) + \mathcal{E}(f) \quad \text{for all } d \in D \text{ and } f \in F \tag{6.10}$$

Suppose we define an index set $\mathbb{W}$, with an interpretation $\mathcal{J}: \mathbb{W} \to \Omega$ for some population Ω, and we specify

$$Y_w = \alpha_w + \beta \cdot X_w(d) + \mathcal{E}_w(f) \quad \text{for all } w \in \mathbb{W} \tag{6.11}$$

Then for each w in $\mathbb{W}$, and thereby for each corresponding element $\mathcal{J}(w)$ of Ω, there are three variables $Y_w, X_w, \mathcal{E}_w$ that are related according to the preceding equation. As we will use such equations here, we will typically consider the distinct letters Y, X, and $\mathcal{E}$ to denote distinct concepts that remain constant across the indices. For example, Y may denote out-of-pocket healthcare expenditures, X may denote income, and $\mathcal{E}$ may denote a combined influence of all other factors, or simply the difference between Y_w and the model $\alpha_w + \beta \cdot X_w(d)$. Even though when indexed by w they denote different functions for each $w \in \mathbb{W}$, thereby interpreted as different function for each $\mathcal{J}(w) = \omega \in \Omega$, they will denote the same conceptual definitions. In this example, in which the index set $\mathbb{W}$ represents a set of people, the preceding equation indicates that for each person in Ω his out-of-pocket expenditures will vary according to the level of income, which, being a variable, is itself allowed to vary.

Note that in the preceding equation the term α_w is a constant, yet it is indexed by w. This means that each w in $\mathbb{W}$ has its own constant; therefore, α_w can vary across $\mathbb{W}$, but it does not vary within w. Being an indexed constant, α_w is a value of a function that has $\mathbb{W}$ as its domain: that is, there is some function $A: \mathbb{W} \to R$ such that $\alpha_w = A(w)$, which according to the interpretation function yields $\alpha_w = A(w) = A(\mathcal{J}^{-1}(\omega)) = A^*(\omega)$, a function with domain Ω as well. Expressing an indexed constant as a function evaluated at the interpretation of the index will be important in translating structural models of variables into probability models of random variables.

Another useful notational maneuver is to apply Occam's Razor to our indices and only use the minimal number of variables required. In the present context, this means that if

$$X_{it} = X_{it'} \quad \text{for all } t \text{ and } t' \text{ in } \mathbb{T} \tag{6.12}$$

then we can create a variable $X_i = X_{it^\circ}$ for any arbitrary $t^\circ \in \mathbb{T}$ and replace each X_{it} for all $t \in \mathbb{T}$ by X_i. Procedurally, this simply means deleting any index across which the variables are the same.

When the variable domains are clear or are not the subject of discussion, we may drop their explicit denotation; for example, we may write $X_i(d)$ simply as X_i, and the preceding equation as

$$Y_i = \alpha_i + \beta \cdot X_i + \mathcal{E}_i \tag{6.13}$$

with the understanding that Y_i, X_i, and $\mathcal{E}_i$ are variables, each having an appropriate domain.

Finally, careful consideration of the preceding discussion will reveal that the following equivalencies hold for appropriate definitions of index sets and domains:

$$Y_i(t) = Y(i,t) = Y_t(i) = Y_{it}(d) \quad \text{for all } d \in D \tag{6.14}$$

with D any domain. For the last term to be equivalent means that the value of Y_{it} at each element of a domain d is constant across all $d \in$ D. Consequently, the strategy for indexing is not part of the logic of mathematics, but only a way of structuring symbols so that they are useful to your purpose. What constitutes a domain or an index set is arbitrary and must be selected for a specific representational purpose.

Suppose we are interested in a person's response to different levels of an intervention (e.g., drug dosages, tax rates, or voucher levels). We define D as the set of possible intervention levels, and for each person population Ω, with index set W, at time t in an index set for time $\mathbb{T}$, and for simplicity defining Ω as its own index set, we define a variable $X_{wt}: D \to \mathbb{R}$ to be the real-valued function of the intervention level and $Y_{wt}: D \to \mathbb{R}$ to be the real-valued function of response. We consider the relationship between these variables to be

$$Y_{wt} = \alpha_w + \beta \cdot X_{wt}(d) + \varepsilon_{wt} \tag{6.15}$$

Both Y_{wt} and X_{wt} are variables for each person w and time t that can take on different values depending on the arbitrary intervention level d. This is a structural specification: it indicates that X can potentially, or hypothetically, vary within w at any time t. Clearly, it would not be an essential characteristic of w such as sex, birthdate, or age; this is because for any given w and t such characteristics could not vary. The constant α_w is a fixed value for each w and may be defined in many different ways; for this example, we could define α_w as

$$\alpha_w = \frac{1}{T} \sum_{t=1}^{T} Y_{wt}(d^0) \tag{6.16}$$

in which d^0 denotes the element of D such that $X_{wt}(d^0) = 0$, that is identified with no intervention (e.g., no drug, no tax, or no voucher). The constant α_w in Equation 6.16 is then the average across time of individual w's responses without intervention. The constant ε_{wt} can be thought of as a deviation at d^0 for all w and t

$$\varepsilon_{wt} = Y_{wt}(d^0) - \alpha_w \tag{6.17}$$

Alternatively, we could define α_w as the value of Y in the condition of no intervention at time $t = 0$,

$$\alpha_w = Y_{w0}(d^0) \tag{6.18}$$

leading to a deviation ε_{wt} of

$$\varepsilon_{wt} = Y_{wt}(d^0) - Y_{w0}(d^0) \tag{6.19}$$

for which $\varepsilon_{w0} = 0$ for all w's.

Using the structural model in Equation 6.15 with the first definition of α_w, let us consider how to apply the notational conventions to the corresponding random variables for two data generating processes.

Example 6.1

Consider a probability space $(\Omega^N, \mathcal{A}^N, P)$ in which P models a data generating process of independently selecting N observations. Consequently, each observation indexed by $i \in I = \{1, 3, \dots, N\}$ has its own probability space $(\Omega, \mathcal{A}, P_i)$, and for any pair (i, j) with $i \in I$ and $j \in I$ such that $i \neq j$, P_i is independent of P_j and $P_i = P_j$ for all $\{w\} \in \mathcal{A}$. Note that the interpretation of I is the set of N occurrences of a data generating process with independent observations.

For simplicity of this initial example, let us consider t to be fixed for all w—this is a repeated measures observational design in which we measure our variables at a fixed set of times (perhaps a baseline and a six-month measure). Define $d_{i,t:w} = D_{i,t}(w)$ as the intervention level for each w measured at the time t. Note that our random variables are defined on $(\Omega, \mathcal{A}, P_i)$ and are thereby functions of the domain Ω and not of D, the domain of the structural model. The following definitions of random variables correspond to our structural variables:

$$Y_{i,t}(w) = Y_{wt}(d_{i,t:w}) \tag{6.20}$$

$$X_{i,t}(w) = X_{wt}(d_{i,t:w}) \tag{6.21}$$

These produce values of Y and X associated with the value d_w that is present at the time of observation. Note that the indices of the random variables are separated by a comma—this indicates that the i index refers to different observations (as determined by the data generating process), whereas the t index refers to different within-observation variables, which in this case are different preset times.

Note that our constants in the structural model vary across indices, which can be expressed as values of variables defined on the corresponding index sets:

$$\alpha_w = A_{i,t}(w) \tag{6.22}$$

$$\varepsilon_w = \mathcal{E}_{i,t}(w) \tag{6.23}$$

However, α_w being constant for each w implies $A_{i,t}(w)$ is the same across all $t \in T$; consequently, we can eliminate the t index and denote it simply as

$$\alpha_w = A_i(w) \tag{6.24}$$

114

The relationship between the random variables $Y_{i,t}$, $X_{i,t}$, A_i, and $\mathcal{E}_{i,t}$ for each $i \in \{1, 3, \dots, N\}$ is therefore

$$Y_{i,t} = A_i(w) + \beta \cdot X_{i,t}(w) + \mathcal{E}_{i,t}(w) \tag{6.25}$$

Intuitively, these are indexed random variables because we are going to engage a data generating process for each $i \in \{1, \dots, N\}$ occasions, and for each w we capture from Ω we will take measurements at times $t \in \{1, \dots, T\}$.

Moreover, if $E(\mathcal{E}_{i,t} \mid X_{i,t} = x) = 0$ for all x, and $E(A_i \mid X_i = x) = \alpha$, a constant, for all x such that

$$A_i(w) = \alpha + \Psi_i(w) \tag{6.26}$$

with $E(\Psi_i) = 0$, then we have

$$Y_{i,t} = \alpha + \beta \cdot X_{i,t}(w) + \mathcal{E}_{i,t}{}^*(w) \tag{6.27}$$

in which $\mathcal{E}_{i,t}{}^*(w) = \Psi_i(w) + \mathcal{E}_{i,t}(w)$ and $E(\mathcal{E}_{i,t}{}^* \mid X_{i,t} = x) = 0$ for all x.

For the convenience of explanation, assume Ψ_i and $\mathcal{E}_{i,t}$ are independent of each other, and assume the conditional variances are the same across values of X. In this case, the variance of $\mathcal{E}_{i,t}{}^*$ is the variance of the sum $\Psi_i + \mathcal{E}_{i,t}$. Because the expected values of Ψ_i and $\mathcal{E}_{i,t}$ are both 0, the variance is

$$\text{Var}(\mathcal{E}_{i,t}^*) = E\left[(\Psi_i(w) + \mathcal{E}_{i,t}(w))^2\right] \tag{6.28}$$

which expanding the square and pushing the expectation through the linear terms yields

$$\text{Var}(\mathcal{E}_{i,t}^*) = E\left[\Psi_i(w)^2\right] + E[2 \cdot \Psi_i(w) \cdot \mathcal{E}_{i,t}(w)] + E\left[\mathcal{E}_{i,t}(w)^2\right] \tag{6.29}$$

Noting that, because Ψ_i and $\mathcal{E}_{i,t}$ are taken to be independent, the expectation of the second right-hand side term of Equation 6.29 is zero, leaving us with the sum of two expectations, each of the square of terms with expectations of zero. The variance on the left-hand side is therefore the sum of two variances:

$$\text{Var}(\mathcal{E}_{i,t}^*) = \text{Var}[\Psi_i(w)] + \text{Var}[\mathcal{E}_{i,t}(w)] \tag{6.30}$$

What is the covariance between $\mathcal{E}_{i,t}^*$ and $\mathcal{E}_{i,t'}^*$, where t and t' are two different arbitrary indices in an index set $\mathbb{T}$? Since both variables are defined for the same observation indexed by i, they will be evaluated at the same element w that is generated by the data generating process. Therefore, the covariance

$$\text{Cov}(\mathcal{E}_{i,t}^*, \mathcal{E}_{i,t'}^*) = E[(\Psi_i(w) + \mathcal{E}_{i,t}(w)) \cdot (\Psi_i(w) + \mathcal{E}_{i,t'}(w))] \tag{6.31}$$

Expanding the square and pushing the expectation through the linear terms of Equation 6.31 yield:

$$\begin{aligned}
\text{Cov}(\mathcal{E}_{i,t}^*, \mathcal{E}_{i,t'}^*) = {} & E[\Psi_i(w) \cdot \Psi_i(w)] + E[\Psi_i(w) \cdot \mathcal{E}_{i,t'}(w)] \dots \\
& + E[\mathcal{E}_{i,t}(w) \cdot \Psi_i(w)] + E[\mathcal{E}_{i,t}(w) \cdot \mathcal{E}_{i,t'}(w)]
\end{aligned} \tag{6.32}$$

in which the arguments for Ψ and $\mathcal{E}$ are the same w because they are both determined by the same observation i, which will thereby have the same w from the data generating process.

Here is where the notational simplification we achieved by dropping indices is helpful. We immediately see that the first right-hand side term of Equation 6.32 is

$$E[\Psi_i(w) \cdot \Psi_i(w)] = E[\Psi_i(w)^2] = V[\Psi_i] \tag{6.33}$$

Without this notational reduction, we would have written $E[\Psi_{i,t}(w) \cdot \Psi_{i,t'}(w)]$, and we would have had to remember, notwithstanding the different indices, that the two indicated variables are the same and, there-fore, the covariance between them is equal to the variance of one of them.

If $\mathrm{Cov}(\Psi_i, \mathcal{E}_{i,t}) = 0$ and $\mathrm{Cov}(\mathcal{E}_{i,t}, \mathcal{E}_{i,t'}) = 0$ for all $i \in \mathbb{I}$ and all $(t, t') \in \mathbb{T} \times \mathbb{T}$ such that $t \neq t'$, then $\mathrm{Cov}(\mathcal{E}_{i,t}^*, \mathcal{E}_{i,t'}^*) = V(\Psi_i)$, that is, the variance of Ψ_i. Otherwise, the covariances among the Ψ_i and $\mathcal{E}_{i,t}$ variables would be included as well.

Next, it is more important to ask what the covariance is between $\mathcal{E}_{i,t}^*$ and $\mathcal{E}_{j,t}^*$ for $(i, j) \in \mathbb{I} \times \mathbb{I}$ and $i \neq j$. In other words, what is the covariance between observations? In terms of the preceding example, we have

$$\mathrm{Cov}(\mathcal{E}_{i,t}^*, \mathcal{E}_{j,t}^*) = E[(\Psi_i(w) + \mathcal{E}_{i,t}(w)) \cdot (\Psi_j(w') + \mathcal{E}_{j,t}(w'))] \tag{6.34}$$

Note the use of distinct symbols w and w' in Equation 6.34 to represent the arbitrary elements of Ω associated with the data generating processes indexed by i and j, respectively. The reason for this is that although $\mathcal{E}_{i,t}^*$ and $\mathcal{E}_{j,t}^*$ have the same domain Ω, they represent two different occurrences of the data generating process and thereby the outcome from Ω obtained for observation i is not necessarily the same as the outcome obtained for observation j.

Expanding the square and pushing the expectation operator through the linear terms of Equation 6.34 give

$$\mathrm{Cov}(\mathcal{E}_{i,t}^*, \mathcal{E}_{j,t}^*) = E[(\Psi_i(w) + \mathcal{E}_{i,t}(w)) \cdot (\Psi_j(w') + \mathcal{E}_{i,t}(w'))] \tag{6.35}$$

which expanding and extending the expectation through the term yields

$$\mathrm{Cov}(\mathcal{E}_{i,t}^*, \mathcal{E}_{j,t}^*) = E[\Psi_i(w) \cdot \Psi_j(w')] + E[\Psi_i(w) \cdot \mathcal{E}_{j,t}(w')] \ldots \\ + E[\mathcal{E}_{i,t}(w) \cdot \Psi_j(w')] + E[\mathcal{E}_{i,t}(w) \cdot \mathcal{E}_{j,t}(w')] \tag{6.36}$$

Consider the first expectation on the right-hand side of Equation 6.36:

$$E[\Psi_i(w) \cdot \Psi_j(w')] = \sum_w \sum_{w'} [\Psi_i(w) \cdot \Psi_j(w')] \cdot P(\{w'\}|\{w\}) \cdot P(\{w\}) \tag{6.37}$$

However, the data generating process is one such that $P(\{w'\}|\{w\}) = P(\{w'\})$ for all $w \in \Omega$ (i.e., the observations are independent). This yields,

$$E[\Psi_i(w) \cdot \Psi_j(w')] = \sum_w \sum_{w'} [\Psi_i(w) \cdot \Psi_j(w')] \cdot P(\{w'\}) \cdot P(\{w\}) \tag{6.38}$$

which, grouping the terms for w', is

$$E[\Psi_i(w) \cdot \Psi_j(w')] = \sum_w \Psi_i(w) \underbrace{\left(\sum_{w'}[\Psi_j(w') \cdot P(\{w'\})]\right)}_{A} \cdot P(\{w\}) \quad (6.39)$$

The summation denoted by A in Equation 6.39 is the expectation of Ψ_j, which is 0; consequently, $E[\Psi_i(w) \cdot \Psi_j(w')]$ is 0. Note that we could just as well have considered the expectation of Ψ_i rather than Ψ_j and obtained the same result.

Here it is important to note that the number of summations corresponds to the number of individual arguments, which in this case is two: one for w and one for w'.

The key to this result is that the data generating process was independent regarding the production of observations for i and j. As discussed in Chapter 4, all random variables across independent observations are independent. Consequently, if we were to investigate the remaining expectations of $E[\Psi_i(w) \cdot \mathcal{E}_{j,t}(w')]$, $E[\mathcal{E}_{i,t}(w) \cdot \Psi_j(w')]$, and $E[\mathcal{E}_{i,t}(w) \cdot \mathcal{E}_{j,t}(w')]$, we will obtain the same result for each—each expectation is 0. The full result is then $\mathrm{Cov}(\mathcal{E}_{i,t}^*, \mathcal{E}_{j,t}^*) = 0$ since observations i and j are independent.

Due to the independence of the observations, the preceding example is uninteresting; however, it points to the usefulness of the notational conventions, particularly regarding dropping indices that do not differentiate variables, and regarding the need to use different notations for arbitrary elements of the random variables' domain across variables (e.g., the use of w and w' above). Let us now consider a slightly different data generating process.

Example 6.2

Consider the same structural model used in Example 6.1,

$$Y_{wt} = \alpha_w + \beta \cdot X_{wt}(d) + \varepsilon_{wt} \quad (6.40)$$

but with a different data generating process. This time the data generating process is one in which we randomly select an individual w and then randomly select two times at which observations are made. We measure the response of the individual to each time. The interesting question is how does this same structural model translate to random variables of this data generating process with random assignment of doses?

The probability space representing a sample of size N each having two randomly selected times is $((\Omega \times T)^{N\cdot2}, \mathcal{A}^{N\cdot2}, P)$. Each observation, and consequent random variable, of this nested data generating process can be indexed by a single observation number. However, in this case it is helpful to use two indices: one being $i \in \{1, \dots, N\}$ representing the part of the process that selects an individual, the other being $j \in \{1, 2\}$ representing the two random selections of times at which measurements are made. The component probability space for an observation indexed by ij is then $(\Omega \times T, \mathcal{A}, P_{ij})$. By inspection, it should be easy to see that this indexing scheme uniquely distinguishes observations and corresponding variables, which is the goal of indexing.

Expressing our relationship between the structural variables,

$$Y_{wt} = \alpha_w + \beta \cdot X_{wt}(d) + \varepsilon_{wt} \tag{6.41}$$

in terms of the corresponding random variables for an arbitrary observation yields

$$Y_{ij} = A_{ij}(w) + \beta \cdot X_{ij}(w,t) + \mathcal{E}_{ij}(w,t) \tag{6.42}$$

The random variable Y_{ij} is measured as just that response for individual w at time t for the intervention dose individual w happens to be subject to at time t, which is $Y_{wt}(d)$ of the structural model; a similar connection exists between the random variable $X_{ij}(w, t)$ and its structural counterpart $X_{wt}(d)$. Note that here, unlike the previous example, the indices for the random variables are not separated by a comma. This is because both indices, together, provide the unique designation of the observational process that will select a pair (w, t) from $\Omega \times T$.

The individual and time-specific constants α_w and ε_{wt} in the structural model can vary across individuals and are therefore random variables $A_{ij}(w)$ and $\mathcal{E}_{ij}(w, t)$ when defined in terms of the probability space $(\Omega \times T, \mathcal{A}, P_{ij})$. Although the full notation of $A_{ij}(w)$ is $A_{ij}(w, t)$, it does not vary across t and therefore t is dropped as an argument. Similarly, we drop the j index from $A_{ij}(w)$ because the variables are the same across j.

If, as in Equation 6.26, we specify

$$A_i(w) = \alpha + \Psi_i(w) \tag{6.43}$$

with $E(\Psi_i) = 0$, then we have

$$Y_{ij} = \alpha + \beta \cdot X_{ij}(w, d) + \mathcal{E}_{ij}^*(w, t) \tag{6.44}$$

in which $\mathcal{E}_{ij}^*(w, t) = \Psi_i(w) + \mathcal{E}_{ij}(w, t)$.

The interesting question is what are the covariances between observations of this data generating process? I will consider two: $\text{Cov}(Y_{ij}, Y_{ij'})$ and $\text{Cov}(Y_{ij}, Y_{i'j})$. The remaining two combinations can be worked out as easily. For ease of presentation, I will consider the variables A_i, X_{ij}, and $\mathcal{E}_{ij}$ to be mutually independent.

The $\text{Cov}(Y_{ij}, Y_{ij'})$ can be expressed as

$$\begin{aligned}\text{Cov}(Y_{ij}, Y_{ij'}) = E[&(\beta \cdot \dot{X}_{ij}(w,t) + \Psi_i(w) + \mathcal{E}_{ij}(w,t)) \\ &\times (\beta \cdot \dot{X}_{ij'}(w,t') \ldots + \Psi_i(w) + \mathcal{E}_{ij'}(w,t'))]\end{aligned} \tag{6.45}$$

This is the same as

$$\begin{aligned}\text{Cov}(Y_{ij}, Y_{ij'}) = \beta^2 \cdot E[&\dot{X}_{ij}(w,t) \cdot \dot{X}_{ij'}(w,t')] + E[\Psi_i(w) \cdot \Psi_i(w)] \ldots \\ &+ E[\mathcal{E}_{ij}(w,t) \cdot \mathcal{E}_{ij'}(w,t')]\end{aligned} \tag{6.46}$$

in which $\dot{X}_{ij}$ denotes the appropriate mean-centered variable. Note the careful use of the w, t, and t'. Both Y_{ij} and $Y_{ij'}$ are based on the same i and will therefore have values determined by the same w that is obtained from that part of the data generating process. However, the variables are based on different indices indicating the two different occurrences of randomly selected times and can therefore produce different times t and t'. Therefore, Y_{ij} will not necessarily be the same as $Y_{ij'}$ due to the different times that observations ij and ij' can produce. Consequently, we use t to indicate the arbitrary time for Y_{ij} and t' to indicate the arbitrary time for $Y_{ij'}$. This is a very important notational convention as it will dictate how the probabilities are applied to the random variables.

Each expectation in the preceding equation is as follows. Regarding the first,

$$E[\dot{X}_{ij} \cdot \dot{X}_{ij'}] = \sum_{w}\sum_{t}\sum_{t'} \dot{X}_{ij}(w,t) \cdot \dot{X}_{ij'}(w,\ t') \cdot P(\{t'\}|\{w\}) \\ \cdot P(\{t\}|\{w\}) \cdot P(\{w\})$$

(6.47)

which, grouping the terms under the summation for t', is

$$E[\dot{X}_{ij} \cdot \dot{X}_{ij'}] = \sum_{w}\sum_{t} \dot{X}_{ij}(w,t) \cdot \left[\sum_{t'} \dot{X}_{ij'}(w,t') \cdot P(\{t'\}|\{w\})\right] \\ \cdot P(\{t\}|\{w\}) \cdot P(\{w\})$$

(6.48)

Here again it is important to note the number of summations correspond to the number of distinct arguments, which in this case is three: there is no sum over a second w' element because both random variables will take on values associated with the same w that is captured in the data generating process.

Because in equation 6.48 the summation with respect to t' is the expected value of $\dot{X}_{ij}$ conditional on $\{w\}$, and similarly the summation with respect to t is the expected value of $\dot{X}_{ij'}$ conditional on $\{w\}$, however these conditional expectations are the same.

Therefore, equation 4.48 can be expressed in terms of the square of either:

$$E[\dot{X}_{ij} \cdot \dot{X}_{ij'}] = \sum_{w} E(\dot{X}_{ij}|\{w\})^2 \cdot P(\{w\}) = \sum_{w} E(\dot{X}_{ij'}|\{w\})^2 \cdot P(\{w\}) \quad (6.49)$$

which is the variance of the conditional expectation plus the expectation of the conditional expectation squared or either random variable $\dot{X}_{ij}$ or $\dot{X}_{ij'}$:

$$E[\dot{X}_{ij} \cdot \dot{X}_{ij'}] = V(E(\dot{X}_{ij}|\{w\})) + E(E(\dot{X}_{ij}|\{w\}))^2 \\ = V(E(\dot{X}_{ij'}|\{w\})) + E(E(\dot{X}_{ij'}|\{w\}))^2$$

(6.50)

However, since the squared terms in equation 6.50 are equal to 0, the first term on the right-hand side of equation 6.46 is simply the squared parameter β multiplied by the variance of the conditional expectation:

$$\beta^2 \cdot E[\dot{X}_{ij}(w,t) \cdot \dot{X}_{ij'}(w,t')] = \beta^2 \cdot V(E(\dot{X}_{ij}|\{w\})) = \beta^2 \cdot V(E(\dot{X}_{ij}|\{w\})) \quad (6.51)$$

Regarding $E[\Psi_i(w) \cdot \Psi_i(w)]$:

$$E[\Psi_i(w) \cdot \Psi_i(w)] = E\left[\Psi_i(w)^2\right]$$

(6.52)

But, given the expected value of $\Psi_i(w)$ is zero, this expectation of its squared value is the variance:

$$E[\Psi_i(w) \cdot \Psi_i(w)] = \text{Var}[\Psi_i(w)] \tag{6.53}$$

and, regarding $E[\mathcal{E}_{ij}(w,t) \cdot \mathcal{E}_{ij'}(w,t')]$:

$$E[\mathcal{E}_{ij}(w,t) \cdot \mathcal{E}_{ij'}(w,t')] = \text{Cov}[\mathcal{E}_{ij}(w,t), \mathcal{E}_{ij'}(w,t')] \tag{6.54}$$

Consequently, regarding random variables across observations that necessarily capture the same person but different times, the covariance is

$$\text{Cov}(Y_{ij}, Y_{ij'}) = \text{Var}[\Psi_i(w)] + \text{Cov}[\mathcal{E}_{ij}(w,t), \mathcal{E}_{ij'}(w,t')] \tag{6.55}$$

However, by the data generating process, $\mathcal{E}_{ij}$ and $\mathcal{E}_{ij'}$ are independent; therefore, $\text{Cov}[\mathcal{E}_{ij}(w,t), \mathcal{E}_{ij'}(w,t')] = 0$ in Equation 6.55 and overall $\text{Cov}(Y_{ij}, Y_{ij'}) = \text{Var}[\Psi_i(w)]$.

Now consider the covariance of random variables across observations that potentially capture different people. The $\text{Cov}(Y_{ij}, Y_{i'j})$ is

$$\text{Cov}(Y_{ij}, Y_{i'j}) = E[(\beta \cdot \dot{X}_{ij}(w,t) + \Psi_i(w) + \mathcal{E}_{ij}(w,t)) \cdot (\beta \cdot \dot{X}_{i'j}(w',t') \dots \\ + \Psi_{i'}(w') + \mathcal{E}_{i'j}(w',t'))] \tag{6.56}$$

which, after expanding the polynomial and pushing the expectation across the linear terms, yields

$$\text{Cov}(Y_{ij}, Y_{i'j}) = \beta^2 \cdot E[\dot{X}_{ij}(w,t) \cdot \dot{X}_{i'j}(w',t')] + E[\Psi_i(w) \cdot \Psi_{i'}(w')] \dots \\ + E[\mathcal{E}_{ij}(w,t) \cdot \mathcal{E}_{i'j}(w',t')] \tag{6.57}$$

Each expectation in Equation 6.57 is as follows. Regarding the first expectation,

$$E[\dot{X}_{ij} \cdot \dot{X}_{i'j}] = \sum_w \sum_{w'} \sum_t \sum_{t'} \dot{X}_{ij}(w,t) \cdot \dot{X}_{i'j}(w',t') \cdot P(\{t\}|\{w\}) \\ \cdot P(\{t'\}|\{w'\}) \cdot P(\{w\}) \cdot P(\{w'\}) \tag{6.58}$$

After grouping the summations for t and t', the expectation is

$$E[\dot{X}_{ij} \cdot \dot{X}_{i'j}] = \sum_w \sum_{w'} \left[\sum_t \dot{X}_{ij}(w,t) \cdot P(\{t\}|\{w\}) \cdot \sum_{t'} \dot{X}_{i'j}(w',t') \cdot P(\{t'\})|\{w'\} \right] \\ \cdot P(\{w'\}) \cdot P(\{w\}) \tag{6.59}$$

Since the summations $\sum_t \dot{X}_{ij}(w,t) \cdot P(\{t\}|\{w\})$ and $\sum_{t'} \dot{X}_{i'j}(w',t') \cdot P(\{t'\}|\{w'\})$ are equal to 0, being the expected value of mean-centered variables, the expectation is 0:

$$E[\dot{X}_{ij} \cdot \dot{X}_{i'j}] = 0. \tag{6.60}$$

In this case, there are four summations in Equation 6.59 because these random variables will take on values associated with potentially different elements of Ω, indicated here as w and w', and potentially different elements of T here denoted as t and t'. The selection of individuals and the selection of times are mutually independent; consequently, the probabilities are those associated with independence. The last equality, by which the expectation is equal to 0, is due to the same argument presented above for $\text{Cov}(Y_{ij}, Y_{ij'})$.

This example shows that the number of distinct arguments for random variables do not necessarily follow the number of distinct indices. Consider, for example, the two variables $\dot{X}_{ij}(w,t)$ and $\dot{X}_{i'j}(w',t')$. Both have the same index j, but different associated arguments t and t'. This is because j is indexing the time-selection process that is nested within the person-selection process. If, for example, $j = 1$, then both random variables are associated with the first occurrence of randomly selecting a time, but since these are different random variables due to being associated with different occurrences of randomly selecting individuals (i.e., i and i'), the resultant randomly selected times can be different for each and are consequently denoted differently as t and t'. It would have a different interpretation if the data generating process was not nested, such as randomly selecting individuals and then randomly selecting two times at which all individuals are measured. In that case, we would have $\dot{X}_{ij}(w,t)$ and $\dot{X}_{i'j}(w',t)$ because both observations would be based on the same randomly selected times. Properly interpreting the current notation requires understanding how it relates to the data generating process—notation alone is not sufficient. We could add more nuance to allow the notation to directly indicate nested versus nonnested processes; for example, we could use parentheses to denote nesting, such as $X_{i(j)}$ to denote j nested within i. However, for the purpose of this text, I will forgo greater notational complexity and depend on our understanding of the data generating process that we are modeling.

Returning to our example, regarding the second expectation of Equation 6.57:

$$E[\Psi_i(w) \cdot \Psi_{i'}(w')] = \sum_w \sum_{w'} \Psi_i(w) \cdot \Psi_{i'}(w') \cdot P(\{w\}) \cdot P(\{w'\}) \qquad (6.61)$$

which, after rearranging the summations is

$$E[\Psi_i(w) \cdot \Psi_{i'}(w')] = \sum_w \Psi_i(w) \cdot P(\{w\}) \cdot \sum_{w'} \Psi_{i'}(w') \cdot P(\{w'\}) \qquad (6.62)$$

and noting that each summation is an expectation equal to 0,

$$E[\Psi_i(w) \cdot \Psi_{i'}(w')] = E[\Psi_i(w)] \cdot E[\Psi_{i'}(w')] \qquad (6.63)$$

the overall expected value is 0, that is, $E[\Psi_i(w) \cdot \Psi_{i'}(w')] = 0$.

Regarding the term $E[\mathcal{E}_{ij}(w,t) \cdot \mathcal{E}_{i'j}(w',t')]$ in Equation 6.57, similar to above, the expectation turns out to be 0 because, again, they are based on independent observations.

Consequently, the covariance between Y_{ij} and $Y_{i'j}$ is 0:

$$\text{Cov}(Y_{ij}, Y_{i'j}) = 0 \qquad (6.64)$$

Examples 6.1 and 6.2 show three important features of the notation used in the remainder of this book: (1) the elimination of those indices and arguments over which a random variable does not vary, (2) distinguishing arguments that correspond to results for different indices (e.g., the use of w and w', and d and d'), and (3) assuring that summation is only taken over those arguments that correspond to the variables under consideration. The indexing notation must be understood based on an understanding of the context of a particular data generating process. Careful attention to these points will allow us to determine the dependence across any pair of random variables.

Random versus Fixed Effects

The terms "random effect," "random coefficient," "random parameter," "hierarchical," and "multilevel" are all commonly (although not exclusively) used to label models of random variables from data generating processes with observations represented by probability spaces such as $(S \times \Omega, \mathcal{A}, P)$ in which elements of Ω are associated by a nonzero P with only one element of S. Assuming our sigma-algebra is the power set, this means that for all elements w of Ω, there is only one element s of S such that $P(\{(s, w)\}) > 0$. In formal logic, assuming the domain of the arguments is understood, this is represented as $\forall w \exists! s(P(\{(s, w)\}) > 0)$, which is to say that for all w's there is exactly one s for which the probability of $\{(s, w)\} \in \mathcal{A}$ is greater than 0. The data generating process is one where an element is sampled from S and then an element is sampled from Ω based on a probability conditional on the result from S. For example, randomly selecting a school from a population of schools (S) and then randomly selecting a student from within the obtained school (the subset of Ω corresponding to student in the selected school), or randomly selecting a physician from a population of physicians (S) and then randomly selecting a patient from the obtained physician's patient panel (the subset of Ω corresponding to the selected physician's patient panel), or randomly selecting an individual (S) and then randomly selecting a time to measure a characteristic (the subset of Ω corresponding to an index set of time). These are examples of nested data generating processes.

It is possible to specify the outcome set with more than two components thereby indicating more elaborate nesting: for example, randomly selecting a hospital from a population of hospitals, and randomly selecting a clinical department within the obtained hospital, then randomly selecting a physician within the selected department, and finally, randomly selecting a patient of the selected physician. Such a process would have an outcome set defined by H × D × P × I in which H denotes the set of hospitals, D denotes the set of clinical departments, P denotes physicians, and I denotes patients. However, for the purposes of this presentation, I will restrict the discussion to the two-level models: more levels are a straightforward extension.

Notwithstanding the above description of a typical random effects model, a more general presentation simply assumes that there is a measurable partition on a product outcome set generated by one of the component sets across which the distribution of random variables under investigation vary. This characteristic alone does not differentiate the partition from other random variables, but as stated above for random and fixed effects models, these partitions typically reflect structure of the data generating process (e.g., clusters in a cluster sampling design). However, as the following sections show, there are other applications as well, each having other reasons to distinguish these partitions from other random variables of interest in our analysis.

Suppose $(S \times \Omega, \mathcal{A}, P)$ is a probability space modeling a data generating process in which S contains K elements. Define $\Pi = \{\pi_1, \pi_2, \ldots, \pi_K\}$ as a measurable partition of $S \times \Omega$ in $\mathcal{A}$ generated by the elements of S. Specifically, an arbitrary element of the partition is defined as $\pi_k = \{(s, w): s = s_k, s \in S, w \in \Omega\}$; consequently, π_k includes all elements that have s equal to s_k. If we have a random variable Y, random vector $\mathbf{X}$ of explanatory variables, and a random vector $\mathbf{Z}$ of indicators of membership in each of the K elements of the partition Π (i.e., for all $(s, w) \in S \times \Omega$, $Z_k((s, w)) = 1((s, w) \in \pi_k)$ for each $k \in \{1, 2, \ldots, K\}$), then the parameter vector $\boldsymbol{\theta} = (\theta_1, \theta_2, \ldots, \theta_K)'$ associated with $\mathbf{Z}$ in the density $f(Y \mid \mathbf{X}, \mathbf{Z}; \boldsymbol{\theta}, \boldsymbol{\phi})$ comprises what are commonly called *fixed effects*. Note that $\boldsymbol{\phi}$ is a vector of remaining parameters of the distribution.

Rather than specifying a vector of indicators $\mathbf{Z}$, we can just as well directly define $\boldsymbol{\theta}$ as Θ a random variable,

$$
\Theta((s, w)) = \begin{cases} \theta_1 & \text{if } (s, w) \in \pi_1 \\ \theta_2 & \text{if } (s, w) \in \pi_2 \\ \vdots & \vdots \\ \theta_K & \text{if } (s, w) \in \pi_K \end{cases} \tag{6.65}
$$

and restate the density as $f(Y \mid \mathbf{X}, \Theta; \boldsymbol{\phi})$. In this case, we consider the random variable Θ as comprising the fixed effects. Note that $\boldsymbol{\phi}$ is not likely to include parameters associated with Θ because Θ likely enters the distribution directly as if it was itself a parameter, which it was in the preceding specification using $\mathbf{Z}$. In this case, if corresponding parameters were included in $\boldsymbol{\phi}$, they would be fixed constants rather than parameters free to be estimated. This second form, that is, including Θ as a random variable, is a common representation for discussing fixed effects and identifying certain types of estimators (e.g., what are commonly called within estimators that ultimately eliminate the fixed effects from the model thereby negating the need to estimate them). The density in terms of $\mathbf{Z}$ is common as a specification for other methods of estimating fixed effects (e.g., methods that include the set of indicators of the partition in the model to be estimated). These two representations are not necessarily identical. Because many elements of the partition may have the same value for Θ, controlling for Θ may be the same as controlling for multiple $\mathbf{Z}$'s.

As a random variable, Θ is called a *random effect* in the joint density $f(Y, \Theta \mid \mathbf{X}; \boldsymbol{\phi})$. In the case where Θ and $\mathbf{X}$ are dependent, then

$$f(Y, \Theta \mid \mathbf{X}; \boldsymbol{\phi}) \, f(Y \mid \mathbf{X}, \Theta; \boldsymbol{\phi}) \cdot f(\Theta \mid \mathbf{X}; \boldsymbol{\varphi}) \tag{6.66}$$

These models are often called *correlated random effects models* because $f(\Theta \mid \mathbf{X}; \boldsymbol{\varphi})$ is taken to be a nontrivial function of $\mathbf{X}$. In the case where Θ and $\mathbf{X}$ are independent, then

$$f(Y, \Theta \mid \mathbf{X}; \boldsymbol{\phi}) = f(Y \mid \mathbf{X}, \Theta; \boldsymbol{\phi}) \cdot f(\Theta \mid \boldsymbol{\varphi}) \tag{6.67}$$

models of this type are typically just called *random effects models*.

Be aware, however, that the labeling of fixed effects and random effects is not consistent across their use; you must be sure that you understand how the terms are specifically being applied when reading any given literature. Fortunately, the underlying characteristics of the relevant distributions are usually the same, notwithstanding the subtle difference in application of terminology.

Perhaps the simplest example of fixed and random effects models is one in which the random variable Y_i is a linear function of random variables Θ_i, $\mathbf{X}_i$, and $\mathcal{E}_i$:

$$Y_i = \Theta_i + \beta \cdot \mathbf{X}_i + \mathcal{E}_i \tag{6.68}$$

Note that here I am using the subscript i as a simple index of the observation and not using a two-index notation that would capture the structure of the data generating process.

If we are interested in the distribution of Y conditional on both random variables X and Θ, then we have a fixed effects model in which the, possibly subset of, elements of Θ that are conditioned on comprise the set of fixed effects. If we are interested in the distribution of Y conditional on X only, then we have a random effects model in which the random variable Θ is a random effect. In both models, the intercept of the linear function is taken to vary across the measurable partition Π and is a random variable—one that we either condition on as a fixed effect or integrate over as a random effect. Note that we could also condition on $\mathbf{Z}$ to obtain a fixed effects model. If the fixed effects associated with each $\mathbf{Z}$ were distinct, then we would have the same model as when conditioning on Θ.

Because Θ is a random variable, conditional distributions are possible and we may express Θ as a function of other variables. For simplicity of exposition, suppose the regression function of Θ is a linear function of measured random variables $\mathbf{W}$. We can model Θ_i as

$$\Theta_i = \varphi \cdot \mathbf{W}_i + \Psi_i \tag{6.69}$$

If we condition on $\mathbf{W}$, the parameters φ are sometimes called fixed effects and Ψ_i is considered a random effect. The corresponding model is a *mixed effect* model. For example, if the partition is indicating hospitals, then the hospital effect Θ_i may be expressed as a function of measured hospital characteristics and a hospital random effect.

Suppose we are interested in two measurable partitions Π_1 and Π_2 defined on an outcome set $S \times Q \times \Omega$ of a probability space $(S \times Q \times \Omega, \mathcal{A}, P)$ for which Π_1 is generated by the elements of S and Π_2 is generated by the elements of Q. If we define corresponding random variables Θ_{i1} and Θ_{i2}, we may condition on each variables (thereby incorporating two fixed effects), or integrate across both (thereby incorporating two random effects), or specify a mixture of the two (thereby obtaining another type of mixed effects model).

Additional constraints apply if one of the partitions is a refinement of the other, for example, Π_2 is a refinement of Π_1 such as indicating physicians (Π_2) within hospital (Π_1), where each physician has privileges at only one hospital. In this case, conditioning on Θ_{i2} fixes the element of Θ_{i1} (e.g., fixing the physician identifies the hospital) and, therefore, we cannot treat Θ_{i2} as a fixed effect while at the same time treating Θ_{i1} as a random effect. However, if $E(\Theta_{i2} | \Theta_{i1}) = \overline{\Theta}_{i1}$, a function of S, then we can model Θ_{i2} as

$$\Theta_{i2}(s,q) = \overline{\Theta}_{i1}(s) + (\Theta_{i2}(s,q) - \Theta_{i1}(s,q)) = \overline{\Theta}_{i1}(s) + \Delta_i(s,q) \tag{6.70}$$

in which $\overline{\Theta}_{i1}$ may be treated as a hospital-level fixed effect, and if the deviation Δ is a physician-level random variable, we can treat as a random effect, again obtaining a mixed effect model. In our hospital example, we would specify a hospital-level fixed effect and a physician-level random effect.

It is also common to consider other parameters as varying across the partition: for example, β. In this case, our function may be specified as

$$Y_i = \Theta_i + B_i \cdot X_i + \varepsilon_i \tag{6.71}$$

and B_i is called a *random coefficient* if B_i is not conditioned on. If B_i is conditioned on, then it comprises a type of fixed effects as well. Note that regardless of whether they are treated as fixed or random effects, Θ_i and B_i can be specified as random variables.

Details of the estimation techniques for these models are outside the scope of this chapter; however, the reason I consider these models in this chapter is that they are often misapplied and the interpretations of parameters and estimation of the standard errors are often wrong due to a lack of understanding what the probability space is modeling. Before discussing these fairly common cases that are often mistakenly specified and interpreted, let us consider a typical simple random effects model.

Problem 6.2

You collect an independent random sample of N states from the United States, and then independently randomly sample M residents from within each of those states. Determine the dependence structure of a model of individual characteristic Y as a linear function of characteristic X with an intercept as a state-level random effect.

Solution: This is an example of a classic random effects model with a nested (or clustered) data generating process. The full probability model is $((S \times \Omega)^{N \cdot M}, \mathcal{A}, P)$ in which S is the set of 50 states and Ω is the population of the United States.

We index the data generating process with $\mathbb{I} = \{1, \dots, N\}$ and $\mathbb{K} = \{1, \dots, M\}$ to identify each marginal space $(S \times \Omega, \mathcal{A}, P_{ik})$ and its random variables. The interpretation of $\mathbb{I}$ is the set of observational processes that randomly select states and the interpretation of $\mathbb{K}$ is the set of observational processes that randomly select individuals from within each state. To be more general and allow for different numbers of observations within each state, we can use a set of index sets $\{\mathbb{K}_i : i \in \mathbb{I}\}$; however, for simplicity we will simply refer to $\mathbb{K}$.

The interpretation of $\mathbb{I}$ is not the set of states S, nor is the interpretation of $\mathbb{K}$ the population Ω. The sets S and Ω are component sets of the product $S \times \Omega$, which is the domain for the random variables. Consequently, a random variable may be denoted such as $Y_{ik}(s, w)$ in which i and k distinguish a particular random variable associated with the data generating process's production of a possible outcome (s, w), and the pair (s, w) is an arbitrary element of the random variable's domain $S \times \Omega$ (i.e., the outcome set).

Rather than develop an underlying structural model, for simplicity in this problem I will create a model for the relationship between the random variables directly. To start, for each $(S \times \Omega, \mathcal{A}, P_{ik})$, I define three variables: $Y_{ik}(s, w)$, $X_{ik}(s, w)$, and $\Theta_i(s)$. The first two, Y and X, denote arbitrary characteristics of interest and Θ denotes an indicator of the elements of S (i.e., Θ is a random variable representing a partition in $\mathcal{A}$ generated by the elements of S). Define another random variable that reflects the expected value of Y within each state among those with $X = 0$:

$$A_i(s) = \mathrm{E}(Y_{ik}|\Theta_i(s), X_{ik} = 0) \tag{6.72}$$

define the regression function for Y as

$$\mathrm{E}(Y_{ik}|\Theta_i, X_{ik}) = A_i(s) + \beta \cdot X_{ik}(s, w) \tag{6.73}$$

and, define the difference between Y and its expected value as

$$Y_{ik} - \mathrm{E}(Y_{ik}|\Theta_i, X_{ik}) = \mathcal{E}_{ik}(s, w) \tag{6.74}$$

Overall then, Y can be expressed as

$$Y_{ik} = A_i(s) + \beta \cdot X_{ik}(s, w) + \mathcal{E}_{ik}(s, w) \tag{6.75}$$

for which $\mathrm{E}(\mathcal{E}_{ik}|\Theta_i, X_{ik}) = 0$.

This is a model in which A_i is a "state-level" random variable reflecting a state's average Y among those with $X = 0$. If we condition on A_i, we have a fixed effects model; if we do not condition on A_i, we have a random effects model. Note that we could replace A_i with a vector of indicators $\mathbf{Z}_{ik}$

comprising dummy variables representing each state and condition on **Z** to obtain another representation of a fixed-effect model. If each state has a distinct value for A_i, these are identical models; if not, these models only slightly vary in that conditioning on A_i may incorporate multiple states.

To evaluate the random effects model in the linear case of Equation 6.75, it is easier to specify $E(A_i) = \alpha$, a constant, and thereby write

$$A_i(s) = \alpha + \Psi_i(s) \tag{6.76}$$

in which $E(\Psi_i) = 0$. We then have

$$Y_{ik} = \alpha + \beta \cdot X_{ik}(s, w) + \Psi_i(s) + \mathcal{E}_{ik}(s, w) \tag{6.77}$$

We can determine the dependence structure of random variables from this specification. For ease of presentation, we will consider the relationships conditional on X assuming Ψ_i and $\mathcal{E}_{ik}$ are independent of X.

First, let us consider the conditional variance of Y_{ik}:

$$V(Y_{ik} \mid X_{ik}) = V(\Psi_i + \mathcal{E}_{ik}) = E\big((\Psi_i(s) + \mathcal{E}_{ik}(s,\ w))^2\big) \tag{6.78}$$

Expanding the polynomial and pushing the expectation operator through the sum yields

$$E\big((\Psi_i + \mathcal{E}_{ik})^2\big) = E\big(\Psi_i^2\big) + 2 \cdot E(\Psi_i \cdot \mathcal{E}_{ik}) + E\big(\mathcal{E}_{ik}^2\big) \tag{6.79}$$

which is

$$E\big((\Psi_i + \mathcal{E}_{ik})^2\big) = V(\Psi_i) + 2 \cdot \mathrm{Cov}(\Psi_i, \mathcal{E}_{ik}) + V(\mathcal{E}_{ik}) \tag{6.80}$$

Equation 6.80 is the variance of the random effect plus the variance of the individual error term plus twice the covariance between them. If the covariance is 0, which is to say the $E(\mathcal{E}_{ik} \mid A_i, X_{ik}) = 0$ for all values of A_i and X_{ik}, as we have specified, then we have

$$V(Y_{ik} \mid X_{ik}) = V(\Psi_i) + V(\mathcal{E}_{ik}) \tag{6.81}$$

The two variances that compose $V(Y_{ik} \mid X_{ik})$ reflect variation due to sampling states $V(\Psi_i)$ and variation due to sampling individuals within state $V(\mathcal{E}_{ik})$.

Next let us consider the conditional covariance of Y_{ik} and $Y_{ik'}$, which represent random variables based on the same selection of state (thereby both indexed by the same element of $\mathbb{I}$, specifically i) but different selection of individual within state (thereby each being indexed by different elements of $\mathbb{K}$, specifically k and k'). To provide greater concision in the presentation, I will denote $\mathrm{Cov}(Y_{ik}, Y_{ik'} \mid X_{ik}, X_{ik'})$ as $\mathrm{Cov}(Y_{ik}, Y_{ik'} \mid X)$. The covariance is

$$\mathrm{Cov}(Y_{ik}, Y_{ik'} \mid X) = E((\Psi_i(s) + \mathcal{E}_{ik}(s, w)) \cdot (\Psi_i(s) + \mathcal{E}_{ik'}(s, w'))) \tag{6.82}$$

Here, it is important to note that random variables with indices that differ will also have different corresponding arguments. Consequently, because $\mathcal{E}_{ik}$

and $\mathcal{E}_{ik'}$ differ in their $\mathbb{K}$ index, they also differ in their corresponding argument associated with Ω: $\mathcal{E}_{ik}(s, w)$ and $\mathcal{E}_{ik'}(s, w')$. This represents the fact that values of both variables will be determined by the same randomly selected state s but potentially different randomly selected individuals w and w'. It is this nuance in notation that will allow us to easily determine dependence.

Expanding the product on the right-hand side of the preceding equation and pushing the expectation through the consequent sum yields:

$$E((\Psi_i + \mathcal{E}_{ik}) \cdot (\Psi_i + \mathcal{E}_{ik'})) = E(\Psi_i^2(s)) + E(\Psi_i(s) \cdot \mathcal{E}_{ik'}(s, w')) + \ldots + E(\mathcal{E}_{ik}(s, w)) \\ \times \Psi_i(s)) + E(\mathcal{E}_{ik}(s, w) \cdot \mathcal{E}_{ik'}(s, w')) \qquad (6.83)$$

The first expectation on the right-hand side is the variance of the random effect: $V(\Psi_i)$. The next two expectations are the covariance terms between the random effect and the individual errors. The last term is the variance of the errors. Considering the first covariance term in Equation 6.83,

$$E(\Psi_i(s) \cdot \mathcal{E}_{ik'}(s, w')) = \sum_s \sum_{w'} (\Psi_i(s) \cdot \mathcal{E}_{ik'}(s, w')) \cdot P(\{w'\}|\{s\}) \cdot P(\{s\}) \qquad (6.84)$$

which, after rearranging the summations, is

$$E(\Psi_i(s) \cdot \mathcal{E}_{ik'}(s, w')) = \sum_s \Psi_i(s) \left[\sum_{w'} \mathcal{E}_{ik'}(s, w') \cdot P(\{w'\}|\{s\}) \right] \cdot P(\{s\}) \qquad (6.85)$$

Noting that the summation on w' is itself an expectation yields

$$E(\Psi_i(s) \cdot \mathcal{E}_{ik'}(s, w')) = \sum_s \Psi_i(s) \cdot E(\mathcal{E}_{ik'}|\Theta_i(s), X_{ik'}) \cdot P(\{s\}) \qquad (6.86)$$

Therefore, the left-hand side of Equation 6.86 is the covariance

$$E(\Psi_i(s) \cdot \mathcal{E}_{ik'}(s, w')) = \text{Cov}(\Psi_i, \mathcal{E}_{ik'}) \qquad (6.87)$$

By a similar argument,

$$E(\mathcal{E}_{ik}(s, w) \cdot \Psi_i(s)) = \text{Cov}(\mathcal{E}_{ik}, \Psi_i) \qquad (6.88)$$

Finally, regarding the last term in Equation 6.83, $E(\mathcal{E}_{ik}(s, w) \cdot \mathcal{E}_{ik'}(s, w'))$:

$$E[\mathcal{E}_{ik} \cdot \mathcal{E}_{ik'}] = \sum_s \sum_w \sum_{w'} \mathcal{E}_{ik}(s, w) \cdot \mathcal{E}_{ik'}(s, w') \cdot P(\{w\}|\{s\}, \{w'\}) \\ \times P(\{w'\}|\{s\}) \cdot P(\{s\}) \qquad (6.89)$$

Noting that the probability of events $\{w\}$ conditional on events $\{s\}$ is independent of $\{w'\}$, the expectation is

$$E[\mathcal{E}_{ik} \cdot \mathcal{E}_{ik'}] = \sum_s \sum_w \sum_{w'} \mathcal{E}_{ik}(s, w) \cdot \mathcal{E}_{ik'}(s, w') \cdot P(\{w\}|\{s\}) \\ \times P(\{w'\}|\{s\}) \cdot P(\{s\}) \qquad (6.90)$$

which is

$$E[\mathcal{E}_{ik} \cdot \mathcal{E}_{ik'}] = \sum_s E(\mathcal{E}_{ik}|\Theta_i(s), X_{ik}) \cdot E(\mathcal{E}_{ik'}|\Theta_i(s), X_{ik'}) \cdot P(\{s\}) \qquad (6.91)$$

the covariance

$$E[\mathcal{E}_{ik} \cdot \mathcal{E}_{ik'}] = \mathrm{Cov}(\mathcal{E}_{ik}, \mathcal{E}_{ik'}) \qquad (6.92)$$

However, the data generating process and model specification is such that $E(\mathcal{E}_{ik}|\Theta_i, X_{ik}) = 0$ and $E(\mathcal{E}_{ik'}|\Theta_i, X_{ik'}) = 0$; consequently, the covariances $\mathrm{Cov}(\Psi_i, \mathcal{E}_{ik'})$, $\mathrm{Cov}(\mathcal{E}_{ik}, \Psi_i)$, and $\mathrm{Cov}(\mathcal{E}_{ik}, \mathcal{E}_{ik'})$ are each equal to 0. Overall, then

$$\mathrm{Cov}(Y_{ik}, Y_{ik'}|X) = V(\Psi_i) \qquad (6.93)$$

This result implies that the covariance between random variables representing the independent selection of individuals within a randomly selected state is the variance of the state-level random effect.

Next, let us consider the conditional covariance of Y_{ik} and $Y_{jk'}$, which represent random variables based on different selections of states (thereby each being indexed by different elements of $\mathbb{I}$, specifically i and j) and different selection of individual within state (thereby each being indexed by different elements of $\mathbb{K}$, specifically k and k'). We have

$$\mathrm{Cov}(Y_{ik}, Y_{jk'}|X) = E[(\Psi_i(s) + \mathcal{E}_{ik}(s, w)) \cdot (\Psi_j(s') + \mathcal{E}_{jk'}(s', w'))] \qquad (6.94)$$

which, upon expanding, is

$$\mathrm{Cov}(Y_{ik}, Y_{jk'}|X) = E(\Psi_i(s) \cdot \Psi_j(s')) + E(\Psi_i(s) \cdot \mathcal{E}_{jk'}(s', w')) \ldots$$
$$+ E(\mathcal{E}_{ik}(s, w) \cdot \Psi_j(s')) + E(\mathcal{E}_{ik}(s, w) \cdot \mathcal{E}_{jk'}(s', w')) \qquad (6.95)$$

Although, as above, we can evaluate each of the expectations on the right-hand side, since ik and jk' index completely independent observations, we know from Chapter 4 that all random variables defined on the marginal space $(S \times \Omega, \mathcal{A}, P_{ik})$ are independent of all random variables defined on $(S \times \Omega, \mathcal{A}, P_{jk'})$ for all $i \neq j$. Consequently, each of the expectations on the right-hand side of Equation 6.95 are 0 and, therefore, the covariance $\mathrm{Cov}(Y_{ik}, Y_{jk'}|X)$ is also 0.

In summary, for the classic nested data generating process described in the problem statement, we can model the intercept as a state-level random effect, which will lead to a conditional variance of the dependent variable equal to the variance of the state-level random effect (Ψ_i) plus the variance of the resident-level error term ($\mathcal{E}_{ik}$). Random variables will be dependent for observations indexed by the same state-level random selection process, having covariance equal to $V(\Psi_i)$, which could be 0, and independent otherwise.

The preceding problem was perhaps the most straightforward implementation of a random effects model to a classic situation. What happens, however, if we consider a different, but also common, situation; one that reflects a slight change in the data generating process. Instead of randomly sampling the state, suppose we use a designated set of states, what then?

Problem 6.3

You collect an independent random sample of N residents from each state in the United States. What is the dependence structure of a model of individual characteristic y as a linear function of characteristic x with an intercept as a state-level random effect modeled as a sampling distribution?

Solution: Suppose we are interested in the relationship between characteristics Y and X on individuals w in the population of people Ω across the 50 states; moreover, we consider for an arbitrary individual w from Ω that the relationship in the following Equation 6.96 holds:

$$Y_w = \alpha_w + \beta \cdot X_w \tag{6.96}$$

By this, we mean that each individual w's level of Y is dictated by the level of some variable X. For notational simplicity in this model, I use Ω as an index set for itself, that is, $\mathcal{J}^{-1} \colon \Omega \to \Omega$. The model implies the slope is the same for everyone, but there is an individual intercept. This constitutes our structural model of individual responses. Note again that the w is indexing an arbitrary element of the population Ω and not an observation of a data generating process.

For comparison with the preceding example, we specify our probability model as follows: let S denote the set of 50 states and Ω the population of the United States; our outcome set for each observation is then $S \times \Omega$, and our set of events $\mathcal{A}$ is the power set of the outcome set. However, and importantly, the data generating process strongly constricts the probabilities on this measurable space. Specifically, each observation is associated with an explicit state; in other words, because we set out to get a sample from each state, the probability of an observation coming from a given state is 1 for that state and 0 for the others. This will have serious consequences in our analysis of dependence for the related random variables and the reason the following results differ from the preceding problem. Our overall probability model is then $((S \times \Omega)^{50 \cdot N}, \mathcal{A}^{50 \cdot N}, P)$, in which N is denoting the sample size within each of the 50 states.

We index the data generating process with $\mathbb{I} = \{1, \dots, 50\}$ and $\mathbb{K} = \{1, \dots, N\}$ to identify each marginal space $(S \times \Omega, \mathcal{A}, P_{ik})$ and its random variables. The interpretation of $\mathbb{I}$ is the set of states in the United States and the interpretation of $\mathbb{K}$ is the set of observational processes that randomly select individuals from the indexed state. As before, we could generalize to a different index set for the observational processes within each state such as $\{\mathbb{K}_i : i \in \mathbb{I}\}$ to be more specific and allow different numbers of observations within each state; however, to minimize notation, we will indicate only one $\mathbb{K}$.

As in the preceding problem, for each $(S \times \Omega, \mathcal{A}, P_{ik})$, I define three variables: $Y_{ik}(s, w)$, $X_{ik}(s, w)$, and $\Theta_i(s)$. The first two, Y and X, denote arbitrary characteristics of interest and Θ denotes an indicator of the elements of S (i.e., Θ is a random variable representing a partition in $\mathcal{A}$ generated by the elements of S, the states). The model specification associated with this data generating process is identical to that of Problem 6.2.

As above, we define another random variable that reflects the expected value of Y within each state among those with $X = 0$ as

$$A_i(s) = E(Y_{ik}|\Theta_i(s), X_{ik} = 0) \tag{6.97}$$

we define the regression function for Y as

$$E(Y_{ik}|\Theta_i, X_{ik}) = A_i(s) + \beta \cdot X_{ik}(s, w) \tag{6.98}$$

and we the difference between Y and its expected value as

$$Y_{ik} - E(Y_{ik}|\Theta_i, X_{ik}) = \mathcal{E}_{ik}(s, w) \tag{6.99}$$

Overall then, Y can be expressed as

$$Y_{ik} = A_i(s) + \beta \cdot X_{ik}(s, w) + \mathcal{E}_{ik}(s, w) \tag{6.100}$$

which by definition has $E(\mathcal{E}_{ik}|\Theta_i, X_{ik}) = 0$.

Here is where we depart from the development in Problem 6.2. The expected value of A_i can be different across indices: in this case, the expectation

$$E(A_i) = \sum_s A_i(s) \cdot P_{ik}(\{s\}) \tag{6.101}$$

has $P_{ik}(\{s\}) = 1$ if $s = \mathcal{I}(i)$ and 0 if not. This is because, for this data generating process in which we set out to obtain a sample from within each state (i.e., the states are not sampled), each observation has a determined state associated with it. Consequently, each observation is for a specific state, with probability 1. Therefore, all elements of the preceding summation are 0, except for the case in which $s = \mathcal{I}(i)$. Given s is a value of the function $\mathcal{I}(i)$, we can denote the specific s associated with a particular i as s_i:

$$E(A_i) = A_i(s_i) \tag{6.102}$$

For ease of presentation, we will denote each of these expectations simply as α_i. Unlike above, the expected value of A_i is not the same across each observation; consequently, A_i cannot nontrivially be expressed as $A_i(s) = \alpha + \Psi_i(s)$, but must remain as $A_i(s_i) = \alpha_i$. By substitution, we then have

$$Y_{ik} = \alpha_i + \beta \cdot X_{ik}(s, w) + \mathcal{E}_{ik}(s, w) \tag{6.103}$$

In determining the dependence structure of random variables from this specification, as in the preceding example, we will consider the relationships conditional on X. First, let us consider the conditional variance of Y_{ik}:

$$V(Y_{ik}|X_{ik}) = E\left[((\alpha_i + \mathcal{E}_{ik}) - (E(\alpha_i) + E(\mathcal{E}_{ik})))^2\right] \tag{6.104}$$

However, since the expected value of α_i is just α_i, and the expected value of $\mathcal{E}_{ik}$ is 0, the conditional variance is

$$V(Y_{ik}|X_{ik}) = E\left[(\alpha_i - \alpha_i) + \mathcal{E}_{ik})^2\right] \tag{6.105}$$

which is simply the variance of $\mathcal{E}_{ik}$:

$$V(Y_{ik}|X_{ik}) = E\left[\mathcal{E}_{ik}^2\right] = V(\mathcal{E}_{ik}) \tag{6.106}$$

Unlike the preceding nested data generating process, which had a variance of $V(Y_{ik}|X_{ik}) = V(\Psi_i) + V(\mathcal{E}_{ik})$, this data generating process, which selects a sample from a fixed set of states, has a variance of $V(Y_{ik}|X_{ik}) = V(\mathcal{E}_{ik})$. The variance is not the same for this data generating process, in which we did not sample states, than for the preceding nested data generating process, in which we did sample states.

Next, let us consider the conditional covariance of Y_{ik} and $Y_{ik'}$, which represent random variables based on the same state (thereby both indexed by the same element i of $\mathbb{I}$) but different selection of individual within state (thereby each being indexed by different elements of $\mathbb{K}$, specifically k and k'):

$$\text{Cov}(Y_{ik}, Y_{ik'}|X) = \text{Cov}((\alpha_i(s) + \mathcal{E}_{ik}(s, w)), (\alpha_i(s) + \mathcal{E}_{ik'}(s, w'))) \tag{6.107}$$

which is simply

$$\text{Cov}(Y_{ik}, Y_{ik'}|X) = E(\mathcal{E}_{ik}(s, w) \cdot \mathcal{E}_{ik'}(s, w')) \tag{6.108}$$

a covariance term equal to 0:

$$\text{Cov}(Y_{ik}, Y_{ik'}|X) = \text{Cov}(\mathcal{E}_{ik}(s, w), \mathcal{E}_{ik'}(s, w')) = 0 \tag{6.109}$$

As with the previous analysis, the $\alpha_i(s)$ term drops out of the covariance because $E(\alpha_i(s)) = \alpha_i(s)$ and, therefore, $\alpha_i(s) - E(\alpha_i(s)) = 0$. Moreover, the covariance $\text{Cov}(\mathcal{E}_{ik}(s, w), \mathcal{E}_{ik'}(s, w')) = 0$ for this data generating process, in which independent samples are taken within each state. Consequently, $\text{Cov}(Y_{ik}, Y_{ik'}|X) = 0$. Again note that this result is different from that of the preceding nested data generating process, which had a covariance of $\text{Cov}(Y_{ik}, Y_{ik'}|X) = V(\Psi_i)$. Within-state random variables are not correlated in the current case, but are correlated in the case of a nested data generating process (if A_i varies across states, otherwise $V(\Psi_i)$ would be 0 in the nested case as well).

Next, let us consider the conditional covariance of Y_{ik} and $Y_{jk'}$, which represent random variables based on different states (thereby each being indexed by different element of $\mathbb{I}$, specifically i and j) and different

selection of individual within state (thereby each being indexed by different elements of $\mathbb{K}$, specifically k and k'). Rather than work out the details,
I will appeal to our understanding from Chapter 4 that random variables
of independent observations are independent; consequently, since the
sampling of individuals from within different states are independent, the
covariance between variables is $\text{Cov}(Y_{ik}, Y_{jk'}|X) = 0$. This is the same as in
the case with a nested data generating process.

   In summary, for independent samples of people taken from each of
a fixed set of states, the random effect variables are a constant and thereby
have a variance of 0. This leads to a variance of $V(Y_{ik}|X_{ik}) = V(\mathcal{E}_{ik})$, a cova-
riance of $\text{Cov}(Y_{ik}, Y_{ik'}|X) = 0$, and $\text{Cov}(Y_{ik}, Y_{jk'}|X) = 0$. These results are dif-
ferent from those of the classic random effects model for nested data sets
in Problem 6.2.

   What happens if we treat the intercept in Problem 6.3 as a random effect
reflecting sampling variation across states as if the data generating process
were nested (i.e., as if the states were randomly selected, which is what is com-
putationally assumed for a typical random effect model in many statistical
analysis software)? Well, we now incorporate variation across the means of
the states into our standard errors as if we were randomly sampling states,
incorrectly using an estimate of $V(Y_{ik}|X_{ik}) = V(\Psi_i) + V(\mathcal{E}_{ik})$ rather than the
correct $V(Y_{ik}|X_{ik}) = V(\mathcal{E}_{ik})$. And, we would mistakenly treat within-state
observations as if they were potentially dependent, incorrectly using
$\text{Cov}(Y_{ik}, Y_{ik'}|X) = V(\Psi_i)$ rather than the correct $\text{Cov}(Y_{ik}, Y_{ik'}|X) = 0$. This would
be a mistake as we are not sampling states. Why would we care to pretend our
estimates could vary according to a process that we did not engage?

Problem 6.4

You collect a random sample of States, and then sample residents from
each of those states. Can you legitimately specify a model of individual characteristic y as a linear function of characteristic x with an intercept as a State-
specific *fixed effect*?

   Solution: Yes. You can always focus on conditional distributions; therefore, you can use a model that conditions on the given states or set of fixed
effects.

   The preceding problems involve data generating processes that either
sample states or define sampling within states. In both cases, we let the data
generating process be our guide. If we forget this, however, and let the data
be our guide, we can be led into a mistaken approach. This can occur if we
mistake data for random variables, and we therefore base our probability
model on the structure of data rather than the structure of the data generating process. Consider the following problem.

Problem 6.5

You are given a data set of N records generated by an independent random sample of people who live in the United States. The data include an indicator of the state in which each person resides. Based on this data structure, can you legitimately analyze the data as if the data generating process were clustered by State?

Solution: It is common for people to face such a data set and think of people being nested (or clustered) within state and to use an analytical strategy that accounts for such "nesting." Results will make the assumptions about the variances and dependence among the random variables as addressed in Problem 6.2. This is, however, mistaken.

To capture the notion of clustering by state, suppose we use the measureable space that we used in Problem 6.2: $(S \times \Omega, \mathcal{A})$. The outcome set comprises the pairs (s, w), representing a state and person combination. If we modeled the probabilities according to a nested design, we would have the same probability space as in Problem 6.2 and the corresponding results. However, if we instead model the actual data generating process, we would have $(\Omega, \mathcal{A}, P_i)$ as the probability space for each observation i in the index set $\mathbb{I}$ having an interpretation of the set of observations to be obtained $\{1, \dots, N\}$. The actual outcome set for this data generating process that samples people from the United States does not include sampling states. The data generating process is not nested.

Each person in Ω is a resident of some state, and therefore we can define an indicator of each possible state of residence as a random variable on the probability space $(\Omega, \mathcal{A}, P_i)$; however, random variables do not imply the structure of the data generating process. State of residence is a random variable just as are age, income, political party, and so on. We should no more perform an analysis clustered by state than we would cluster by age, income, or other random variable.

State of residence is irrelevant to defining the probabilities of this data generating process. The corresponding distribution of random variables is determined by the independent random sampling of people having sampling probabilities defined by nationwide independent sampling. This example highlights the need to carefully consider the proper definition of the probability space underlying the random variables that generate data.

This mistake can easily arise when researchers are analyzing data that they did not collect, particularly observational data from natural data generating processes. For example, when a researcher is provided a data set for analysis; observes many patient records with the same physician or many student records with the same school, or any other similar "nesting" structure; and considers that physicians would drive some patient responses or schools would drive student responses, he mistakenly engages a strategy of analysis for a nested data generating process. Here the researcher is mistaking data for random variables and/or random variables for the data generating process that define their underlying probabilities: as has been stated throughout the book, they are not the same. When taking a Frequentist approach to modeling random variables, it is the data generating process that makes the variables random and not the data. The phrase "nested data" is not statistically meaningful in this context.

The preceding problems pose questions about how to properly account for the data generating process when using probability to model this source of uncertainty. The next problem poses a question regarding the scientific merit of always modeling the full data generating process as opposed to ignoring at least part of it.

Problem 6.6

You run a large multisite clinical trial of patients, in which you are able to recruit 100 clinics to participate. Can you treat clinic as a random effect? *Should* you treat clinic as a random effect?

Solution: The answer to the first question is, arguably, yes. You can treat the fact that your recruitment strategy had a less than perfect chance of convincing any given clinic to participate so that if you had repeated the process you might have obtained a different set of willing clinics. By this argument, you might model the uncertainty in the clinic participation generating process with a probability measure and proceed with a random effects analysis as in Problem 6.2. This is a common approach for multisite trials with a large number of sites.

However, *should* you use such a random effects analysis? The answer is, arguably, no. This is a question of scientific utility and not one of mathematical probability. First, suppose that you were to use a clinic-specific fixed effects model. In this case, you can obtain legitimate estimates conditional on the given set of clinics. Generalizability to the overall population of clinics cannot be addressed by statistical arguments and must be based on arguments about clinic homogeneity. The standard errors are interpreted in accordance with the sampling variation due to patients that show up at the clinics. This allows us to understand how the estimates could vary due to the people we happen to have obtained in each clinic. Next, suppose you use a random effects model to account for the sampling of clinics. Unfortunately, due to the idiosyncratic selection process, the parameters of the probability measure modeling the researchers' ability to recruit clinics are not likely identified with the parameters of an interpretable population model of the clinics. Consequently, in the absence of knowing (or having good estimates of) the recruitment probabilities of clinics, generalizability to the overall population of clinics still cannot be addressed by statistical arguments and again must be based on appeals to clinic homogeneity. However, now the standard errors incorporate variation due to the idiosyncratic clinic recruitment strategy, which makes them much less clear in their interpretation. In this case, the random effects model has no scientific advantage over the fixed effects model (i.e., it has no greater statistical generalizability), yet muddles the interpretation of the standard errors.

Inherent Fixed Units, Fixed Effects, and Standard Errors

In this section, we consider the combination of the preceding two sections. We look at how understanding the underlying probability space can help us understand what standard errors we wish to calculate.

Problem 6.7

You have a sample of residents from each of the 62 counties in New York State of the United States. You are interested in the linear relationship across counties of the counties' proportions of hospitalizations and the counties' proportions of poor. You use a least-squared errors algorithm to estimate the quantity of interest. What is the standard error?

Solution: Here the counties are inherently fixed: the counties are what they are, and your data generating process was to get a sample of records from each county—there is no sampling of counties. Using the data from each county, you calculate the proportion of hospitalizations (y) and the proportion of poor (x) for each county. You are interested in $b = (X'X)^{-1}(X'y)$, the OLS estimator (X has a row for each of the 62 counties, and columns for x and a constant). You calculate the linear regression parameter b of y on X by ordinary least squares in your favorite statistical package. How would you interpret the reported standard error of b?

The usual reported standard errors are meaningless! The statistical program assumes that your counties are from a probability sample and report standard errors that use the variation in estimates across counties to calculate standard errors for b associated with a process of sampling counties: a process that did not generate the data and therefore did not produce sampling variation in the estimator.

If you had the true population values for y and x for each county, then b would be *the* linear relationship across counties without variation. So, in the case using samples of individuals within each county, is there a standard error associated with b? Yes. Both y and x for each county are estimated by the samples taken from within each county; different samples within county would produce different y and x values.

We can see this by tracking the probabilities that underlie the distribution of the estimator b. These are a set of probabilities as shown in Figure 6.1. Line 1 of Figure 6.1 presents the individual data generating processes for each of the 62 counties. The outcome set for each county comprises the product of the county population (Ω_s for arbitrary county s) N_s times: for example, $\Omega_s^{N_s} = \Omega_s \times \ldots \times \Omega_s$ in which there are N_s replicates of Ω_s, one for each observation in the sample.

Line 2 of Figure 6.1 shows the two random variables, proportion of hospitalizations and proportion of poor, defined on each of these county-specific probability spaces. Each of these random variables presents a

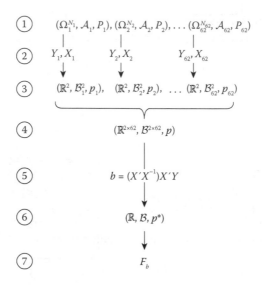

FIGURE 6.1
Tracking probabilities from the initial data generating process to the distribution of the least squared errors estimator.

proportion across the set of N_s individuals that can be captured in the data generating processes. Hence, Y_1 is the proportion of the N_1 individuals from county indexed as 1 who are hospitalized, and X_1 is the corresponding proportion of individuals who are poor. Each pair of random variables map their domain to a subset of the real plane (R^2), specifically to the unit square—see line 3 of Figure 6.1. The probability measure, p_s, that defines the joint distribution of each pair is derived from the probability representing the data generating process of each county (i.e., the P_s in line 1); therefore, the variation in these variables derives from the process of sampling individuals from within each county.

All probability spaces representing the pairs of county-specific random variables shown in line 3 can be combined into the single probability space shown in line 4. This is a product space reflecting the $62 \times 2 = 124$ random variables. Assuming independence of variables across counties, the probability p is the simple product of the p_s probabilities. The distributions of the random variables, such as b in line 5, defined on this space are defined in terms of p, which is derived from the p_s measures, which are in turn derived from the P_s probabilities reflecting sampling. Therefore, as before, the variation in such random variables derives from the original data generating process. The estimator b is a random variable defined on the probability space of line 4. It has a probability measure p^* in line 6 that underlies its sampling distribution F_b in line 7. The variation in the distribution F_b derives from p^*, which is derived from p, which ultimately is derived from the original 62 probabilities P_s.

Consequently, the standard error of b is a function of the within-county data generating processes. Note that the number of counties is irrelevant to the standard error—the logic represented in Figure 6.1 is not changed by considering an arbitrary number of counties (so long as b as defined can be calculated).

The proper standard error for b is the variance associated with $(X'X)^{-1}(X'y)$ in which each measurement of y and x is taken to vary by the data generating process of observed individuals within each county. Because it makes little sense to condition on the observed x values, which are themselves estimates, one would probably calculate the full variance of b and not the variance of b conditional on X.

Note that this has serious ramifications regarding the sample size and power: the number of counties is irrelevant, except to identify the functional relationship (e.g., we would need at least 2 counties for a linear relationship). The number of counties does not impact our sample size considerations. It is the number of individuals sampled within each county that dictates the precision of the county's estimate and thereby impacts the standard error of b. As the sample sizes of individuals within counties go to infinity for all counties, the standard error of b goes to zero, whether you have 2 counties or 62 counties.

The preceding problem addresses using aggregated data within fixed units to study those fixed units. A more common situation is when a smaller unit of analysis is the target of study and samples are obtained from a set of fixed larger units. An example is expressed in the following problem.

Problem 6.8

You have an equal probability sample of residents (with replacement) from each of the 62 counties in New York. You are interested in the relationship between individual-level variables (i.e., measurements on the people of each county). Can you combine the data? What are the standard errors?

Solution: This problem is essentially same as Problem 6.3; however, in that problem I skipped over an important issue, which will be addressed here. Specifically, you have 62 separate data generating processes—one for each county. You can consider a measurable space associated with each county c from the set C of 62 counties as $(\Omega_c, \mathcal{A}_c)$, that is, you would define the 62 measurable spaces $(\Omega_1, \mathcal{A}_1)$, $(\Omega_2, \mathcal{A}_2)$, ..., $(\Omega_{62}, \mathcal{A}_{62})$ that each one represents the residents of a particular county. However, since probability measures can assign nonempty sets the value of zero, you can more simply use a common measurable space $(\Omega, \mathcal{A})$ in which Ω denotes the set of New York State residents and $\mathcal{A}$ is an appropriately rich sigma-algebra (let's just say the power set for convenience). The different data generating processes of the different counties are indicated by their probability measures

P_c which assigns nonzero sampling probabilities to residents of county c and assigns zero to residents of other counties. Your probability spaces are then $(\Omega, \mathcal{A}, P_c)$ for each county $c \in C$.

Because each county has a different probability space, without further assumptions, there is no *a priori* reason to assume that the random variables with corresponding probability spaces $(\mathbb{R}, \mathcal{B}, P_c)$ have the same distributions F_c or shared characteristics (e.g., a regression function). Consequently, without further assumptions, there is no *a priori* reason to believe that $F_c = F_d$ (or any shared distribution characteristics) for any arbitrary pairs of counties c and d; therefore, there is no reason to believe that data from one county provide information about the distribution of random variables for any other county, and the data from the different counties cannot be combined in analysis!

Suppose, however, that it is reasonable to assume the distribution of random variables for each county is of the same parametric family and differs across counties solely by their parameterization. Then you can write each distribution F_c as F_{θ_c}, a distribution indexed by a county-specific parameter θ_c rather than merely by the county, thereby indicating that the distribution varies only in its parameterization and not in its family. If all parameters are distinct across counties, which some would call a fully interacted model, you have gained very little by this reduction because your analysis would be the same as assessing each county's data separately. On the contrary, if some of the parameters in θ are considered to be the same across counties, you are in a position to use the combined data to inform your estimates.

To make this point clear, suppose you are interested in the conditional distribution of random variable Y given values of random variable X, and further suppose it is reasonable to model this distribution as being a member of the normal family of distributions in which the mean is a linear function of X. Then for each county, $Y_c \sim N(\alpha_c + \beta_c \cdot X, \sigma_c^2)$. As stated above, without further assumptions we have gained little in terms of combining the data, but if it is plausible to assume the conditional variance is the same across counties, then $\sigma_c^2 = \sigma^2$ for all counties c, and $Y_c \sim N(\alpha_c + \beta_c \cdot X, \sigma^2)$. In this case, you can combine the data and estimate the county-specific parameters α_c and β_c (by the judicious use of dummy variables as county indicators—assuming you have a large enough sample size) and the common parameter σ^2. This will provide a more precise estimate of σ^2 (since one can use all data to inform this parameter), which will improve your standard error estimators for the remaining parameters.

Suppose it is also reasonable to assume $\beta_c = \beta$ for all counties c. Then our distribution becomes $Y_c \sim N(\alpha_c + \beta \cdot X, \sigma^2)$ and you have the classic fixed effects model in which the intercepts α_c are allowed to vary across counties and can be estimated by combining the data and including county dummy variables in the model, and again greater efficiency is achieved by combining the data.

Other restrictions are available as well: for example, it might be reasonable to also assume $\alpha_c = \alpha$ but $\beta_c \neq \beta$ across counties thereby using the combined data and interacting X with county dummy variables. Or, perhaps it is reasonable to consider all parameters as being the same across counties and thereby allowing the combined data to be analyzed without concern for county-specific effects.

The assumptions in this example are overly restrictive; for example, if it is reasonable to assume that regression equations have common parameters (as was done above), then, with enough data to appeal to large-sample results, one can often combine the data and use method of moments or generalized method of moments to estimate parameters without requiring the distributions be from the same family. In other words, it might be that $F_c \neq F_d$ for arbitrary pairs c and d of counties, but $E(Y|X) = \alpha + \beta \cdot X$ for all counties (or with at least one of the parameters a constant).

The main point of the preceding problem is that you started with separate data generating processes that imply different distributions for random variables, without further assumptions there is no justification for combining the data. However if it is reasonable to make certain assumptions, then common parameters may be identified that warrant using all the data in estimation. The standard errors for these estimators will be the typical ones calculated for fixed effects models.

Inherent Fixed Units, Random Effects, and Standard Errors

The preceding problems may lead you to conclude that random effects cannot be applied when a data generating process includes inherent fixed units. But this conclusion is mistaken. Random effects can be applied in such cases; however, you must be careful and understand what the probability space underlying the random effects is modeling and construct standard errors accordingly.

Problem 6.9

Consider Problem 6.8 again. You have an equal probability sample of residents (with replacement) from each of the 62 counties in New York. You are interested in the relationship between individual-level variables (i.e., measurements on the people of each county). Can you meaningfully treat the inherent fixed-unit county effects as a random effect?

Solution: We have observations from all 62 New York counties, and the counties do not compose a sample of counties. As discussed above, in terms of sampling uncertainty, the county-level should not be modeled as a random effect based on sampling probabilities; if it is, it is trivial.

However, suppose we can set up the problem, as above, in terms of the model $Y \sim F(\alpha_c + \beta \cdot X, \sigma^2)$ for some distribution F. The α_c parameters are fixed for each county, but across the counties there is a population distribution of this parameter and we can use a probability space to model this distribution. In other words, since each county has its own α_c, there must be a mean α_c across the counties and a likely variation across the α_c's, and, in general, some distribution of α_c across the population of counties. In this case, it is helpful to use $\Omega \times C$ as our outcome set in which Ω denotes the population of New York and C denotes the set of counties in New York. We can then define $(\Omega \times C, \mathcal{A}_\Omega \otimes \mathcal{A}_C, P)$ as our probability space. Here we describe P as $P = P(A_\Omega | A_C) \cdot P(A_C)$ in which $P(A_C)$ is defined to produce a model of the normalized histogram of county characteristics (such as α_c), and $P(A_\Omega | A_C)$ is modeling the patient data generating process within each county. Consequently, α_c can be considered a latent variable with a distribution associated with $P(A_C)$ as a population model of counties, and we can estimate its parameters, such as the mean and variance of the fixed-unit effects across the counties. For example, we might base our analysis on the mixture model

$$f(y|x; \beta, \theta) = \int f(y|x, \alpha; \beta) \cdot f(\alpha; \theta) \cdot d\alpha \qquad (6.110)$$

This model treats α (our county effect) as a random variable in which $f(\alpha; \theta)$ is its density associated with $P(A_C)$. After specifying our distributional families, we can estimate the model parameters, including θ, which describe the distribution of the fixed-unit effects across the counties.

We want our standard errors to only reflect sources of sampling uncertainty, and the standard errors must therefore be constructed so as not to include the variation related to the population model $P(A_C)$ as if it were sampling variation. For some models, it might be possible to work out an equation for the standard error or a Taylor series approximation of it, but it might be easier to bootstrap the standard error in which bootstrap samples are taken from within each county (i.e., a county-stratified bootstrap sampling method). In this way, we take into account the variation due to the within-county patient data generating process, but do not inappropriately account for across-county variation as if it were due to sampling. Such models can be very useful when eliminating the fixed effects is not possible and there are too many parameters to directly model. In such a case, the preceding random effects approach reduces the number of parameters from one fixed effect per county to only those describing the distribution of fixed effects.

For statistical software that allows stratified bootstrapped standard errors, estimating this model is quite easy: assuming the bootstrap algorithm is appropriate for the within-county patient data generating process, simply run a random effects model with county random effects using county-stratified bootstrapped standard errors. The results are directly interpretable, and the usual random effects assumptions apply.

Treating Fixed Effects as Random

In Problem 6.4, above, we declared that fixed effects are certainly possible for the classic nested data generating process. However, Problem 6.9 admits a modification, presented below in Problem 6.10, that allows us to treat such fixed effects, which are not due to inherently fixed units, as random effects that are not modeling the nested sampling design.

Problem 6.10

You collect a random sample of 1000 hospitals in the United States and then sample patients from each of those hospitals. Can you legitimately specify a model of individual characteristic y as a function of characteristic x with an intercept as a random effect modeling the distribution of the sampled hospitals specific effects?

Solution: Yes. You can condition on the hospitals in your sample yet model the normalized histogram of these specific hospital effects as if it were a population model. The approach is identical to that presented for Problem 6.8; however, the interpretation is different.

As mentioned above, in this approach the standard errors must only account for the within-hospital variation; however, since the distribution of hospital-specific effects is a distribution across the hospitals in the sample only, the corresponding parameters are to be interpreted accordingly. The advantage of this strategy, rather than merely using a fixed effects model, is to allow for a distribution of such effects when there are too many fixed effects to include in the model and elimination of the fixed effects is not possible, or when one is interested in the association of the outcome with hospital-level characteristics.

Conclusion

Note that the nonstandard random effects models presented in this chapter are subject to the same assumptions required for identification that apply to the standard random effects models. However, in testing these assumptions, it is important to use the correct standard errors for the nonstandard models. For example, if you run your software's usual Hausman test for random effects, your software is likely to mistakenly assume that the distribution of random effects is reflecting sampling variation. The proper standard errors for specification tests must be based on the sampling variance alone, just as the other standard errors discussed above.

Additional Readings

In this chapter, I focused primarily on problems derived from various uses of fixed effects and random effects models. I did not, however, focus on estimation of these models. Estimation procedures can be found across the many fields of applied research. For example, in econometrics, see Greene's book *Econometric Analysis*, seventh edition (Prentice Hall, 2012), Cameron and Trivedi's book *Microeconometrics: Methods and Applications* (Cambridge University Press, 2005), and Davidson and KacKinnon's book *Econometric Theory and Methods* (Oxford University Press, 2004) for just a few out of many books that address these models.

These models are also addressed in the literature on hierarchical models and multilevel models. Of the numerous books, see for examples of introductory books, Raudenbush and Bryk's *Hierarchical Linear Models: Applications and Data Analysis Methods* (Sage, 2002) and Snijders and Bosker's *Multilevel Analysis: An Introduction to Basic and Advanced Multilevel Modeling*, second edition (Sage, 2011). Also, random effect models are a type of mixed model and that literature addresses estimation as well. See, for example, Demidenko's book *Mixed Models: Theory and Applications* (Wiley, 2004).

Note, however, that each of the above referenced books as well as other books that I am aware of treat these models presupposing a cluster (nested) data generating process. Consequently, the problematic issues discussed in this chapter are not typically addressed in these books, and therefore the proper interpretation and standard errors of model parameters and estimators are not necessarily as presented in these references and related literature if the underlying probability measure is not solely representing variation in a data generating process.

Bibliography*

Bear, H. S. (1997). *An introduction to mathematical analysis*. New York: Academic Press.

Billingsley, P. (1995). *Probability and measure* (3rd ed.). New York: Wiley.

Cameron, A. C. & Trivedi, P. K. (2005). *Microeconometrics: Methods and applications*. Cambridge, UK: Cambridge University Press.

Davidson, J. (1994). *Stochastic limit theory: An introduction for econometricians*. Oxford: Oxford University Press.

Davidson, R. & MacKinnon, J. G. (2004). *Econometric theory and methods*. New York: Oxford University Press.

Demidenko, E. (2004). *Mixed models: Theory and applications*. Hoboken, NJ: Wiley-Interscience.

Dhrymes, P. J. (1989). *Topics in advanced econometrics: Probability foundations*. New York: Springer-Verlag.

Eagle, A. (Ed.). (2011). *Philosophy of probability: Contemporary readings*. New York: Routledge.

Earman, J. (1992). *Bayes or bust?: A critical examination of Bayesian confirmation theory*. Cambridge, MA: MIT Press.

Gillies, D. (2000). *Philosophical theories of probability*. New York: Routledge.

Greene, W. H. (2012). *Econometric analysis* (7th ed.). Boston, MA: Prentice Hall.

Hall, A. R. (2005). *Generalized method of moments*. Oxford: Oxford University Press.

Kolmogorov, A. N. & Fomin, S. V. (1970). *Introductory real analysis*. New York: Dover.

Kyburg, H. E., Jr. & Thalos, M. (Eds.). (2003). *Probability is the very guide of life: The philosophical uses of chance*. Chicago, IL: Open Court.

Mayo, D. G. (1996). *Error and the growth of experimental knowledge*. Chicago, IL: University of Chicago Press.

Mayo, D. G. & Spanos, A. (2011). *Error and inference: Recent exchanges on experimental reasoning, reliability, and the objectivity and rationality of science* (1st paperback ed.). New York: Cambridge University Press.

Mellor, D. H. (2005). *Probability: A philosophical introduction*. New York: Routledge.

Raudenbush, S. W. & Bryk, A. S. (2002). *Hierarchical linear models: Applications and data analysis methods* (2nd ed.). Thousand Oaks, CA: Sage.

Resnick, S. I. (1999). *A probability path*. Boston, MA: Birkhauser.

Schervish, M. J. (1995). *Theory of statistics*. New York: Springer-Verlag.

Snijders, T. A. B. & Bosker, R. J. (2012). *Multilevel analysis: An introduction to basic and advanced multilevel modeling* (2nd ed.). Los Angeles, CA: Sage.

Spanos, A. (1999). *Probability theory and statistical inference: Econometric modeling with observational data*. Cambridge, UK: Cambridge University Press.

Sprecher, D. A. (1970). *Elements of real analysis*. New York: Dover.

---

* This bibliography provides the full citations for the works presented in the Additional Readings sections of each chapter.

Stoll, R. R. (1979). *Set theory and logic*. New York: Dover.
Suppes, P. (2002). *Representation and invariance of scientific structures*. Stanford, CA: CSLI.
Taper, M. L. & Lele, S. (2004). *The nature of scientific evidence: Statistical, philosophical, and empirical considerations*. Chicago, IL: University of Chicago Press.

Index